Dissociative Identity Disorder

WILEY SERIES IN GENERAL AND CLINICAL PSYCHIATRY

Series Editor
MAURICE R. GREEN
New York University
Medical School

The Broad Scope of Ego Function Assessment
Edited by Leopold Bellak and Lisa A. Goldsmith

The Psychological Experience of Surgery
Edited by Richard S. Blacher

Presentations of Depression: Depressive Symptoms in Medical and Other
Psychiatric Disorders
Edited by Oliver G. Cameron

Clinical Guidelines in Cross-Cultural Mental Health
Edited by Lillian Comas-Diaz and Ezra E. H. Griffith

Sleep Disorders: Diagnosis and Treatment (Second Edition)
Edited by Robert L. Williams, Ismet Karacan and Constance A. Moore

Multiple Personality Disorder: Diagnosis, Clinical Features,
and Treatment
Colin A. Ross

Stressors and the Adjustment Disorders
Edited by Joseph D. Noshpitz and R. Dean Coddington

Russian/Soviet and Western Psychiatry
Paul Calloway

Psychotherapeutic Drug Manual (Third Edition, Revised)
Edited by Julie Magno Zito

Unbearable Affect: A Guide to the Psychotherapy of Psychosis
David A. S. Garfield

DISSOCIATIVE IDENTITY DISORDER

Diagnosis, Clinical Features, and Treatment of Multiple Personality

Second Edition

Colin A. Ross, M.D.

John Wiley & Sons, Inc.

New York • Chichester • Brisbane • Toronto • Singapore • Weinheim

Library of Congress Cataloging-in-Publication Data:
Ross, Colin A.
    Dissociative identity disorder : diagnosis, clinical features, and treatment of multiple personality / by Colin A. Ross. — 2nd ed.
       p.   cm.
    Rev. ed. of: Multiple personality disorder, c1989.
    Includes bibliographical references and index.
    ISBN 0-471-13265-9 (cloth : alk. paper)
    1. Multiple personality. I. Ross, Colin A. Multiple personality
disorder. II. Title.
    [DNLM: 1. Multiple-Personality Disorder.   WM 173.6 R823d 1996]
RC569.5.M8R65 1996
616.85′236—dc20
DNLM/DLC
for Library of Congress   96-23334

Printed in the United States of America

10 9 8 7 6 5 4 3 2

Preface

The purpose of this book is to give the reader a comprehensive and detailed grounding in the history, diagnosis, and treatment of dissociative identity disorder (DID). It is not to create diagnosticians or therapists de novo out of untrained individuals. The assumption throughout is that trained professionals must provide the treatment for DID, based on general principles of psychotherapy. Having said that, I must acknowledge that I launched into my first case in 1979 without adequate training or supervision: I hope that this book will be helpful for clinicians who find themselves in a similar situation. The book is also aimed at the more experienced clinician.

In August 1979, I was a third-year medical student at the University of Alberta in Edmonton. A few weeks into my first clinical rotation, I was assigned to do an admission history and physical on a woman with amnesia. This patient provided me with my first opportunity to diagnose and treat dissociative identity disorder. Although I worked with her therapeutically for only a short time, I learned that dissociative disorders were my area of subspecialty.

I submitted an account of the case to the *International Journal of Clinical and Experimental Hypnosis,* which had a history of publishing papers on DID. By chance, the editor, Martin Orne, was looking for one more paper for a special issue on DID, and mine was accepted (Ross, 1984). This was my first experience with editorial comment from a psychiatric journal, although I had published previously in a medical journal (Ross, 1981). The detailed and helpful editing steered me more strongly into the dissociative disorders.

Since then, I have received support from a number of people and institutions whose contributions to my career, and indirectly to this book, I wish to acknowledge. The Fee Pool of the Department of Psychiatry at St. Boniface Hospital in Winnipeg, Canada, supported my work for three years from 1988 to 1991, despite inadequate resources and other pressing priorities. I received research grants from the Manitoba Mental Health Research Foundation, the Manitoba Health Research Council, and the National Health Research Development Program, as well as the B.Sc. Med. Program of the Faculty of Medicine at the University of Manitoba.

A source of indirect support during those years was a number of drug companies that employed me as an investigator on clinical trials of their products. I diverted substantial amounts of money from these projects to otherwise unfunded aspects of dissociative research, including an epidemiological study (Ross, Joshi, & Currie, 1990). Dr. Ron Norton was of great assistance in the planning and analysis of my research in Canada.

Two colleagues contributed more than any others to my work in Winnipeg: Geri Anderson and Pam Gahan. Together, the three of us learned many difficult lessons. At the beginning of November 1991, I moved to Dallas, Texas, to become the Medical Director of a fledgling Dissociative Disorders Program at Charter Behavioral Health System of Dallas, and I have been there since. I was recruited to Dallas by Gay Fite, who has provided much support and assistance for over four years now. Charter Behavioral Health System of Dallas, a private for-profit freestanding psychiatric facility, has provided me a workshop in which to refine my skills and deliver clinical service to more than 500 patients in four years.

I have also received support and encouragement from the International Society for the Study of Dissociation and its members, and was honored to serve as president of the organization in 1994. In 1995, I formed the Colin A. Ross Institute for Psychological Trauma, which was created to provide education, conduct research, and deliver clinical service, with a focus on psychological trauma and the dissociative disorders. My goal is that the Institute will establish trauma programs elsewhere in the United States, conduct training workshops, and fund research in the future. Creation of the Institute was possible because of the hard work and assistance of Gay Fite, Joan Ellason, Tere Kole, and Dale Whitmer.

I would like to thank Tom Rourke, CEO of Charter Behavioral Health System of Dallas for his ongoing support of my work and writing, and now of the Ross Institute. Aleen Davis, who was the administrator at Charter for the first three years I was there, also supported my work in many ways, and I thank her. This kind of support and interest were not forthcoming in Canada within the structure of the Canadian healthcare system. Charter has provided an environment in which I have been able to conduct research, acquire a large volume of clinical experience, and complete and publish three further books since the first edition of this book appeared in 1989: *The Osiris Complex: Case Studies in Multiple Personality Disorder* (1994); *Satanic Ritual Abuse: Principles of Treatment* (1995); and *Pseudoscience in Biological Psychiatry* (1995), of which I wrote about one third.

As always, my greatest debt is to the patients. They are my teachers. I have learned infinitely more from these courageous survivors of unimaginable childhoods than from all other patients, books, and colleagues put together.

COLIN A. ROSS

Dallas, Texas
August 1996

Introduction to the Second Edition

The second edition of this book, like the first, is meant for mental health professionals from all disciplines. Its purpose is to provide a broad yet detailed grounding in the recognition and treatment of multiple personality disorder, renamed *dissociative identity disorder* (DID) in the fourth edition of the *Diagnostic and Statistical Manual of Mental Disorders* (*DSM-IV*; American Psychiatric Association, 1994a). Why bother writing or reading such a book? I believe, based on my clinical experience and the existing research evidence, that DID is quite common and that dissociation is a common feature of many other psychiatric disorders, just as anxiety and depression occur in many illnesses that are not primarily anxiety or mood disorders. DID can teach the general psychiatrist a great deal about mental illness.

Working with DID patients and consulting with nonmedical community-based therapists have taught me about the limitations of diagnostically based assessment and therapy. As a psychiatrist, I have available to me a variety of highly differentiated treatment modalities, and it is important for me to make specific psychiatric diagnoses. It makes a big difference, in terms of the treatment plan and its outcome, whether I diagnose someone as suffering from panic disorder, schizophrenia, bulimia, or DID. I need to be able to make valid and reliable diagnostic discriminations between these disorders.

In a community-based agency that provides counseling and psychotherapy services for disturbed individuals, however, there is less need for differential diagnosis. Diagnostic labeling may, in fact, be countertherapeutic in such settings. In addition, the people seeking the services of such agencies have often had unpleasant contacts with hospital-based psychiatry and feel strongly that the diagnostic process works against their interests, rather than in favor of them.

In general, I think that an adult woman who has been sexually abused as a child, whether or not she has DID, has better odds of getting helpful treatment from a nonmedical community-based agency than from an academic department of psychiatry. I hope that therapists outside the psychiatric domain of the mental health system will be able to benefit from this book and will not be put off by its medical flavor.

The diagnosis of DID does not imply that there is anything fundamentally wrong with the person who has the disorder. There is no evidence to date that there is anything wrong with the brains, or the genes, of people who have DID. Although it is likely that the psychobiology of extreme, chronic childhood trauma involves alterations in brain function, nothing conclusive to this effect has been demonstrated in DID. Nor does the diagnosis imply that the person is "hysterical" or in any way bad, inferior, or weak. DID is, however, a true psychiatric disorder. It has an etiology, phenomenology, treatment, and prognosis that differentiates it from any other disorder.

DID is based not on defect but on talent and ability. The patients have used their ability to dissociate to cope with overwhelming childhood trauma, which usually involves both physical and sexual abuse. The problem with adult DID is that, like any survival strategy gone wrong, it creates more problems than it solves. If this were not so, the person wouldn't come for treatment. The treatment involves unlearning an overreliance on dissociation and learning more varied, flexible, and adaptive ways of coping with life.

Nonmedical therapists could easily incorporate the assessment and treatment techniques described in this book into their practices without ever having to use the term dissociative identity disorder or referring to the dissociated parts of their clients as "personalities." I make these remarks because I am aware that many therapists might reject a book like this on the assumption that it medicalizes the consequences of childhood abuse, labels the victims as deviant, and perpetuates a variety of prejudices against abused children, battered wives, and women in general. I don't think that is true.

There is a big gap between academic psychiatry and nonmedical community-based therapy in North America, which DID patients might help to bridge. They do have a specific psychiatric disorder, and they can benefit from hospitalization in a specialty unit that can deal with them effectively. Better liaison between hospital and community would work to the benefit of the mental health system and the DID patient or client.

There is still a great deal of resistance to DID in North America, especially in academic psychiatry, despite the exponential growth in the diagnosis and treatment of the disorder since 1980. Consequently, I have tried to provide a broad historical and conceptual discussion: It is important to know how to think about DID, not just what diagnostic and therapeutic techniques to use. Once one learns to think dissociatively, the world changes, and the plan of treatment falls into place more easily. The opening historical section of the book is directly relevant to therapy.

I have decided not to attempt an exhaustive referencing of the literature for two reasons. First, the literature up until 1992 is available in a comprehensive bibliography (Goettman, Greaves, & Coons, 1992). Second, the literature is now too large for any one person to read all of it. The major sources of ongoing references are the journal *Dissociation,* edited by Richard P. Kluft, M.D., and the *Newsletter of the International Society for the Study of Dissociation* (ISSD): Both may be obtained through the ISSD head office at 4700 West Lake Avenue, Glenview, IL 60025-1485 (phone 708-375-4718; fax 708-375-4777).

I have adopted a number of conventions in this second edition. I will refer to the therapist as male and the patient as female in most cases, and I will refer to the patient interchangeably as a patient or client, since persons with DID receive treatment under both designations.

I have tried to clarify for the reader when my discussion has a base in clinical experience, when it is based on research data, and when it runs beyond experience and data into conjecture. I may appear, at times, to speak with unwarranted certainty about the etiology, phenomenology, and treatment outcome of DID; I think that research and clinical findings will accumulate over the next decade supporting my views. However, I do not expect the skeptical reader to be immediately convinced by everything I say. Psychiatry has suffered from too many fads and transient enthusiasms, and I hope that DID will not be one more of these.

DID is not a metaphor for guiding therapy; it is not exclusively an iatrogenic artifact; and it is not an epiphenomenon of other psychiatric disorders. It is a legitimate and real psychiatric disorder with a specific treatment. It is not just another way of describing an amorphous, heterogeneous group of people who have been called "borderline," "as-if personality," and a variety of other terms.

There is a large group of disturbed individuals who do not fit into the psychiatric diagnostic system very well and for whom conventional treatments are not very helpful. These people tend to be polysymptomatic and to receive numerous different diagnoses. Only some people within this group have DID, but many have histories of serious childhood trauma. Those with DID are fortunate because they have a chance for complete recovery if they can find a therapist and can tolerate the difficult work of therapy.

DID occurs within a cluster of diagnoses and symptoms including depression, borderline personality disorder, panic disorder, somatization disorder, substance abuse, Schneiderian first-rank symptoms of schizophrenia, extrasensory perception experiences, secondary features of DID, and DID itself. The cluster is strongly associated with severe, chronic childhood trauma: the study of DID, I believe, will eventually result in a reorganization of the *DSM* diagnostic system around the theme of trauma.

DID is an important disorder, about which all mental health professionals should be knowledgeable, because it is common and treatable, and because it illustrates with great clarity and intensity the consequences of the childhood physical, sexual, and emotional abuse epidemic in our society.

Those are the assumptions on which I have based this account of the diagnosis, clinical features, and treatment of DID, a disorder thought to be extinct only four decades ago.

The second edition is much expanded and revised. I have added three new chapters on epidemiology, a critique of the skeptics, and the problem of attachment to the perpetrator and the locus of control shift. The discussion of four pathways to DID in Chapter Five is new thinking, and is based on accumulated reading, research, clinical experience, experience as an expert witness, and analysis of the problem of false memories. Since the first edition appeared in 1989, the major change in our society concerning childhood sexual abuse has been the false memory controversy: Current treatment of DID must consider the problem of false memories in a thorough and detailed fashion. Throughout the book, I have updated the discussion to reflect new research.

A second edition was required because the field has expanded rapidly in the last seven years. Treatment of DID must now be based on an understanding of the error-prone and reconstructive nature of memory. The standard of care for mental health professionals regarding memory has evolved significantly since the late 1980s, and the treatment of DID must keep pace with these developments. It is impossible to learn any therapy solely from a book, and reading this one will not create a fully qualified DID therapist. It will, however, provide a comprehensive understanding of people who have used dissociation in a complex, intricate way to cope with years of childhood physical, sexual, and emotional abuse. There are many such individuals in our culture.

Contents

PART ONE

The History of Dissociative Identity Disorder

. . . gods, strange gods, come forth from the forest into the clearing of my known self, and then go back.

    D. H. Lawrence, Studies in Classic American Literature

  Dissociative identity disorder (DID) is a complicated clinical disorder. Treating it effectively requires a number of different perspectives. The practitioner cannot take a narrow or "purist" point of view, but must understand in an historical and cultural context. The treatment of DID in the 1990s represents the attempts of therapists to relieve the suffering of a group of people whose disorder exists in a particular historical context. DID was not diagnosed very often only 15 years ago, and it is rarely diagnosed in many countries today.

  Because we are in a period of exponential increase in the rate of diagnosis of DID in North America, the Netherlands, Turkey, Norway, Japan,

Australia, New Zealand, and other countries, it is particularly important to be aware of the history of dissociation. In all countries where the diagnosis is made, the majority of DID patients have a dissociative disorder because of childhood sexual and physical abuse; in other cultures or times, the trauma provoking the dissociation might be war, famine, religious persecution, or natural disaster, and the symptoms and treatment might therefore be different.

It is important to understand that the cultural and historical aspects of DID do not make it less serious, less worthy of treatment, or less a legitimate subject of scientific study than any other psychiatric disorder. Panic disorder and schizophrenia did not exist as diagnoses prior to the twentieth century, and their phenomenology varies with culture. DID is not a biomedical disease in the sense that bacterial pneumonia is a disease, but it is a major public health problem, and it is often treatable. Untreated, DID imposes great suffering on the patient and a great drain on societal resources.

The first step in understanding DID is to review the history and to place the disorder in a broad context. By studying the past, we can learn a great deal about the range of dissociative phenomena, and variations in symptomotology. Practitioners can pick up numerous clinical tips and ideas from the nineteenth century specialists in dissociative disorders. A perusal of the history of dissociation shows that many recent findings were already known 100 years ago.

In this historical review of DID, I will be pursuing a number of interrelated ideas. In the first chapter, I will review developments up to and including Freud, beginning with ancient history. The chapter will conclude with a discussion of Breuer and Freud's *Studies on Hysteria* (1895/1986), and the peak of interest in dissociation in the early twentieth century. In the second chapter, I will describe the decline and discrediting of DID after about 1910, the gradual picking up of interest after World War II, and then the exponential increase in the diagnosis of DID in the 1980s.

The interrelated ideas in this historical review are these:

1. Dissociative phenomena can be recognized throughout history. DID is embedded in a universal historical context and is not a transient aberration.

2. Themes of the fragmentation of self and the transformation of identity are likewise universal.

3. The switching of executive control of the body from one psychic entity to another has occurred throughout history.

4. By reading case histories, one can chart a gradual evolution of demon possession into DID in the Western world, with the final transition in the nineteenth century.

5. In the nineteenth century and up until 1910 or so, the study of dissociation was in the mainstream of Western psychology and psychiatry,

and received attention from many major figures of the field such as Freud, Jung, Charcot, Janet, Binet, James, and Prince. The study of dissociation had clinical, experimental, and theoretical components.

6. DID and dissociation fell into disrepute after 1910 due to Freud's repudiation of the seduction theory and the new diagnosis of schizophrenia.

7. Also, DID fell into disrepute because of major flaws in the leading theories of dissociation.

8. The upsurge in the diagnosis of DID since 1980 provides an opportunity for modern scientific study of dissociation. This could result in dissociation being reestablished in the mainstream of psychiatry, on equal footing with anxiety and depression. Alternatively, dissociation could fall into disrepute again, repeating the events of the late nineteenth and early twentieth centuries.

To write a complete history of dissociation would require a large book in itself. A number of books provide elements of the history. These include *Hysteria: The History of a Disease,* by Ilza Veith (1965); *Multiple Man: Explorations in Possession and Multiple Personality,* by Adam Crabtree (1985); *From Mesmer to Freud: Magnetic Sleep and the Roots of Psychological Healing,* by Adam Crabtree (1993); *The Passion of Ansel Bourne: Multiple Personality in American Culture,* by Michael G. Kenny (1986); *Split Minds Split Brains,* edited by Jacques M. Quen (1986); *Multiple Personality, Allied Disorders, and Hypnosis,* by Eugene Bliss (1986); and *Multiple Personalities, Multiple Disorders: Psychiatric Classification and Media Influence,* by Carol North, Jo-Ellyn Ryall, Daniel Ricci, and Richard Wetzel (1993). These are the books I have found the most valuable. From them and from other sources, I have drawn together the preceding eight points.

Towering above these books and demanding separate mention is *The Discovery of the Unconscious,* by Henri F. Ellenberger (1970). This work of amazing scholarship is very clear and persuasive, and should be read by all students of dissociation.

CHAPTER ONE

The History Prior to and Including Freud

Dissociative identity disorder (DID) is not a transient aberration, peculiar to twentieth-century North America. Examples from ancient history show that the fragmentation of self and the transformation of identity have been recognized by all races. Examining dissociation in different cultures will give a sense of the universality of these themes. The purpose of this discussion is to demonstrate that the basic building blocks of DID have been present in most cultures throughout history. DID has gradually evolved from its prehistoric origins, through intermediate phenomena, to its modern form.

THE FRAGMENTATION OF SELF IN ANCIENT EGYPT: THE OSIRIS COMPLEX

The history of ancient Egypt is organized into three kingdoms, each of which is subdivided into dynasties. The Old Kingdom (3400–2445 B.C.) included Dynasties I–VIII; the Middle Kingdom (2445–1580 B.C.) included Dynasties IX–XVII; the New Kingdom (1580–332 B.C.) and included Dynasties XVIII–XXX. Dynasties XXVII–XXX (525–332 B.C.) are called the Persian Dynasties because during this period Egypt was ruled by Persian kings. The Persian Dynasties came to an end in 332 B.C. when Alexander the Great occupied Egypt.

The Egyptian myth that I have chosen to illustrate the fragmentation of self is that of Isis and Osiris (Ross, 1994b). The cult of Isis reached its peak just after the end of the Thirtieth Dynasty, at which time it was centered on the island of Philae in the Nile River. A temple to Isis had been built on that location in the Thirtieth Dynasty.

After the 4th century B.C., the cult of Isis spread from Alexandria throughout the Hellenic world. It entered Greece in combination with the cults of Horus, who was the son of Isis, and Serapis, which was the Greek name for Osiris. Herodotus apparently identified Isis with Demeter, the Greek goddess of earth, agriculture, and fertility.

The myth entered the Roman world as a tripartite cult of Isis, Horus, and Serapis in 86 B.C., when it was brought in by the consul Lucius Cornelius Sulla, and became one of the most popular branches of Roman mythology. The last Egyptian temples to Isis were closed in the 6th century A.D. Thus the cult and its theme of fragmentation were widely influential throughout the civilized Western world for centuries, attesting to the compelling importance of fragmentation. DID is the most extreme modern manifestation of the fragmentation of self.

In Egyptian mythology, only the ocean existed at first. Then Ra, the sun, was born from an egg that appeared on the surface of the ocean. Ra in turn gave rise to two gods, Shu and Geb, and two goddesses, Tefnut and Nut. Geb and Nut had two sons, Set and Osiris, and two daughters, Isis and Nephthys. Osiris married his sister Isis and succeeded Ra as king of the earth. However, his brother Set hated him. Set killed Osiris, cut him into many pieces, and scattered the fragments over a wide area.

Isis gathered up the fragments, embalmed them, and resurrected Osiris as king of the nether world, king of the land of the dead. As king of the dead, Osiris, aided by 42 assistants, judged the dead and assigned them to thirst and hunger, or dismemberment, on the one hand, or to the fields of Yaru, which were paradise, on the other. According to Egyptian belief, it was the person's *ka* that survived death and was judged by Osiris. The *ka* could only survive if the dead physical body survived on earth, however. It was this belief that gave rise to embalming, mummification, and the pyramids. The dead person's corpse was embalmed according to the original ritual embalming of Osiris by Isis.

Isis and Osiris had a son, Horus, who defeated Set in battle and became king of the earth. Thus in this myth we see the fragmentation, death, healing, and resurrection of the self in a new form. This is the cycle through which the successfully treated DID patient must pass. In our culture, the original agent of the fragmentation of self does not always receive divine retribution and is not always dethroned from his position of temporal power, resulting in perpetuation of the myth, which in our world takes the form of continued child abuse, and transmission of the abuse to future generations.

The DID patient suffers from an Osiris complex in addition to an Oedipus complex. The cause of her disorder is not conflicted incestuous fantasies, as Freud theorized was true of his patients. The DID patient has a fragmented self caused by real physical, sexual, and psychological assault. Her fragmentation represents a creative strategy for coping with and surviving this assault. DID requires treatment because, like all defenses gone wrong, it causes more suffering than it prevents, especially when the victim has become an adult and the original abuse is no longer occurring.

To say that the DID patient suffers from an Osiris complex in addition to an Oedipus complex is not to propose a complete break with Freud. Osiris was murdered by his brother and healed by a woman who was both his wife and sister. His parents were brother and sister. There is no shortage of oedipal conflict in the Osirian family. The crucial difference is that the victim of the Osiris complex was actually sexually abused. Her resulting complex is the inevitable and normal consequence of this abuse in a highly dissociative individual, and is not due to any intrinsic defect or abnormality in the victim. As I will explain in later chapters, the abusive events are traumatic in and of themselves, but they also give rise to *the problem of attachment to the perpetrator.* This inescapable problem of ambivalent attachment to the perpetrator is a core focus of the cognitive-behavioral treatment of DID. It is the cognitive-behavioral analog of the oedipal conflict.

There is no need to illustrate the theme of the fragmentation of self with further examples. Like any universal human theme, the Osiris myth is subject to variation and permutation from culture to culture. A myth is a stylized embodiment of living human themes, problems, and aspirations. In that sense, DID is a mythic disorder. It embodies in a profound and dramatic way the struggle of the self to maintain its integrity in the face of severe violation. That is a struggle in which we are all engaged to varying degrees.

The point of these remarks is to establish that DID is not a curiosity or an incomprehensible aberration. It is a commonsense disorder, and its features are familiar from myth, legend, religion, and literature. Many aspects of DID are represented in our popular culture in secular form today, in comic books, movies, and elsewhere.

THE THEME OF THE TRANSFORMATION OF IDENTITY IN HAIDA MYTHOLOGY

Before the arrival of the white explorers, the North American Indians varied as much in physique, economy, and culture as the Europeans. Two North American Indians could be as different as a Sicilian and a Swede. One of the most intense foci of native North American civilization is in the Pacific Northwest, and one of the tribes living in this area is the Haida.

The myth of the beginning of the Haida world (Clark, 1960), illustrates the theme of the transformation of identity, which is also one of the diagnostic criteria for DID. In the beginning of the Haida world, when in fact there was no world, Sha-lana ruled in a kingdom in the clouds. Raven, who was his chief servant, fell into disfavor and was cast forth from the celestial realm. It was Raven who created our world through a series of transformations.

First, by beating his wings, Raven transformed part of the primordial ocean into rock, from which sand and then trees gradually appeared, thereby creating the Queen Charlotte Islands. Raven created the human race by piling up clam shells and transforming them into two human females. Because of complaints by the two women, he then transformed one of them into a male. Unfortunately for Raven, however, seeing the two humans together made him lonely, so he decided to make a visit to Cloudland.

In Cloudland, Raven transformed himself into a bear and managed to be accepted by his chief as a playmate for the chief's son. In Cloudland, the children, as well as Raven, would transform themselves into animals in order to play. One day, Raven stole the chief's three children, who were in the form of bears, and also stole the sun. Transforming himself into an eagle, Raven flew off with the three bear-children and the sun. The people of Cloudland gave chase, but Raven dropped the three children, who were safely recovered. Sha-lana ordered the people not to pursue Raven to the earth because he was afraid that this might cause the ruler of the lower world to come to the celestial world. Sha-lana therefore created a new sun for Cloudland and allowed Raven to take the original sun to earth. Raven had stolen a fire stick at the same time, and this is why we have sunlight and fire in our world.

There are countless myths and legends from around the world that make use of transformation of identity. Citing more examples would not strengthen the point. Children in our culture are familiar with transformation of identity from comics, movies, television, and books. Who has not watched a child zooming around on the sidewalk or in the backyard, imagining that he is a superhero? Who can doubt the child's intensity of imaginative involvement in this transformation? I think it is reasonable to say that the normal child partially believes in this transformation on a transient basis.

We don't have to wonder where the DID child gets the idea of creating someone else inside to cope with the abuse. The strategy of transformation of identity to gain strength, coping power, and even invulnerability is readily available in the child's environment. Because this theme is universal, it would be surprising if DID occurred commonly in North America but rarely elsewhere. The building blocks of DID must be present in most if not all cultures. The most thorough study of dissociation in other cultures and its relationship to DID is *Trance and Possession in Bali: A Window on Western Multiple Personality, Possession Disorder, and Suicide,* by Suryani and Jensen (1993).

Suryani and Jensen's book and book chapters by Golub (1995), Krippner (1994), Kirmayer (1994), and Lewis-Fernandez (1994) explore dissociation as a theme in transcultural psychiatry.

DISSOCIATION AND TRANCE STATES IN CIRCUMPOLAR SHAMANISM

Except for five months when I was in Edmonton, I lived in the Northwest Territories from 1970 to 1975. The Northwest Territories are Canada's equivalent of Alaska. During this period, I read extensively about North American Indians, Eskimos, and circumpolar shamanism. For this reason, and because circumpolar shamans are, geographically and historically, the closest representatives of cultivated dissociation, I have chosen the shamans as illustrative of dissociative phenomena.

There is a controversy in the anthropological literature about whether shamans were mentally ill (Eliade, 1964). There is debate, for example, about whether they were hysterics or schizophrenics. This is an unproductive debate because it is not based on an adequate definition of schizophrenia, or recognition of the complexity and heterogeneity of chronic psychoses. The same is true for allegations that shamans are hysterics. DID patients are frequently misdiagnosed as schizophrenic, or dismissed as hysterics, so it is not surprising that anthropologists make similar conceptual errors about shamans.

As far as I can tell, most shamans did not suffer from any mental disorder. With variations of emphasis, they functioned as weather forecasters, doctors, priests, hunting consultants, and conveyors of oral tradition. Their professional activities were adaptive, culturally integrated, and planned. They undertook a long period of training and mastered a large number of techniques as well as an esoteric technical vocabulary. They were masters of self-hypnosis and used their ability to enter trances and altered states of consciousness in their work. Except for Siberian use of the hallucinogenic mushroom *amanita muscaria* (Wasson, 1973), the circumpolar shamans did not make extensive use of drugs, unlike their more southerly counterparts (Harner, 1973).

Clements (1932, cited in Ellenberger, 1970) listed five types of psychic illness treated with psychotherapy in preindustrial culture, each of which was treated by the shamans. They were:

1. Disease-object intrusion.
2. Loss of soul.
3. Spirit intrusion.
4. Breach of taboo.
5. Sorcery.

Each of these illnesses, with its corresponding specific modality of treatment, was within the expertise of the circumpolar shaman. I have encountered modern equivalents of loss of soul, spirit intrusion, breach of taboo, and sorcery in DID patients. Many DID patients feel that one or more of their alters are discarnate entities, intruders from the outside, and many feel that their original self is far away, lost, and unavailable for contact with the outside world. This is our equivalent of soul loss. The majority of DID patients report breach of the incest taboo. I have been told by DID patients about the effects of Satanic cults (Ross, 1995a), which are the modern form of black sorcery, and in a sense have encountered disease-object intrusion. In shamanism disease-object intrusion was concrete and was treated by the shaman sucking out the object through the patient's skin. In the DID patient, the intruding object is usually "bad feelings" that the patient "gets out" with help from the therapist through verbal techniques and rituals.

The shamans are interesting because they exhibit many of the dissociative features of the DID patient. They differ from the DID patient in that the shamans were healthy and used their dissociation in a culturally integrated way. The DID patient tends to be dysfunctional and socially isolated. This difference between the circumpolar shaman and the DID patient is one reason that DID is a disorder. Dissociation is not intrinsically pathological. Any given dissociative phenomenon may be functional or dysfunctional, healthy or a sign of illness, depending on its context. As well as resembling the DID patient, the shaman has much in common with the DID therapist, a theme that must be left to a later work.

In his book, Eliade presents the equation "shamanism = technique of ecstasy." This could as easily read "shamanism = technique of dissociation." I will describe 11 dissociative features of the shaman's work, all of which illustrate the presence of dissociation in other cultures.

Structured, Meaningful Hallucinations

Like the DID patient, the shaman heard voices and saw visions. For the shaman, these were not chaotic or meaningless symptoms of psychosis, however, as they are not for the DID patient. The shaman deliberately induced special states of being in which he could communicate with the spirits, hear their voices, and visually enter their worlds. For example, the shaman might travel to the underworld to negotiate with spirits that controlled the animals, asking the spirits to allow his people success in the hunt. Although it is a matter of philosophical axiom whether the shaman's experiences were hallucinations or perceptions of actual reality, for the DID patient similar experiences are clearly dissociative and psychologically meaningful.

Trance States

The shamans conducted public ceremonies in which, with the help of drumming, chanting, and ritualized movements, they entered trance states. While in trance, they exhibited many of the phenomena of modern hypnosis, including talking as if they were another person or an animal spirit (Spanos, Weekes, Menary, & Bertrand, 1986). The trance state was an essential prerequisite for communication with the spirits and temporary incarnation of spirits in the shaman's body. DID patients frequently enter trance.

Hypnotic Anesthesia

The shamans often demonstrated their power by public feats of hypnotic anesthesia such as holding hot objects, walking naked in the cold, or piercing themselves with sharp objects. According to tradition, the old shamans, prior to the decline of shamanism in recent centuries, could perform feats that were beyond the limits of modern hypnotic trance, such as drying several wet sheets by wrapping them on their naked bodies during an arctic blizzard, or holding extremely hot objects for long periods without discomfort or injury. DID patients often report anesthesia for the pain of abuse or self-inflicted pain.

Symbolic Dreams

The shamans were also specialists in spirit dreaming. They had dreams that resulted in the finding of game, foretold the future, helped the souls of dead people find their way in the afterworld, and performed other functions. Such dreams were sources of information about the real world, and in them the shamans carried out deliberate, conscious actions just as they would in the waking world. The DID patient frequently has dreams in which information about past abuse, the organization of the personality system or other knowledge is transmitted from alter personalities to the waking personality. The graduated recovery of abuse memories through dreams can be contracted for by the therapist. There are no studies concerning the historical accuracy of memories recovered initially as dreams, however, so such techniques must be used with caution.

Ritual Dismemberment

One way that the shamans could be initiated into their profession was through a ritual dismemberment reminiscent of the death of Osiris. This involved specific ceremonies and the spiritual fragmentation of the self. The DID patient, by definition, has undergone a dismemberment of the self for a specific purpose, in her case not to become a shaman but to survive severe childhood trauma.

Possession by the Souls of Ancestors

During ceremonial trances, the shamans would often deliberately become possessed by the souls of dead ancestors. The ancestors would speak through the body of the shaman for a variety of purposes, which might include practical advice or consolidation of social structure and tradition.

Alter personalities claiming to be dead relatives of the patient occur in 20.6% of cases of DID (Ross, Norton, & Wozney, 1989).

Possession by Helping Spirits

Another entity that frequently took possession of the shaman during rituals was the helping spirit. This might be an animal or a spirit entity. The shaman had a special relationship with his helpers, with whom he was on familiar terms. DID patients almost always have helper personalities, some of whom claim to be from other dimensions, or to be spirits. The helpers have usually been active prior to diagnosis and treatment, and also cooperate with the therapist for the patient's benefit.

Exhaustion Following Strenuous Trance Work

Following a particularly rigorous ceremony, during which a great deal of dancing might occur, and during which the shaman might perform numerous athletic feats, there was often a period of exhaustion that could last several days. This can also happen following an intense DID treatment session. The patient may feel drained and may lie down in bed for several hours, not fully recovering that day.

Stimulating Dissociation through Intoxication

The shamans by and large did not use hallucinogens in their work. Eliade feels that mushroom intoxication, when it was used, was "a mechanical and corrupt method of reproducing 'ecstasy,' being 'carried out of oneself'; it tries to imitate a model which is earlier and belongs to another plane of reference" (1964, p. 223). The principal hallucinogen used was the mushroom *amanita muscaria,* also known as fly agaric, which is the red toadstool with white flakes on it depicted in fairy tales. The later shamans held amanita parties that lacked structure or cultural purpose and indicate the deterioration of the shamans' dissociative skills (Harner, 1973). DID patients frequently abuse substances to achieve chemical dissociation, and also switch to substance-abusing alters to be in a more permissive state before drug ingestion. They use drugs to escape from pain, but the technique is crude and self-destructive compared with psychological dissociation.

Out-of-Body Experiences

One of the skills of the shaman was astral projection, or out-of-body travel. The shamans would ascend to the sky world or descend to the underworld to carry out various tasks. As well, they sent spirit helpers out into the landscape searching for game. Many DID patients have had out-of-body experiences, which originally occurred during childhood abuse. The little girl would float up to the ceiling and count the dots in the plaster, or travel to another location to play with dolls or friends. Later in life, such experiences can become more complex and can occur independently of traumatic events.

Transformation of Identity

During ceremonies, the shamans would deliberately induce a state of possession. When the animal spirit entered the shaman's body, it could then use his voice and gestures to communicate directly with the audience. The shaman, however, wasn't simply invaded by a foreign object. The possession state involved a reciprocal relationship between the two beings in which the shaman became the spirit and the spirit became the shaman. Thus there was a transformation of identity on the part of the shaman. This was controlled and transient. When the ceremony was completed, the shaman transformed back into his human self, and the spirit continued to exist as an independent entity outside him. This process is similar to the switching of alters in DID patients, but not identical.

I have described these dissociative experiences of circumpolar shamans to demonstrate that such experiences have occurred in many cultures throughout history. Any given dissociative event may be part of a disorder, a culturally normal ceremony, or simply an individual experience. There is a universal group of experiences involving trance, auditory hallucinations, and transformation of identity that has different meanings in different cultures. The DID patient has drawn on this region of human experience and ability to deal with chronic childhood trauma.

THE EVOLUTION OF DEMON POSSESSION INTO DISSOCIATIVE IDENTITY DISORDER

A full account of this history would require a book in itself. I am going to rely heavily on a book that has already done much of the work, *Possession Demoniacal and Other,* by T. K. Oesterreich (1974), first published in 1921. In Oesterreich's book, the reader can trace the evolution of demon possession into modern DID, although the author doesn't make that an explicit theme.

Like DID, demon possession is in many aspects an exaggeration of normal psychology. Oesterreich believes that there is a continuum from normality through obsessive states to possession, and that possession is a hypnotic phenomenon. With the possible exception of paranormal events associated with possession, all its phenomena can be reproduced in modern hypnotic trance.

Possession states share many of the properties of DID. For example, possession is subdivided into two categories depending on the presence or absence of one-way amnesia (see Chapter Four). In DID, one-way amnesia is said to occur if the presenting personality is amnesic for periods when alter personalities are in control of the body. In such cases, the alters are fully aware of the main or presenting personality. There was debate about the status of amnesia as a diagnostic criterion for DID prior to its inclusion in the *DSM-IV* criteria set, and there is likewise some controversy as to whether amnesia is required for true possession.

In fact, the diagnostic criteria for possession do not differentiate it from DID. These are the criteria of Nevius quoted in *Demon Possession* (Montgomery, 1976) by Wilson (1976, p. 224):

1. The chief differentiating mark of so-called demon possession is the automatic presentation and the persistent and consistent acting out of a new personality.
   a. The new personality says he is a demon.
   b. He/she uses personal pronouns; first person for the demon, third person for the possessed.
   c. The demon uses titles or names.
   d. The demon has sentiments, facial expressions, and physical manifestations that harmonize with the above.
2. Another differentiating mark of demon possession is the evidence it gives of knowledge and intellectual power not possessed by the subject.
3. Another differentiating mark of demonomania intimately connected with the assumption of a new personality is that with the change of personality there is a complete change of moral character (aversion and hatred to God and especially to Christ).

I have integrated alter personalities that met all these criteria using purely psychological methods, with no need for theological interpretations. In fact, personalities identified as demons occur in 28.6% of contemporary cases of DID (Ross, Norton, & Wozney, 1989). These diagnostic criteria for demon possession are culture-bound, because in other cultures neither priest, patient, nor demon would have heard of Jesus, and the behavioral response to the name Jesus would not occur.

In Chapter Seven, I will discuss the close link between dissociative disorders and obsessive-compulsive disorder (Ross & Anderson, 1988). This linkage is present in Oesterreich's analysis of possession states as well. He believes that possession may occur by one of two pathways, the first of which involves the elaboration of an obsessive state. The two forms of classical possession are *lucid possession* and *somnambulistic possession*. Lucid possession is similar to DID without amnesia, while somnambulistic possession is similar to DID with amnesia between alters.

Lucid possession occurs when the possessed person does not experience amnesia. The victim of lucid possession remembers everything the demon said and did while in control of his body. The lucidly possessed person feels a separate being inside him controlling his speech and actions, and struggles to regain control of his body. In somnambulistic possession, the possessed person is amnesic for everything the demon or spirit does during the periods of active possession. During treatment of DID, as the amnesia barriers are dismantled, the patient passes in reverse order to a stage of lucid possession and then to a normal integrated state.

According to Oesterreich, possession may arise in two ways. The first pathway to possession begins with a state of clinical obsession. Through an undefined process Oesterreich calls *condensation,* which is strongly influenced by cultural factors, the obsessed person progresses to a state in which he experiences an increasing sense of internal dividedness. This process may involve identification with someone in the environment or the past, hypnotic suggestion, or reinforcement by other people. The person then progresses to a state of lucid possession, in which he believes that his thoughts and impulses come not from himself but another being inside him.

As shown in Figure 1.1, from lucid possession the person may progress to somnambulistic possession, with amnesia, or to one of two other possibilities: successful fusion of the dissociated states or psychological deterioration.

The other starting point for the development of possession, according to Oesterreich, is the existence of two incompatible emotional states that are not fully dual, such as are experienced by all people. In a culture in which one of the states is defined as morally bad, the drive to possession will be greater. Thus, as shown in Figure 1.2, the person, under the influence of his culture, progresses to possession, which may be either lucid or somnambulistic, depending on how hypnotizable the person is, and the expectations of the culture. Somnambulistic possession, according to Oesterreich, requires a deeper level of autohypnosis than the lucid form, an idea consistent with modern scales of hypnotizability, in which the capacity for posthypnotic amnesia defines the highly hypnotizable individual.

If the culture does not endorse the possibility of demon possession, then one would expect the process diagrammed in Figure 1.2 to lead to a secular version of demon possession, which in our world is DID. Thus as our civilization evolved from the Middle Ages to the late twentieth century, there was a decline in demon possession and a rise in DID.

In medieval Europe, there was a dissociation of certain elements of being based on theological disapproval of those elements. Oesterreich remarks that there is no demon possession in Homer, a poet thought by Nietzsche (1956)

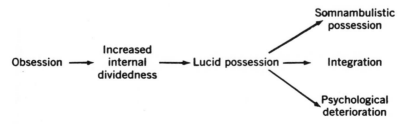

Figure 1.1. The First Pathway to Possession States

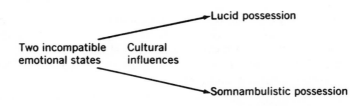

Figure 1.2.   The Second Pathway to Possession States

to be purely Apollonian. An Apollonian culture depends on dissociation of the Dionysian elements of being from public life, the Dionysian elements being sensuality, spontaneity, fertility, a pagan sense of religion, and physical ecstasy. These elements were punitively dissociated by the medieval church, as I describe in more detail in *Satanic Ritual Abuse: Principles of Treatment* (Ross, 1995a).

Though dissociated, the Dionysian was not absent. It was present as an incompatible set of impulses and knowledge in nuns, monks, peasants, and other medieval folk. When the dissociation broke down, the spontaneous sensual being regained control in a caricatured form as a demon. According to Oesterreich, exorcism reestablished the dissociation through hypnotic suggestion, although Oesterreich did not use the term *dissociation*.

The cases of classical demon possession were stereotyped and always conformed to cultural expectations. The exorcists engaged in theological debates and battles with the demons, but made no attempt to understand the phenomena psychologically. Also, demon possession was highly contagious: Epidemics could be prevented by physical isolation of the first case, a measure actually undertaken at times.

The transition from classical demon possession to DID occurred in four overlapping stages, for each of which I will give a case example.

Classical Demon Possession

In classical demon possession, the dissociated state identified itself as a Christian demon and uttered blasphemous statements. The exorcist engaged in theological debates with the demon, as well as using threats and commands prior to formal exorcism. The roles and attitudes of both demon and exorcist were highly structured and inflexible. In Christian culture, demons might identify themselves as Leviathan or Beelzebub, but this, I assume, never happens in non-Christian cultures in which neither exorcist nor possessed person has heard of these particular demons.

There was invariably a strong contrast between the character of the possessed person and that of the demon, with the person being devout and polite, and the demon irreverent and insulting. This is similar to the dual personalities of the nineteenth century and modern popular entertainment, in which the alters are polar opposites, such as quiet depressed housewife and promiscuous partygoer.

Oesterreich (1921/1974) quotes a typical case of classical demon possession occurring in 1714:

At the unexpected rumor that two possessed women had been brought into the workhouse of that place, I followed the dictates of my pastor's conscience and went to the workhouse on the evening of the 14th of December, 1714. After . . . the paroxysm began in one of the possessed women, and Satan abruptly hurled this invective at me by her mouth: "Silly fool, what are you doing in this workhouse? You'll get lice here," etc. I made him this answer: "By the blood, the wounds and the martyrdom of Jesus Christ, thou shalt be vanquished and expelled!" Thereupon he foamed with rage and shouted: "If we had the devil's power we would turn the earth and heaven upside down, etc. . . . What God doesn't want is ours!"

In the morning, towards 11 o'clock, this possessed woman came at my request, but not willingly, into the church of the place. There, in order that I might inform myself of her most wretched state, I began to sing the canticle: "May God the Father be with us," and after such preparation as I judged necessary I read from the pulpit the two remarkable passages concerning possession in the fifth and ninth chapters of St. Mark, so earnestly and for so long that Satan who was in the possessed cried to me from below the pulpit: "Won't you soon have done?" After I had replied: "When it is enough for God it will be enough for thee, demon!" Satan broke into complaints against me: "How dost thou oppress, how dost thou torment me! If only I had been wise enough not to enter thy church!" As he cried out impudently: "My creature must now suffer as an example!" I closed his mouth with these words: "Demon! the creature is not thine but God's! That which is thine is filth and unclean things, hell and damnation to all eternity." When at last I addressed to him the most violent exhortations in the name of Jesus, he cried out: "Oh, I burn, I burn! Oh, what torture! What torture!" or loaded me with furious invectives: "What ails thee to jabber in this fashion?"

During all these prayers, clamourings, and disputes, Satan tortured the poor creature horribly, howled through her mouth in a frightful manner and threw her to the ground so rigid, so insensible that she became as cold as ice and lay as dead, at which time we could not perceive the slightest breath until at last with God's help she came to herself . . .

Although the possessed once more recovered her reason on this occasion without being able, be it noted, to remember what Satan had said by her mouth, he did not leave her long in peace after my departure; he tormented her as before . . . . (p. 9)

In his book *Ecstatic Religion: An Anthropological Study of Spirit Possession and Shamanism,* I. M. Lewis (1971) argues very persuasively, with examples from many cultures, that spirit possession often serves a social function. For example, women living in cultures in which they are politically powerless can acquire power, influence, autonomy, and partial satisfaction of thwarted needs through possession. In one culture, there may be a special women's cult that exorcises the possessed; in another, possession may confer relief from unpleasant duties. Demon possession in western Europe made possible the ritualized expression of Dionysian impulses and opinions that were politically or theologically dangerous and that could not be stated directly, or even consciously acknowledged by the possessed person.

Demon possession was not always an effective strategy for the politically or theologically oppressed since it could be dealt with by witch-hunt and Inquisition (Ross, 1995a).

Early Transitional Demon Possession

By 1830, possession states no longer invariably met the classical features. Instead of being possessed by demons, folk could be overtaken by dead neighbors or relatives, and the exorcists had shifted toward a psychological theory of possession. The social context of the possession had become more prominent in the narratives, but from reading them one could not form psychological hypotheses about identification, secondary gain, or other factors that might be operative.

The following case was observed in 1830 (Oesterreich, 1921/1974):

The first woman possessed in the Biblical manner with whom I became acquainted, writes the Swabian poet and physician Justinus Kerner, I owe to the confidence of Doctor . . . He had sent her to me for cure, informing me that all treatment by ordinary methods had been fruitless when applied to this woman.

The patient was a peasant-woman of thirty-four years. . . . Her past life up to this time had been irreproachable. She kept her house and showed due regard for religion without being especially devout. Without any definite cause which could be discovered, she was seized, in August, 1830, by terrible fits of convulsions, during which a strange voice uttered by her mouth diabolic discourses. As soon as this voice began to speak (it professed to be that of an unhappy dead man), her individuality vanished, to give place to another. So long as this lasted she knew nothing of her individuality, which only reappeared (in all its integrity and reason) when she had retired to rest.

This demon shouted, swore, and raged in a most terrible fashion. He broke out especially into curses against God and everything sacred.

Bodily measures and medicines did not produce the slightest change in her state, nor did a pregnancy and the suckling which followed it. Only her continual prayer (to which moreover she was obliged to apply herself with the greatest perseverance, for the demon could not endure it) often frustrated the demon for a time.

During five months all the resources of medicine were tried in vain. . . . On the contrary, two demons now spoke in her; who often, as it were, played the raging multitude within her, barked like dogs, mewed like cats, etc. Did she begin to pray, the demons at once flung her into the air, swore, and made a horrible din through her mouth.

When the demons left her in peace she came to herself, and on hearing the accounts of those present, and seeing the injuries inflicted upon her by blows and falls, she burst into sobs and lamented her condition. By a magico-magnetic (that is to say, hypnotic) treatment . . . one of the demons had been expelled before she was brought to me; but the one who remained only made the more turmoil. (p. 10)

A number of features of modern DID and its treatment are beginning to appear by 1830. First, the possessed person is classified as a *patient* and is treated by a physician. A number of traditional medical approaches are tried unsuccessfully, as often happens in DID, and then treatment progress is made with hypnosis. There is a hint of a conception of possession as a form of hysteria, in that hysteria was thought to be treatable with marriage, sexual activity, and motherhood in at least some cases. As well, by remarking that the possession state began "without any definite cause," the narrator implies that some possession cases have discernible secular causes, which in turn implies that they are psychological not theological in nature.

The full transition to late twentieth-century DID has not been made in this case, however, because the demon is treated by expulsion. This conception has lingered in muted psychological form into the 1990s, in the sense that undesirable (in the eyes of the therapist) alters were expelled, suppressed, or otherwise banished by some therapists to ensure that the "real" self gained control.

Late Transitional Demon Possession

In late transitional demon possession, the conception of the therapist is purely psychological and so is the treatment. The patient complains of being demon possessed, but the demon is considered by the physician to be a dissociated psychic entity, and its purpose is psychological. The psychological theory and the therapeutic interventions are subtle and complex, and the case is related to a wide range of dissociative phenomena, other cases, multiple personality, and a theory of dissociation.

An excellent example of late transitional demon possession is the case of Achille, treated by Pierre Janet at the Saltpetriere, where a great deal of work on hypnosis, hysteria, and dissociation was done. The case is quoted at length by Oesterreich, so I will summarize it.

Achille had no psychiatric problems until 1890 when, at the age of 33, he had a brief affair while away from his wife and child on a business trip. On his return, he rapidly fell into a depression, which progressed to a state of demon possession, with the devil assuming executive control spontaneously. The devil made statements such as "Cursed the Trinity, cursed the Virgin!" and "Priests are a worthless lot!" A priest was called who diagnosed Achille as mad and in need of medical treatment. The transition from classical possession to DID was accompanied both by medicine taking over responsibility for these cases and by the church relinquishing responsibility.

Janet devised a treatment strategy derived from his knowledge of multiple personality and experimental work on automatic writing (Janet, 1901/1977,

1907/1965). He allowed the demon to "rave and rant as he pleased" and while standing behind him quietly ordered him to make certain movements. This is an experimental technique for eliciting dissociated behavior that was used extensively in nineteenth-century French psychology. By automatic writing, the demon entered into a conversation with Janet, during which he tricked the devil into cooperating with him. "To force the devil to obey me I attacked him through the sentiment which has always been the darling of devils—vanity."

Janet tricked the devil into a demonstration of his power: The devil placed Achille in a hypnotic trance, which Janet himself had been unable to do. Once this was achieved, Janet was able to discover the extramarital affair, which had not been disclosed. He then began a systematic process of hypnotically transforming Achille's memories, thoughts, and feelings about the event, with the goal of relieving his guilt. Janet's summary of the treatment, which resulted in complete and lasting cure, is as follows:

> If we wished to cure our unhappy Achille, it was completely useless to talk to him of hell, demons and death. Although he spoke of them incessantly, they were secondary things, psychologically accessory. Although the patient appeared possessed, his malady was not possession but the emotion of remorse. This was true of many possessed persons, the devil being for them merely the incarnation of their regrets, remorse, terrors and vices. It was Achille's remorse and the very memory of his wrong-doing which we had to make him forget. This was far from being an easy matter—forgetting is more difficult than is generally supposed.
>
> . . . The memory of his transgression was transformed in all sorts of ways thanks to suggested hallucinations. Finally Achille's wife, evoked by a hallucination at the proper moment, came to grant complete pardon to her spouse, who was deserving rather of pity than of blame. (p. 116)

I have called this a case of late transitional demon possession for several reasons, the first being that the dissociated state identified itself as a demon. More important, the treatment consisted of a refined psychological exorcism not of the demon but of the memory that resulted in creation of the demon. Few contemporary therapists would advocate such an approach except in exceptional cases, and most would strive for integration of the memory into the main body of consciousness, possibly with adjunctive marital therapy. The case is late transitional, also, because the demon makes stereotypically demonic denunciations of Christian religion.

Since the final transition to modern DID, demon possession has been viewed in purely psychological terms by most physicians and psychotherapists. For example, a few years ago while covering for a colleague on vacation, I interviewed an inpatient he was treating for a psychotic depression. She had stated that she was possessed by the devil, prior to her responding to antidepressant and antipsychotic medication. Like her attending psychiatrist, I viewed the belief in demon possession as a depressive delusion. As a teaching exercise for the resident and medical students, I reviewed the differential diagnosis between possession states occurring as dissociative disorders, and ideas of possession arising from cognitive errors made by the patient. A delusion is an extreme form of cognitive error.

In this case, the patient concluded that she must be possessed as an explanation for the obsessive thoughts she had been having. These had started after the onset of her depression. Since the thoughts were uncharacteristic of her normal thinking and felt ego-alien, she concluded that they must not be coming from her. At no time did she have a sense of the palpable presence of an alien entity within her, she did not hear the voice of the devil, and she did not talk like a demon. She readily accepted my explanation that obsessive thoughts can be a symptom of depression, and my reassurance that they should go away with further resolution of her depression, which was in partial remission.

There was no hint of anyone on the ward considering exorcism. Demon possession, in such cases, in 1988, had been attenuated to the status of a delusional idea, with little or no behavioral manifestations. It really exists only as an ideational remnant of past culture. However, demon possession is still accepted as an actual possibility by some theologians and clinicians, which gives rise to postdemonic possession.

Postdemonic Demon Possession

In the modern world, Christian religion no longer exists as the organizing principle, or guiding core of most medical and therapeutic practice. Most psychotherapy is agnostic or atheistic. In professional journals and books, there are no techniques, theories, or viewpoints it would make sense to call *spiritual*. Not surprisingly, there is also no demon possession. In this cultural climate, any alleged cases of demon possession can therefore be described as postdemonic, from the perspective of the mainstream.

Such cases are reported in a book called *Demon Possession* (Montgomery, 1976). This is a collection of papers arising from a conference on demon possession held by the Christian Medical Society at Notre Dame University in 1975. Several cases of possible demon possession are presented that are indistinguishable from secular dissociative disorders, and that would be considered part of the regular caseload on any service specializing in dissociative disorders.

One of these is described by a physician (Wilson, 1976):

This 32-year old twice-married female was brought in because of falling spells which had been treated with all kinds of anticonvulsant medication. She was examined on the neurological service and after all examinations including EEG, brain scan, and a pneumoencephalogram were negative, she was transferred to the psychiatric service. Her mental status examination was unremarkable and all of the staff commented that she seemed normal until she had her first "spell."

> While standing at the door of the day room she was violently thrown to the floor bruising her arm severely. She was picked up and carried to her room all the while resisting violently. When the author arrived, eight persons were restraining her as she thrashed about on the bed. *Her facial expression was one of anger and hate.* Sedation resulted in sleep. During the ensuing weeks, the patient was treated psychotherapeutically and it was learned that there was considerable turmoil in her childhood home, but because she was "pretty," she was spoiled. She married the type of individual described by Jackson Smith as the first husband of a hysterical female. She was a "high liver" and after her separation and divorce, she was threatened with rejection by her parents. She remarried and her second husband was a "nice" but unexciting man. She continued to associate with her "high living" friends. When her husband demanded that she give up her friends and her parties, she started having the "spells." (p. 225)

My hypotheses about this woman are that the "turmoil" in her childhood was paternal incest; that the angry state was an alter who remembered the abuse; that there was at least partial amnesia for the "high living," which was carried out by a promiscuous alter; that there had been auditory hallucinations and amnesic periods prior to the recent "spells"; and that the patient was a "hysterical" female because she was a victim of childhood sexual abuse. Further, the "acceptance of Christ" described in a paragraph subsequent to those quoted did not represent a real religious conversion of her whole being: it was a pseudo-acceptance that reinforced the amnesia for the incest. If this is correct then the patient would inevitably relapse.

My distrust of the "theological" hypothesis about this case is compounded by a statement that appears shortly after the case history: "Other examples of possible 'hysterical' demon possession meeting the criteria of Nevius may be found in the *Three Faces of Eve,* by Cleckley, and in *Sybil,* by Schreiber." Such clinico-theological "treatment" reinforces silence about the sexual abuse of girls, and blaming of the adult survivor, who is said to be either hysterical, possessed, or both.

The hypothesis of demon possession in this case is an attempt to impose an out-of-date worldview on secular phenomena that have superseded the old Christian culture. I say that as someone who is willing to believe that demon possession may actually occur, and who sees the fragmentation and secularization of our society as cultural decay. Actually it is important for both clinical and religious reasons not to interpret dissociative disorders as possession, because such misinterpretation is both bad medicine and bad religion. It doesn't make sense to exorcise dissociative states, not because there are no demons, but because dissociative states are part of the whole person.

Perhaps it would make sense to leave the last word on demon possession to a patient of mine. This woman, who had been sexually abused by her father, wrote the following passage in her diary after I had seen her once in consultation, and several months before I started working with her psychotherapeutically:

Where do these feelings stem from the Religious beliefs that were so hypocritical and confusing that caused two different sides between the parts good/evil how from childhood they were taught to honor the mother and father no matter how abusive they are to you how that they must always be good and confess their sins or the devil will get them being that in the form of the father. What sins does a child have when growing up except for the ones that they were made to believe in. They were so instilled with miracles that they waited for miracles to happen to them because of all the suffering that they deserved one and when they didn't receive them they became angry with God and possible created an evil part as a form of revenge not only on men but on God as well.

SCIENTIFIC STUDY OF DISSOCIATION IN THE NINETEENTH CENTURY

The authors I mentioned earlier in this chapter, especially Ellenberger (1970), have detailed much of this history in books that are readily available, so I need only mention some of the main figures. When I speak of the nineteenth century, I really mean the period until about 1910.

Especially in France and the United States, a great deal of work was done on dissociation in the nineteenth century. There were case studies of DID and fugues, experimental studies of automatic writing and hypnosis, and theoretical treatises. Cases of DID were reported from a number of centers. The main figures included Janet, Charcot, Bernheim, Liebault, Freud, Jung, Prince, James, and others.

In his *Principles of Psychology* (1983), first published in 1890, William James discussed multiple personality in a theoretical chapter on the consciousness of self. He spoke of a plurality of selves in the normal individual, which included the material, social, and spiritual selves, and the pure ego. These selves could undergo various derangements, some resulting in DID. Thus the leading American psychological theoretician took DID seriously, advocated further empirical study of the disorder, and believed that it had numerous theoretical implications for the field. There was no question of DID being dismissed as unworthy of serious study.

Sidis and Goodhart published a case study of a patient called Hannah under the title *Multiple Personality* (1905) with a dedication to William James. Boris Sidis also coedited the *Journal of Abnormal Psychology* with Morton Prince, who wrote extensively on DID. Prince's case study, *The Dissociation of a Personality* (1905/1978), is still widely referred to and has recently been reprinted. The leading figures of the day were interlinked both personally and professionally by their interest in dissociation.

Jung studied mediums and spiritism and presented case histories containing numerous dissociative phenomena in a treatise called "On the Psychology and Pathology of So-Called Occult Phenomena" (Jung, 1902/1977). Jung's interest in parapsychology was one of the factors that led to his eventual split with Freud. If we think of Jung's interest in the paranormal as intertwined with his study of dissociation, we realize that to stay with Freud, Jung would have had to abandon his study of dissociation and related phenomena. It is well known, for example, that Freud repudiated the use of hypnosis.

Before discussing Freud, I want to do two things: first, outline the major flaws in the two leading approaches to dissociation in nineteenth-century psychology, and second, discuss Alfred Binet and F. W. H. Myers, two neglected but major figures in the history of dissociative studies. The flaws in dissociative theory probably contributed to its being abandoned as a field of serious study after 1910.

Janet is a chief representative of one approach. He believed that dissociation originates from real trauma. He also held, however, that dissociation, like mental illness in general, is based on a biological predisposition. That is reasonable, except that the predisposition was called "mental degeneration," a term derived from Morel. Patients were thought of as mental degenerates. They fell victim to dissociation, basically, because of weakness and an inability to *associate* psychic elements normally. Their disorders were based on incapacity. According to this view, one would develop DID in response to childhood trauma because of an intrinsic biological defect. Such a theory is not able to account for the phenomena adequately, because integrated DID patients do not display signs of degeneracy.

The idea that patients with posttraumatic dissociative disorders are tainted with "mental degeneracy" contributed to the discrediting of DID. With the appearance of the diagnosis of schizophrenia, DID patients were rediagnosed as schizophrenic, which really meant that they were viewed as suffering from an organic brain syndrome (see Chapter Two). If Janet had thought of the biological predisposition as a talent or ability, which I believe it is, it might not have been so easy for DID to be swallowed up by organic mental disease.

Morton Prince made the other major error in the field, and Thigpen and Cleckley repeated it in *The Three Faces of Eve* (1957). They decided that the best way to treat DID is to force the disappearance of most alters, and to back the ascendancy of one. Such treatment consists of trying to get rid of the "bad" alters and keep the "good" or "real" ones. This does not work because the "bad" alters have a function, only appear to be bad when not understood, and are a necessary part of the whole. This kind of treatment is a secular version of exorcism that does not heal the pain, resolve the conflicts, or lead to integration, and that reinforces the dissociation.

These flaws in the theory of dissociation and its treatment made it easier for the field to fall into disrepute by weakening its foundations.

The theoretical, experimental, and clinical study of dissociation in the nineteenth century is exemplified by Alfred Binet, who, like other early figures, has been overlooked in the recent revival of interest in Janet (Haule, 1986; van der Hart & van der Velden, 1987).

The Work of Alfred Binet

Alfred Binet was born in Nice in 1857 and died in 1911. Besides his interest in intelligence, he wrote two major treatises on dissociation. *On Double Consciousness* (1977b) was published in 1890, while *Alterations of Personality* (1977a) appeared in 1896. Both have recently been reprinted (Binet, 1977a, 1977b). The two volumes contain a wealth of theory, clinical observation, and experimental evidence on multiple personality and dissociation.

Binet noted that experimental alters can be produced in normal highly hypnotizable subjects, thus anticipating work by Spanos et al. (1986) and others who do not refer to Binet. He also observed that these alter personalities were transient and incomplete analogs of full DID.

Binet viewed the doubling of consciousness as a common clinical mechanism in a variety of psychiatric disorders, including somatization disorder, conversion disorder, and dissociative disorders, as classified in *DSM-III* (American Psychiatric Association, 1980), *DSM-III-R* (American Psychiatric Association, 1987), and *DSM-IV* (American Psychiatric Association, 1994a). He demonstrated that amnesia, muscle paralysis, auditory hallucinations, automatic writing, obsessive thoughts, and many other phenomena were associated with double consciousness and that this doubling was the basic mechanism in forming these symptoms.

Binet performed experiments to demonstrate the leakage of information across amnesia barriers. These experiments have only been revived in the past decade or two, without acknowledgment of Binet. He also studied Hilgard's hidden observer (Hilgard, 1977, 1984) in a large series of experiments, acknowledging Richet as the first person to identify the hidden observer. The term "hidden observer" was not used in the nineteenth century, but it is the same experimental phenomenon. Binet said of Richet, "He has brought out the fact, that in hysterical persons and in a great many individuals reputed normal, there exists a sort of permanent semi-somnambulism; in other words, there is, in these subjects, an unconscious ego, an unconscious activity, which is constantly on the watch, which contemplates, which gives attention, which reflects, which forms inferences, and lastly which performs acts—all unknown to the conscious ego."

Some of Binet's experiments were simple, some complicated. I will describe a simple one. Binet took a person he called hysterical, hypnotized him or her, and induced an experimental anesthesia in one hand. He then had the person read an eye chart, and adjusted the distance between the person and the eye chart so the person could just read the largest letters. The subject was then asked to read smaller letters on the chart, but could not do so. The subject had not seen these smaller letters during the earlier phase of the experiment. In the next step, Binet placed a pen in the anesthetic hand, without changing the distance between the eye chart and the subject. The person was still unable to read the smaller letters, but the anesthetic hand was now able to write them down accurately. The subject denied any conscious awareness of the activity of the hand.

This was basically a hidden observer experiment. Binet used numerous experimental procedures, and worked with pain, touch, hearing, memory, and other faculties. By the standards of modern experimental psychology, his work was crude, but it was pioneering. His findings were entirely consistent with those of Hilgard. Binet also made a number of other interesting observations. He repeated Janet's observation that the naming of an alter personality "crystallizes" it, making it more formed and definite.

Binet stated that alters created experimentally can only be called out by the person who created them, whereas autohypnotic alters can be called out by anyone. This crucial observation, which has been lost for 100 years, needs to be studied. It is an observation that strikes to the heart of the field, and bears directly on the controversy about iatrogenic influence in DID.

This brief summary of Binet's work highlights that there was a great deal of clinical and experimental study of dissociation in the nineteenth century. We have suffered a nearly complete discontinuity with that work and have started to repair it only in the past two decades.

F. W. H. Myers

F. W. H. Myers was born on February 6, 1843, in Keswick, Cumberland, and died in Rome on January 17, 1901. He won numerous honors and awards while a student at Trinity College, Cambridge, and worked closely with leading Cambridge intellectuals including Henry Sidgwick, who was instrumental in creation of the English Department at Trinity College (Leavis, 1968). Myers, who published a monograph on William Wordsworth, was a man of broad interests and scholarship. He was one of a small group of men who founded the Society for Psychical Research in 1882, which was devoted to the study of paranormal phenomena of all kinds. Henry Sidgwick was the first President of the Society.

Myers published *Human Personality and Its Survival of Bodily Death* posthumously in 1903; my copy is an abridged version published in 1920. It is a wonderful book. Myers presents a theory of normal human psychology based on dissociated parallel tracks of consciousness, with various interactions between the two tracks or selves. He uses this theory to tie together and account for many phenomena studied by Janet and Binet including motor automatisms, hypnosis, possession states, and alternations of personality. He includes telepathy and phantasms of the dead in the range of human experience accounted for by his theory.

Myers describes a *subliminal self,* which roughly corresponds to the unconscious mind, and a *supraluminal self,* which corresponds to the conscious self. In his scheme the subliminal self is not unconscious, however; it is dissociated but conscious and can intrude on the supraluminal self in many ways through automatisms, paranormal intrusions, possession, trance states, alternations of personality, and the insights of genius. Myers says:

Perceiving (as this book will try to show) that these submerged thoughts and emotions possess the characteristics which we associate with conscious life, I feel bound to speak of a *subliminal* or *ultra-marginal consciousness*—a consciousness which we shall see, for instance, uttering or writing sentences quite as complex and coherent as the supraluminal consciousness could make them. Perceiving further that this conscious life beneath the threshold or beyond the margin seems to be no discontinuous or intermittent thing; that not only are these isolated subliminal processes comparable with isolated supraluminal processes (as when a problem is solved by some unknown procedure in a dream), but that there is also a continuous subliminal chain of memory (or more chains than one) involving just that kind of individual and persistent revival of old impressions, and response to new ones, which we commonly call a Self—I find it permissible and convenient to speak of subliminal Selves, or more briefly of a subliminal Self. I do not indeed by using this term assume that there are two correlative and parallel selves existing always within us. Rather I mean by the subliminal Self that part of the self which is commonly subliminal; and I conceive that there may be—not only *co-operations* between these quasi-independent trains of thought—but also upheavals and alternations of personality of many kinds, so that what was once below the surface may for a time, or permanently, rise above it. (p. 15)

Although in theory the subliminal and supraluminal selves are not independent parallel tracks of consciousness, in practice, they are usually highly dissociated, and the supraluminal self experiences the intrusion of the subliminal self as ego-alien—as a possession state, for instance.

Myers was a great theoretician of the dissociated structure of the normal mind, and also a collector of countless anecdotes and examples. The richness of nineteenth-century literature on dissociation, hypnosis, trance, possession, and the paranormal is in part due to the case histories it contains. Myers should be remembered as one of the great figures of nineteenth-century dissociation theory, on a par with Janet, although he was not a clinician and therefore doesn't compare with Janet in that dimension. Nor was he an experimentalist like Binet. Nevertheless, Myers is a major precursor of late twentieth-century writers on dissociation.

Breuer and Freud's Studies on Hysteria

Breuer and Freud published *Studies on Hysteria* (1986) in 1895. The book consists of their case histories of female patients as well as several theoretical chapters. All the women described in the case histories had dissociative disorders, and most had been sexually abused. Anna O., the subject of the most famous case history in the book, clearly had DID. Up until 1895, Freud considered these patients to be suffering from the adult consequences of real childhood abuse. His treatment took the reality of the trauma into account both technically and theoretically.

Within a few years of publishing *Studies on Hysteria,* however, Freud repudiated the seduction theory. There are probably personal, social, and intellectual reasons behind this major shift in Freud's thinking. Several of them are apparent in Ernest Jones's biography of Freud (1953). For one thing, it would have been awkward for Freud to state publicly that his patients had been sexually abused as children. Many of the abusive fathers were part of his own social circle.

Anna O.'s family lived one street away from Freud. In 1880, they had moved to Vienna to a neighborhood called Liechtensteinerstrasse, which was one block away from a street called Bergasse, where Freud had both his home and office from 1891 to 1938. Anna O. was a friend of Freud's wife and visited in the Freud home more than once. Later, Anna and Freud's wife, Martha, became related by marriage.

We know that the sexual aspects of Anna O.'s symptomotology made Breuer very uncomfortable. The relationship between Breuer and Anna O. ended when she developed a hysterical pregnancy, for which Breuer was the father. The last time Breuer saw her was on a house call, during which she was in hysterical labor. Jones writes, "Though profoundly shocked, he managed to calm her down by hypnotizing her, and then fled the house in a cold sweat. The next day he and his wife left for Venice to spend a second honeymoon, which resulted in the conception of a daughter; the girl born in these curious circumstances was nearly sixty years later to commit suicide in New York" (p. 247). The timing of the second honeymoon and the conception of Breuer's daughter is aprocryphal (Pollock, 1984), but Jones's account captures his understanding of the psychodynamics at work.

Breuer's wife had been jealous of her husband's preoccupation with Anna O. and the amount of time he spent with her. According to Jones, Martha Freud "identified herself with Breuer's wife, and hoped the same thing would not ever happen to her, whereupon Freud reproved her vanity in supposing that other women would fall in love with *her* husband: 'For that to happen one has to be a Breuer'" (p. 247).

Freud's repudiation of the seduction theory was a great misfortune for psychiatric patients. It resulted in a repudiation of the clinical realities of both abused children and adult survivors of childhood abuse. To "explain" the symptoms of his patients, in what he thought was the absence of any actual trauma, Freud invented a complex metapsychology. Despite this false premise, he was then able to construct valuable and lasting theory.

At the time of *Studies on Hysteria,* Freud was working with patients similar to those of Binet, Janet, and Prince. His ideas were consistent with their tradition, and with a large body of experimental data. Following his repudiation of the seduction theory, however, Freud embarked on a metapsychological digression: A second aspect of Freud's genius was his ability to create a socially acceptable theory that denied the reality of childhood sexual abuse.

Anna O. had DID. There is no evidence that she was sexually abused by her father. If she was, though, that would explain her conflict about nursing her father while he was dying. The diagnosis of DID was made by Freud and Breuer, and also by Ernest Jones, who said, "More interesting, however, was the presence of two distinct states of consciousness: one a fairly normal one, the other that of a naughty and troublesome child, rather like

Morton Prince's famous case of Sally Beauchamp. It was thus a case of double personality" (p. 246). It was actually a case of triple personality.

Anna O.'s DID has been retrospectively diagnosed by Walter Stewart, a contemporary psychoanalyst (1984), who wrote, "As a next line of defense she developed a double personality. In the normal state, she was oriented but depressed and anxious. In the *condition seconde,* she was abusive, rebellious, moody, and naughty. The split in personality was an attempt to isolate the angry aspect of her character" (p. 50). The question is, what was Anna O. so angry about?

F. W. H. Myers also thought that Anna O. had DID: "The condition of extreme instability thus induced, varying from hour to hour, gave rise at times to a secondary personality which lay outside the primary memory. We thus have a very direct transition from isolated disturbances to a cleavage of the whole personality" (p. 33).

Loewenstein (1993a, 1993b) reformulated Anna O. as a case of DID and provided an exhaustive symptom checklist comparing her profile with that established in published series of DID cases.

To establish beyond doubt for readers of this book that Anna O. had DID, I will quote a number of passages from *Studies on Hysteria.* I have used the Pelican edition because it is more readily available to readers who want to study the entire case history.

Breuer noticed Anna O.'s DID immediately, prior to any use of hypnosis, other treatment interventions, or the formation of a transference relationship:

> It was while the patient was in this condition that I undertook her treatment, and I at once recognized the seriousness of the psychical disturbance with which I had to deal. Two entirely distinct states of consciousness were present which alternated very frequently and without warning and which became more and more differentiated in the course of the illness. In one of these states she recognized her normal surroundings; she was melancholy and anxious, but relatively normal. In the other state she hallucinated and was "naughty"—that is to say, she was abusive, used to throw the cushions at people, so far as the contractures at various times allowed, tore buttons off her bedclothes and linen with those of her fingers which she could move, and so on. At this stage of her illness if something had been moved in the room or someone had entered or left it (during her other state of consciousness) she would complain of having "lost" some time and would remark upon the gap in her train of conscious thoughts. (p. 76)

These are classical signs and symptoms of DID (see Chapter Six), including ongoing amnesia for current events that is far outside the range of ordinary forgetfulness. Anna herself offered the diagnosis of DID: "At moments when her mind was quite clear she would complain of the profound darkness in her head, of not being able to think, of becoming blind and deaf, of having two selves, a real one and an evil one which forced her to behave badly, and so on" (p. 77). The amnesia barrier between the two states is commented on repeatedly in the text, as is the switching from one state to another. There were several interesting features, including the two states speaking different languages, and the second state believing that the correct date was one year earlier than the actual date.

On page 92, there is an excellent description of the second state, or *condition seconde,* waking up disoriented. This kind of disorientation, which in Anna O. was caused by her second state thinking it was 1881 when it was actually 1882, occurs commonly in DID:

> The following incident, among others, illustrates the high degree of logical consistency of her states. During this period, as has already been explained, the patient was always in her *condition seconde*—that is, in the year 1881—at night. On one occasion she woke up during the night, declaring that she had been taken away from home once again, and become so seriously excited that the whole household was alarmed. The reason was simple. During the previous evening the talking cure had cleared up her disorder of vision, and this applied also to her *condition seconde.* Thus when she woke up in the night she found herself in a strange room, for her family had moved house in the spring of 1881.

On page 100, there is a clear description of the phenomenon of copresence, which is similar to lucid possession. Copresence occurs when an alter personality in the background takes joint control of the body without displacing the primary personality, or when it influences the primary personality's mental state from the background:

> Throughout the entire illness her two states of consciousness persisted side by side: the primary one in which she was quite normal psychologically, and the secondary one which may well be likened to a dream in view of its wealth of imaginative products and hallucinations, its large gaps in memory and the lack of inhibition and control in its associations. In this secondary state the patient was in a condition of alienation. The fact that the patient's mental condition was entirely dependent on the intrusion of this secondary state into the normal one seems to throw considerable light on at least one class of hysterical psychosis. Every one of her hypnoses in the evening afforded evidence that the patient was entirely clear and well-ordered in her mind and normal as regards her feeling and volition so long as none of the products of her secondary state was acting as a stimulus "in the unconscious." The extremely marked psychosis which appeared whenever there was any considerable interval in this unburdening process showed the degree to which these products influenced the psychical events of her "normal" state. It is hard to avoid expressing the situation by saying that the patient was split into two personalities of which one was mentally normal and the other insane.

One can see here the same error that Morton Prince made: One personality is thought to be "bad," "insane," or "delirious," while the primary personality is viewed as desirable and normal. In psychoanalytic terms, this is a major countertransference distortion of the reality of the patient.

Anna O. had a third state as well, which today would be called a hidden observer, internal self-helper, or center. This was an entity described as follows: "a clear-sighted and calm observer sat, as she put it, in a corner of her brain and looked on at all the mad business" (p. 101). If Breuer had been able to enlist this state as a cotherapist, he might have uncovered earlier childhood trauma and provided a more effective treatment.

Anna O.'s real name was Bertha Pappenheim. She became one of the first social workers in Europe. Pappenheim's work was recognized in a commemorative German stamp issued in 1954. She was also an early feminist, whose achievements involved the establishing of homes for prostitutes and unwed mothers. It is possible that, in psychoanalytic terms, this career was an undoing of her own childhood sexual trauma, and of the failure of any person in authority to validate its reality, or offer comfort. We might have a strange historical irony: Freud repudiated the seduction theory, thereby making effective treatment of sexually abused women less likely, but based on that repudiation he went on to develop theory that accurately explains much of Bertha Pappenheim's career drive.

The other case histories in *Studies on Hysteria* (Breuer & Freud, 1895/1986) are written by Freud. His patient Emmy Von N. had a dissociative disorder for sure, and almost certainly had DID. She was an excellent hypnotic subject. In his first session with her, Freud observed alternating states, one of which was probably a child alter personality that had been abused.

He writes, "What she told me was perfectly coherent and revealed an unusual degree of education and intelligence. This made it seem all the more strange when every two or three minutes she suddenly broke off, contorted her face into an expression of horror and disgust, stretched out her hand towards me, spreading and crooking her fingers, and exclaimed, in a changed voice, charged with anxiety: "Keep still—Don't say anything!—Don't touch me!" She was probably under the influence of some recurrent hallucination of a horrifying kind and was trying to keep the intruding material at bay with this formula" (p. 104). We have here the embryonic beginnings of Freud's theory of obsession. I suggest that the intruding material was actually an abuse memory. Put another way, I suggest that the formula was communicating real trauma, and that it was not an obsessive defense against conflict and fantasy.

Emmy Von N. had a history of past unsuccessful treatments, which is common in DID. Freud understood her symptoms to be due to the "associative inaccessibility" of certain ideas and feelings. If psychic content is associatively inaccessible, that means it has been dissociated: Freud was saying that this patient had a dissociative disorder. He spoke of the patient's "mnemonic symbols," which are equivalent to the "somatic memories" common in DID (Kluft, 1987b). These are physical symptoms that symbolically express and communicate past trauma too painful to remember. Thus Freud was partly on track but was already forming theories that would lead away from a full understanding of the etiology of his patients' disorders.

On page 157, Freud notes that there was an amnesia barrier between Emmy Von N.'s two states. On one occasion, the *condition seconde* claimed to be a woman from the previous century, a claim sometimes made by contemporary alter personalities. Emmy Von N. displayed many of the primary and secondary features of late twentieth-century DID.

The case of Miss Lucy R. contains dissociative features as well, and in it Freud refers to "the splitting of consciousness in these cases" (p. 188). Katherina, another case, had dissociative features secondary to attempted paternal incest, but not DID. Fraulein Elisabeth Von R. had a dissociative disorder that seemed to be based on adult conflict rather than childhood trauma. Freud said that her symptoms arose because "the incompatible idea had been forced out of her associations" (p. 227), which is to say, dissociated. Another case, Fraulein Rosalia H., is mentioned briefly; she had symptoms arising from attempted paternal incest.

The cases in *Studies on Hysteria* represent a range of dissociative disorders including some cases of full DID. Not all patients had experienced childhood sexual abuse, but some had.

In the theoretical sections of the book, both Freud and Breuer build a theory of trauma-driven dissociation. There are numerous references to splitting of consciousness, dissociated states, autohypnosis, and a spectrum of increasing severity and complexity of dissociation. On page 63, Breuer and Freud write jointly, in italics:

> The longer we have been occupied with these phenomena the more we have become convinced that *the splitting of consciousness which is so striking in the well-known classical cases under the form of* "double conscience" *is present to a rudimentary degree in every hysteria, and that a tendency to such dissociation, and with it the emergence of abnormal states of consciousness (which we shall bring together under the term "hypnoid"), is the basic phenomenon of this neurosis.* In these views we concur with Binet and the two Janets, though we have no experience of the remarkable findings they have made on anesthetic patients.

Freud nearly decided that dissociative symptoms can arise from a rational, intelligent sphere of consciousness, equivalent to the subliminal self of Myers. He spoke of his "impression of there being a superior intelligence outside the patient's consciousness which keeps a large amount of psychical material arranged for particular purposes and has fixed a planned order for its return to consciousness. I suspect, however, that this unconscious intelligence is no more than an appearance" (p. 356). He puts it a different way on page 273: "The pathogenic material appears to be the property of an intelligence which is not necessarily inferior to that of the normal ego. The appearance of a second personality is often presented in the most deceptive manner."

If Freud had pursued this line of thinking, his topographical and structural models of the mind would have been very different. With the repudiation of the seduction theory, however, it became necessary for the "unconscious" to have certain properties. One of these could not be rational memory of actual abuse. We learn from DID patients that the "unconscious" is not unconscious. One can converse directly with the alter personalities who hold the memories. The alters commonly control the rate of release of traumatic memories to the primary personality, and in fact I contract with them for this staged recovery of memory.

Concerning the "superior" intelligence of the dissociated ego in DID patients, I want to say a couple of things. Some skilled therapists feel that the patient's inner observer embodies a superior spiritual knowledge (Comstock, 1987). It is my experience that inner self helpers can be excellent cotherapists, but they do not have transcendental abilities: In Myers's terms, the subliminal self may be equal to the supraluminal in IQ, but is not necessarily more intelligent. I will discuss the extrasensory experiences and paranormal powers of DID patients in Chapters Six and Nine.

Freud's repudiation of the seduction theory contributed to the discrediting of DID. When he repudiated the reality of his patients' childhood trauma, Freud, given his genius, felt compelled to create an original theoretical explanation of their symptoms. Although this theory contained much truth, it was founded on an essential error that needs correction. The dissociative patients treated after the repudiation of the seduction theory were not understood as suffering from the adult consequences of real childhood trauma. They were misclassified diagnostically, and their symptoms were misunderstood in terms of incorrectly applied psychoanalytical theory. As a result, they received the wrong treatment.

This historical error cannot be corrected by a repudiation of Freud because he contributed too much that is lasting and therapeutically useful. Corrected psychoanalytic theory can easily accommodate posttraumatic dissociation into its thinking and therapy (Paley, 1988). Breuer was right when he said, "It is certain that we have only taken the first steps in this region of knowledge, and our present views will be substantially altered by further observations" (p. 316). The insight of *Studies on Hysteria* needs to be rescued from Freud's later distortions. Why? So that Anna O. can be correctly remembered as "the best known and clearest example of major hysteria with manifest *"double conscience"* (p. 316). She was only partially treated.

DID disappeared early in the twentieth century for two major reasons: Its traumatic origins were repudiated; and Freud assigned properties to the unconscious mind that were incompatible with dissociation theory, as exemplified by Myers. The unconscious was not allowed to hold accurate memories, perform adult cognitive functions, or assume rational executive control of the body. In the first decade of the twenty-first century, dissociated executive control may once again become a core construct in psychiatry and psychology. It appears unlikely that the dissociative disorders will vanish from professional awareness again, as they did early in the twentieth century, because of developments to be described in the next chapter.

CHAPTER TWO

Freud to the Present

Studies on Hysteria (Breuer & Freud, 1986) was published in 1895. The decline in diagnosis and study of DID had set in by about 1910. As I proposed in the preceding chapter, Freud's repudiation of the seduction theory was probably a major force in the discrediting of DID. Patients with trauma-driven dissociative disorders were understood as suffering from unresolved incestuous fantasies. Their treatment did not take the true etiology of their symptoms into account and would be described as an elaborate form of blaming the victim, in any feminist analysis (Rivera, 1987, 1988, 1989, 1991).

When Freud repudiated the seduction theory, he simultaneously repudiated hypnosis and Jung's interest in the paranormal. Since DID, sexual abuse, autohypnosis, and extrasensory experiences are closely linked (see Chapters Six and Nine), Freud effectively banned a large area of psychic reality from serious study. People who came to physicians and nonmedical therapists with dissociative posttraumatic stress disorders could not receive treatment that took the cause of their problems into account.

Along with the discrediting of hypnosis in the early twentieth century, for which Freud was not solely responsible, there was an ascendancy of the view that DID is an artifact. The artifact was thought to be the result of an interaction between a naive diagnostician and a gullible, hysterical patient. Hypnosis, it was held, amplified and entrenched the artifact. Both hypnosis and DID were thrown out.

The work of Pavlov was another factor contributing to the decline of DID and dissociation. Professional energy and ideological commitment that did not flow into psychoanalysis were channeled into behaviorism. Hilgard (1987) has mentioned this aspect of the history, which I won't consider any further.

In this chapter, I am going to discuss the history of DID from 1910 to 1995. I will concentrate on events from 1980 onward, because this is when most of the important developments have occurred. During the period 1910 to 1980, we see DID vanish from serious study, mentioned only in a few case reports and two review articles. Then in the 1970s, a resurgence begins. Starting in 1980, there is an exponential takeoff in the number of diagnoses of DID in North America.

The next major landmark is 1984. In this year, the field began to become politically organized and, in publications, began a transition from a prescientific to a scientific literature. By 1990, this transition was complete, and the field was in the phase of early scientific development.

THE ROLE OF SCHIZOPHRENIA IN THE DECLINE OF DISSOCIATIVE IDENTITY DISORDER

Those DID patients who were not classified as oedipal hysterics after 1910 were likely to be called schizophrenic. In this instance, it was not the patient's conflicts that were blamed for the symptoms, but her brain. Rosenbaum (1980) has documented the role of the term *schizophrenia* in the decline of diagnoses of DID. His work is valuable but should be followed up with a detailed scholarly analysis of the relationship between DID and schizophrenia in the twentieth century: Gainer (1994) has initiated this line of study. Schizophrenia was called *dementia praecox* until Bleuler introduced the term schizophrenia. Dementia praecox is actually a better name for this group of disorders than schizophrenia, while schizophrenia is a better name for DID than multiple personality disorder. Schizophrenia means "split mind" from the Greek *schizo,* split, and *phren,* mind, while dementia praecox means a dementia of early onset. It is actually DID which is characterized by a split mind. This confused terminology has given rise to popular confusion about schizophrenia, which is often thought to be the same as split personality. It is schizophrenia which is characterized by dementia-like symptoms, now called negative symptoms.

The consensus in modern psychiatry is that schizophrenia is not one illness but a group of related illnesses. Schizophrenia is widely assumed to be a physical disorder of the brain, although this hasn't been proven. There is no evidence that it responds to individual insight-oriented psychotherapy, but it does respond to medication. The medication suppresses the so-called positive symptoms such as delusions, hallucinations, and disturbed behavior. However, the medications have no effect on the negative symptoms of emptiness, lack of drive, inner deadness, and deteriorating occupational and social function. The medications never cure the illness.

Today, schizophrenia is viewed as a form of organic brain syndrome. We don't classify it as an organic brain syndrome only because we have not identified the specific physical causes of schizophrenia. Schizophrenia is more closely related to Alzheimer's disease than to DID, in contemporary psychiatric thought. It makes some sense to call schizophrenia dementia praecox, but no sense at all to call it split mind disorder, in Greek or English. Perhaps *dementia psychotica juvenalis* would appeal to some. Setting that neologism aside, the point is that schizophrenia is almost undoubtedly a disease of the brain requiring physical treatment. There is no evidence that anything is structurally or physiologically wrong with the DID brain. There is in fact no sound conceptual reason to suppose that there is a primary physical disturbance of the brain in the *DSM-IV* dissociative disorders (American Psychiatric Association, 1994a).

The effect of renaming dementia praecox *split mind disorder* was to absorb many DID patients into the organic brain syndromes. Over the past 100 years, there has been an ideological dichotomy in psychiatry that is not yet resolved. Initially, on one side were the Freudians, on the other the "biological" psychiatrists. The unitary Freudian camp has since been replaced by a welter of diverse schools. Some biological psychiatrists have a strong desire to be accepted as respectable medical scientists, and never to be mistaken for psychoanalysts. The reciprocal morbid phobia is also in place. Where has this left the DID patient?

With the same presenting features, he or she may be consigned to ineffective biological treatments, on the one hand, or ineffective psychological treatments on the other. In one case, the diagnosis is schizophrenia, or, fancier, schizoaffective disorder, with an assumed organic etiology. In the other, the diagnosis is borderline or hysterical personality disorder, with an assumed metapsychological etiology.

Rosenbaum has shown that there were more diagnoses of DID made in North America from 1914 to 1926 than of schizophrenia. During that period, 15 cases of DID and 10 of schizophrenia were reported in the literature. Rosenbaum says that the diagnosis of schizophrenia "caught on" in the United States in the late 1920s and early 1930s. Following this catching on, there was a sharp increase in diagnoses of schizophrenia and a sharp decline in diagnoses of DID. How are we to understand this?

It is commonly said today that DID is an iatrogenic artifact and a transient diagnostic fad. What about schizophrenia? Could it be that many diagnoses of schizophrenia are incorrect, leading to negative iatrogenic complications? Could it be schizophrenia that is the fad, driven by biological reductionism (Ross, 1986a; Ross & Pam, 1995)? Why should this not be the case? Why is DID singled out for the criticism of iatrogenesis by mainstream psychiatry, but not schizophrenia? Because of data? No. Because of ideology.

Many dissociative posttraumatic stress disorders are misdiagnosed as schizophrenia in North America today (see Chapter Eight). In a series of 236 cases of DID reported to me by 203 clinicians throughout North

America (Ross, Norton, & Wozney 1989), 40.8% had a previous diagnosis of schizophrenia, while in a second series of 102 cases assessed with the Dissociative Disorders Interview Schedule (Ross, Miller, Reagor, et al., 1990), 26.5% had received prior diagnoses of schizophrenia, and 55.9% had received antipsychotic medication.

There is, I believe, a group of related organic brain syndromes that present with delusions, hallucinations, and deteriorating occupational and social function, as defined by the term schizophrenia in *DSM-IV*. The problem in contemporary psychiatry is the inability of many psychiatrists to make an accurate diagnostic discrimination between two groups of illnesses (organic brain syndromes and posttraumatic dissociative disorders) that have different etiologies, treatments, and prognoses.

Another factor contributing to the decline of DID after 1910 was probably the name of the disorder. The name multiple personality disorder led to incredulity and arguments about whether the disorder is "real." Much of the argument was based on assumptions generated in the minds of adherents and skeptics by the term multiple personality disorder. The term suggests that it is necessary to debate whether or not one person can "really" have more than one personality, or, put more extremely, whether there can "really" be more than one person in a single body. Of course there can't. Nevertheless, DID is a real disorder.

It may be, on the other hand, that the name of a disorder is irrelevant, as long as it is properly conceptualized, diagnosed, and treated. The fact that a group of organic brain syndromes has been misnamed *split mind disorder* in the twentieth century has not resulted in any systematic research attempting to show that schizophrenia is an expression of oedipal conflict. The field is steadily moving toward an organic theory and treatment of schizophrenia, undistracted by the inappropriate name given to the illness. If it appears to be unnecessary to rename schizophrenia, why did we rename multiple personality disorder?

I personally advocate retaining the terms schizophrenia and dissociative identity disorder, but classifying one as a presumed organic brain syndrome and the other as a posttraumatic dissociative disorder. There is much better evidence in favor of the posttraumatic nature of DID than in favor of the organic etiology of schizophrenia. What is needed is sound empirical research on the overlap and distinctions between trauma-driven dissociative symptoms and organic/psychotic symptoms. I will discuss these points in more detail in Chapter Eight. For now, it is sufficient to note the role of the term schizophrenia in the decline of diagnoses of DID.

REVIEW ARTICLES IN 1944 AND 1962

Two bibliographies of the DID literature (Boor & Coons, 1983; Damgaard, Van Benschoten, & Fagan, 1985) provided a comprehensive list of publications on the subject in the 1980s. A more recent and more comprehensive bibliography is the one by Goettman, Greaves, and Coons (1992), which also includes summaries and citations for many relevant legal cases. I am going to highlight only a couple of landmarks between 1910 and 1980.

The first of these is a review article by Taylor and Martin (1944) that begins, "Morton Prince, who founded this JOURNAL, made much of multiple personality. In articles, books, and lectures, he described cases and grouped them into types; he told how some of the cases were caused and how some were cured; he encouraged other authors to contribute like observations, particularly to this JOURNAL; and throughout his professional life he seemed to think of abnormal psychology, psychotherapy, and mental hygiene largely in terms of multiple personality."

One of the features of the article is a list of 76 cases of DID taken from the entire literature available to the authors: of these, 57% were American, 18% French, 16% British, and the rest German and Swiss. Each case is listed by reporting professional, name of the patient, number of personalities, and references in which the case appears. As well, Taylor and Martin typed the cases according to a clearly defined classificatory scheme.

The classificatory system included such items as whether the case displayed mutual amnesia (two-way amnesia), one-way amnesia, coconsciousness, and other structural features. In addition, certain qualities of the alters were tabulated including sex, being of different ages, and general temperament. Many of these terms are consistent with or identical with Braun's (1986a) terminology.

A striking difference between this inventory of 76 cases and contemporary series (Putnam, Guroff, Silberman, Barban, & Post, 1986; Ross, Norton, & Wozney, 1989) is the much smaller number of personalities in the older cases. Of the 76 cases listed by Taylor and Martin, 49 were dual personality, and only 6 had more than five alters. The average number of personalities was 2.9, while the median was 2.0. In contrast, in our series of 236 cases the mean number of alters was 15.7, and the median was 8.0. In Putnam's series of 100 cases, the mean was 13.3 personalities, and the median was 9.0.

Just as demon possession evolved into DID, DID has continued to evolve over the past 100 years. Because the face of DID may undergo transformation again before current students of dissociation finish their careers, we need to find historical constants in the phenomonology of dissociation. Another major feature of contemporary DID, besides the larger number of alters, that does not appear in Taylor and Martin's review, is sexual abuse. The authors include no discussion of a traumatic etiology for DID. The possible causes of DID apparent in 1944 were, "head injury, marked intoxication, extreme fatigue, lowered general energy, unbalanced urges, severe conflicts, and excessive learnings and forgettings."

Although less than 50 years old, that list is quaint for a contemporary clinician who has listened to DID abuse histories. Several possible ways of accounting for the smaller number of alters, and the absence of abuse histories in the older cases are apparent. First, it is likely that few of the clinicians seriously considered or inquired about sexual abuse. These older DID patients may have had dual personality without an abusive etiology, and therefore may not have needed to create a large number of alters to cope with severe, chronic trauma. Alternatively, the older cases may have had severe abuse histories that were remembered by undetected alters.

Advocates of iatrogenesis will say that DID hysteria has escalated in recent years as clinicians feed into the charade. The most likely hypothesis, I believe, has three interrelated aspects: Since 1944, DID has evolved into a syndrome with a posttraumatic etiology, whereas before it tended to have less severe external precipitants; our society has gotten sicker, and the abuse of children more bizarre; earlier clinicians missed the abuse history in many DID patients, which was not as severe, on average, as that experienced by contemporary patients.

The incidence of DID, then, is an indicator of the amount of child abuse occurring in Western society. Taylor and Martin made a concluding observation with which I agree: "The mechanisms of multiple personality are those of normal personality working under abnormal conditions." I have listened to a child alter describe an incident in which her father came into her bedroom dressed in women's clothing. Before having intercourse with her, according to her retrospective account in adulthood, he stuffed live spiders into her vagina. Although this sounds unbelievable, there is no scientific way to determine simply from listening to the account whether it is historically accurate or not. The key issue in the etiology of contemporary DID is not iatrogenesis, it is the degree of confabulation in the abuse histories.

If the abuse histories are real, then iatrogenesis becomes a minor influence for which one nevertheless has to be vigilant. If the abuse never happened, the disorder may be driven by other conflicts I will describe in Chapter Three, but there is no more reason to think that it is primarily iatrogenic. In either alternative, iatrogenesis is a secondary issue.

The second review paper appeared in 1962 in the *International Journal of Clinical and Experimental Hypnosis,* a journal with a tradition of publishing papers on DID. The authors, Sutcliffe and Jones, refer to Taylor and Martin's paper and present a bar graph of the number of cases reported from 1800 to 1940, based on the 1944 series of 76 cases. This graph shows very clearly a sudden increase in the number of cases reported between 1880 and 1900, then a decline from there. The decline in publications on DID was accompanied by the disappearance of publications on all aspects of dissociation: Hilgard (1987) has pointed out that *Psychological Abstracts* shows 20 abstracts on dissociation from 1927 through 1936, 8 from 1937 through 1946, 2 from 1947 through 1956, and 3 from 1957 through 1966.

Sutcliffe and Jones divide the history of DID into three periods: Period 1, hazy beginnings, up until 1880; Period 2, establishment and elaboration of DID, from 1880 until 1900; Period 3, full maturity and a falling off of theoretical elaboration, from 1900 on. There was some overlap between periods. They describe what they call "notable" cases from each of these periods, which in Period 3 include Miss Beauchamp (Prince, 1905/1978) and Eve White (Thigpen & Cleckley, 1957). I would say that Period 3 lasted from 1910 until 1980, followed by Period 4, resurgence of interest in DID; and I would extend Period 2 until 1910.

It is difficult to set an end to Period 4, but I would place it in 1984. After this begins Period 5, modern scientific study of dissociation. Thus the revised chart of the history of DID is as follows:

Period 1. Up until 1880. Hazy beginnings.

Period 2. 1880–1910. Establishment and elaboration of DID.

Period 3. 1910–1980. Full maturity and rapid decline.

Period 4. 1980–1984. Resurgence of interest in DID.

Period 5. 1984–present. Modern scientific study of DID.

Sutcliffe and Jones conduct a lengthy and subtle discussion that deals with iatrogenesis, diagnostic habits, false positive diagnoses, philosophical climate, psychological theories, and a number of other factors affecting the reporting of cases of DID.

They make criticisms suggesting that the number of true cases in Periods 1 through 3 may have been less than the number reported. They point out that diagnostic criteria were vague to nonexistent, and that some of the classical cases might be more accurately diagnosed as organic brain syndrome, epilepsy, or schizophrenia. Actually, there were probably more false positive diagnoses in the opposite direction (see Chapter Eight); in other words, cases of DID misdiagnosed as schizophrenia, brain damage, or epilepsy. Nevertheless, Sutcliffe and Jones are probably right that enthusiasm to report a case of DID led to incorrect diagnoses.

The most convincing example of a false positive diagnosis of DID is the Sargeant of Bazeilles (Binet, 1896/1977a), who had damage to his left parietal lobe from a war injury. This man does not belong to the diagnostic category of contemporary DID, because he did not have psychologically coherent alters, an abuse history, or a psychological rationale for the development of DID. In their discussion of iatrogenesis and the influence of hypnosis, Sutcliffe and Jones conclude that neither can account fully for the phenomena. However they take the influence of suggestion, therapist expectations, subtle cuing by the therapist, and demand characteristics in general very seriously. This is a necessary scientific attitude today.

The major feature of Sutcliffe and Jones' review that I want to highlight is the complete absence of trauma in the discussion. They discuss Janet's psychological theory of dissociation, and make several pointed criticisms of the circularity of much of Janet's reasoning, but they never focus on sexual or physical abuse. It is as if *Studies on Hysteria* had never been written.

After the repudiation of the seduction theory by Freud, an amnesia set in among psychologists and psychiatrists. Freud's evidence and argument about the traumatic origins of dissociation were lost. This occurred so suddenly that it cannot be attributed to passive scholarly forgetting. In fact, the field developed a dissociative disorder, an active dismissal and forgetting of the role of sexual abuse and other childhood trauma in the formation of DID. This was a convenient intellectual maneuver for the abusive patriarchy.

Overall, little new work was done on DID in the period 1910 to 1980. As Sutcliffe and Jones point out, any further cases accumulated did not add new theory or understanding to the field (Alexander, 1956; Brandsma & Ludwig, 1974; Congdon, Hain, & Stevenson, 1961; Copeland & Kitching, 1937; McKee & Wittkower, 1962; Winer, 1978). DID had sunk so far into oblivion that Eve White was thought to be the only living case in the late 1950s. The book and the movie *The Three Faces of Eve* were thought to be about an extravagantly rare curiosity.

Before moving on to the modern scientific study of dissociation, I want to describe work done by the psychologist G. H. Estabrooks: This work bridges Binet, Myers, and contemporary writers such as myself and Crabtree (1985, 1993).

G. H. ESTABROOKS

George H. Estabrooks was born in St. John, New Brunswick, Canada, on December 16, 1895. He completed his BA at Acadia University, in Wolfville, Nova Scotia, then was a Rhodes Scholar at Oxford and Exeter from 1921 to 1924. After completing a PhD in psychology at Harvard University, he moved to Colgate College in Hamilton in upper New York State in 1927, where he remained the rest of his career, and where he died on December 30, 1973. Estabrooks wrote a textbook entitled *Hypnotism* (1943, 1957) that went through a series of editions, as well as other books and articles, including an article "Hypnosis Comes of Age" (1971) published in *Science Digest.*

In his book *Spiritism,* Estabrooks (1947) refers repeatedly to Myers, and quotes him many times. The book is an examination of mediums, mental telepathy, automatic writing, dreams, ghosts, hypnotic trance, spiritism, and related topics from a scientific and psychological viewpoint. Chapter Four is entitled "Multiple Personality" and contains a review of famous cases including Miss Beauchamp (Prince, 1905/1978) and Hannah (Sidis & Goodhart, 1905).

Like Myers, Estabrooks reviews all this material to support a general psychological theory based on the assumption of a second or subliminal self. He writes, "Strange as it may seem, all of us appear to have another person living within our bodies besides ourselves. This other person, this unconscious mind, is quite as capable of handling our bodies as we are, and does so in the most startling manner" (p. 30).

Estabrooks agrees with Myers that the so-called unconscious mind is not really unconscious: according to Myers and Estabrooks, the properties ascribed to the unconscious by Freud and subsequent writers, and revealed by trance mediums, could not exist unless the unconscious was in fact a dissociated consciousness. Estabrooks states this more fully:

> We cannot solve a problem in mathematics while we are unconscious nor can we write a book in that state. To be sure many a psychologist has demonstrated that we can do all these things while in hypnotism or in various trance states—when we actually *are* unconscious so far as ordinary language is concerned. But Dr. Morton Prince has ably demonstrated that even in these states we are conscious—or rather that there is existing what he terms a "co-conscious state." This state is quite similar to those existing in multiple personality. In other words, when we are hypnotized it would appear that there was really a secondary personality doing the work. We are not unconscious but another consciousness takes over the running of the body—quite a different thing. This other consciousness is frequently present in our ordinary life, but it is submerged. We know nothing about it. Yet it does exist, for all that. It is co-conscious with our ordinary self, has all the information of this self and so can do mathematics or write poetry quite as the normal "we." In other words, it seems that even when we do work in an "unconscious" condition, such as hypnotism, we are not really unconscious. Another consciousness takes over the running of the body. (p. 230)

During the middle third of the twentieth century, when serious interest in DID had almost disappeared, Estabrooks viewed DID as genuine, and thought it illustrated many principles of normal psychology. Rather than debunking multiples as really being like all the rest of us, Estabrooks reversed the argument: He rejected the illusion of a single executive self, and held that we are all more multiple than our culture acknowledges. This was Myers half a century later.

Estabrooks was not only a theorist, however. He is also the only writer to describe systematically creating DID for military intelligence agencies, and the use of these individuals in covert operations. He describes this under a subheading "The Super Spy" in a chapter entitled "Psychological Warfare" in the 1957 edition of *Hypnotism,* and also in his *Science Digest* article (1971).

In an obituary in the *Syracuse Herald American,* January 6, 1974, Richard Case writes, "Once I felt he was ready to tell me about his experiences in the war, how hypnotism might have been used, in early *Manchurian Candidate* fashion, as a weapon of psychological warfare, but then he drew back to the style of conversation that stops just short of major revelations."

Estabrooks presents a number of case histories of Army and Marine personnel serving in World War II in whom artificial DID was created for use in courier and infiltration operations. Although he is vague about the techniques by which the DID was created, he says that the procedure required months of intensive conditioning and hypnosis. He describes the insertion of verbal access codes so that the alter personality holding classified information could be called out by personnel at the far end of a courier mission. The insertion of access codes to breach hypnotically implanted amnesia barriers in subjects is also described in PROJECT ARTICHOKE documents I obtained from the CIA through the Freedom of Information Act. PROJECT ARTICHOKE and PROJECT BLUEBIRD were covert CIA programs which ran from 1951 to 1953 before they were rolled over into MKULTRA, which then ran from 1953 to 1963, before it was in turn renamed MKSEARCH (Marks, 1979). MKSEARCH was operational until 1973.

Estabrooks writes in his 1971 article:

> During World War II, I worked this technique with a vulnerable Marine lieutenant I'll call Jones. Under the watchful eye of Marine intelligence, I split his personality into Jones A and Jones B. Jones A, once a "normal" working Marine, became entirely different. He talked communist doctrine and meant it. He was welcomed enthusiastically by communist cells, was deliberately given a dishonorable discharge by the Corps (which was in on the plot) and became a card-carrying party member.

> The joker was Jones B, the second personality, formerly apparent in the conscious Marine. Under hypnosis, this Jones had been carefully coached by suggestion. Jones B was the deeper personality, knew all about the thoughts of Jones A, was a loyal American and was "imprinted" to say nothing during conscious phases.

Estabrooks calls the product of this military mind control "multiple personality" and compares his subjects with classical DID cases in the literature. He also refers to work by Harriman (1942a, 1942b), which describes the creation of DID by hypnosis: Harriman was a military psychiatrist. There were two documented independent military programs for the creation of DID in the 1940s, although Harriman did not describe any operational use of his subjects. The amount of other work that was done by military and civilian intelligence agencies—and when it stopped—is unknown, as is the degree to which subjects were used in operations and the variety of tasks they carried out.

Estabrooks's description of the creation of enduring and secure amnesia barriers and secondary personalities is important for several reasons. It shows that iatrogenic DID actually can occur. At the same time, the work suggests that creating artificial DID in adults requires a lot of time, control, and persuasion. This would appear to set the threshold for creation of iatrogenic DID rather high, a subject I will return to in Chapter Three.

Like Binet, Estabrooks has been overlooked in the revival of interest in Janet. He deserves to be remembered as an important theorist of DID and dissociation, and he should be thanked for documenting the creation of artificial DID by military intelligence agencies. Without Estabrooks, this fact would still be hidden. Estabrooks provides a link between the late nineteenth century and the late twentieth century.

1980: A MAJOR LANDMARK IN THE HISTORY OF DISSOCIATIVE IDENTITY DISORDER

The situation had begun to change in the late 1970s prior to the next major landmark in the history, which is the year 1980. A major event of the 1970s was Hilgard's publication of *Divided Consciousness* (Hilgard, 1977). This book inaugurates the serious modern study of dissociation. Valuable as it is, and despite its devoting over 20 pages to DID, the book is not based on clinical experience with dissociative patients. Instead, it is based on experimental psychology and therefore is not directly a part of the history I am outlining. I will discuss Hilgard's neodissociation theory in Chapter Three.

Three other factors contributed to the resurgence of clinical interest in DID in the 1970s. One was the revival of interest in hypnosis after World War II: The level of interest in hypnosis and DID have always been intertwined and have covaried. The second factor was the Vietnam War, which brought with it an increased understanding of and emphasis on the role of trauma in psychiatric disorders. The third was the Women's Movement, which helped to bring child abuse, and particularly incest, out of the closet. Each of these factors and their interrelationships need to be studied in more detail.

By the late 1970s, a gradual increase in clinical experience with DID began to be visible to a small number of specialists. Cornelia Wilbur treated a case described in the book *Sybil* (Schreiber, 1973), as well as a number of other cases. She and a group of clinicians including George Greaves, Richard Kluft, Bennett Braun, Ralph Allison, Eugene Bliss, David Caul, and others participated in an oral tradition that was transmitted partly through annual workshops at the American Psychiatric Association meetings.

When I diagnosed my first case as a medical student in 1979 (Ross, 1984), this oral tradition was unknown to the psychiatric mainstream. None of my supervising psychiatrists in medical school had read a single paper on DID, nor could they advise me where to look other than in general textbooks. I found the references for my 1984 paper describing my first case by a hand search of the *Index Medicus.* The point is not that my supervisors were poorly educated—they weren't—but that DID was an obscure curiosity for mainstream psychiatry at that time.

The year 1980 is a landmark in the history of DID because in that year the disorder was given official diagnostic status in *DSM-III.* As well, four important papers were published (Bliss, 1980; Coons, 1980; Greaves, 1980; Rosenbaum, 1980) in leading psychiatric journals. I will discuss Bliss's paper in Chapter Seven, and have already reviewed Rosenbaum's article. The exponential takeoff in diagnosis of DID in North America began in about 1980.

George Greaves (1980) wrote a paper that summarized the clinical experience with DID of the previous 10 years. This paper is a landmark both because of its quality and because it is the last major review surveying an anecdotal DID literature. Reviews after this take into account the results of large clinical series and preliminary scientific studies.

Greaves counted 33 cases of DID reported from 1901 to 1944, and only 14 from 1944 to 1969. In his paper, however, he tabulates 50 cases either known to him personally or reported in the literature during the decade 1971 to 1980. This he regarded as a remarkable increase. Braun (1986a) estimated that 500 cases of DID had been identified by 1979. According to Braun's estimates, this number had increased to 1,000 by 1983, and 5,000 by 1986. Coons (1986c) estimated that 6,000 cases had been diagnosed in North America by 1986. These estimates, even though they are only educated guesses, indicate an exponential increase in the rate of diagnosis since 1980.

In his paper, Greaves discusses the trauma-driven nature of dissociation, unlike the reviewers before him, which is a major advance. But he hasn't quite brought the severity or the frequency of the childhood abuse into focus. This is not a criticism of Greaves, rather it is an observation about the state of the field in 1980. In a 1972 paper entitled "The Etiology of Multiple Personality," for example, Horton and Miller note the occurrence of incest in their case, but do not discuss trauma in a list of four DID dynamics.

Greaves seems to imply that the abuse experienced by Sybil was unusually severe even for an DID patient. Anyone working with DID patients today, including George Greaves, has heard many patients tell equally horrific stories. Some patients have experienced trauma far beyond that inflicted on Sybil. In 1980, even leading experts in the field had not yet grasped the frequency or severity of the abuse experienced by DID patients.

Coons (1980) made a clear statement of the role of trauma as a general cause of DID. His discussion of the etiology of DID focuses on childhood trauma, with a minimum of metapsychological speculation. Coons was an early exponent of empirical study of the role of trauma in DID. He refers to two earlier cases (Schreiber, 1973; Stoller, 1973) that dramatically illustrate the role of childhood abuse in the formation of DID, and gives one of his own. Coons's paper is usually referred to because of his statement that amnesia is an essential diagnostic criterion for DID. His early emphasis on trauma should not be overlooked.

In his discussion of the treatment of DID, Greaves, for the first time in the history of the field, is able to draw on the extensive clinical experience of a group of contemporaries. He quotes principles of treatment enunciated by Bowers et al. (1971), Allison (1974), and Wilbur (Schreiber, 1973), which I will discuss in Chapter Eleven, and is able to say that integration can be achieved in an average of 2 to 5 years by a skilled therapist. More rapid integration he holds to be possible only for a handful of particularly expert therapists.

The year 1980 thus marks the beginning of the resurgence of interest in DID. At least half a decade of preparatory work by a small number of clinicians was required before the exponential increase in diagnosis could really take off. I am not able to give an inside account of the political work needed to get DID into *DSM-III,* but this must have required a big effort against even bigger resistance. In the next period, 1980 to 1984, the field began to organize politically in preparation for transition from a prescientific to a scientific body of knowledge.

THE PERIOD 1980 TO 1983

Much more took place in the study of DID during this period than is evident from publications. In terms of my own personal development, I was in residency training from 1981 to 1985. During this period, I did not receive a single lecture, handout, reference, or other didactic material on DID. I did not meet anyone else who had diagnosed a case of DID, never heard DID considered in the differential diagnosis of a patient, and never heard anyone mention DID in a lecture or seminar. DID didn't come up any more often in professional conversation than it did outside work. I diagnosed and treated one more case myself, but I kept fairly quiet about it.

One important paper in this period was that by Myron Boor (1982), titled "The Multiple Personality Epidemic: Additional Cases and Inferences Regarding Diagnosis, Etiology, Dynamics, and Treatment." Boor went over the literature and found 29 more cases of DID in 16 papers published between 1970 and early 1981, some of which had been missed by Greaves (1980). Boor added these 29 cases to the 76 described by Taylor and Martin (1944), and found that the overall female/male ratio was 8 : 1. He also noted the increased number of alters in recent cases, occurrence of headache in 17 of the 29 recent cases, suicide attempts in 22 of the 29, and high rates of childhood abuse.

Concerning etiology, Boor echoed Greaves's statement that trauma and "environments that foster extreme ambivalence" were the two main factors. He also speculated that the preponderance of females in DID might be because the males are in prison. This is an important but unresolved question in the literature. Boors's paper advanced the field by urging it toward analysis of large series of cases. This was a necessary step in the development from speculation based on single cases to scientific inquiry. Confer and Ables (1983) published a book on DID during this period that does not appear to have had a major influence on the field, and that is rarely cited.

Frank Putnam and coworkers (1986) made the next step when they presented a series of 100 cases of DID at the American Psychiatric Association meeting in 1983. This was the first large series reported in a single study. Putnam's analysis of these 100 cases provided a great deal of detail on the clinical phenomenology of DID, which I will discuss in Chapter Five. The 100 cases were reported to Putnam by 92 clinicians responding to a questionnaire. Such studies have methodological limitations, but they are a necessary step in the evolution of any field. The provide a bridge between anecdote and valid, reliable diagnosis and clinical assessment.

The next event was the publication of a special issue of the *American Journal of Clinical Hypnosis* on DID in October 1983. Although this was an important contribution to the field, the editors somewhat inconvenienced future historians by not holding the issue back till 1984. In 1984, three other psychiatric journals published special issues on DID, in which the transition from a prescientific to a scientific literature occurred. The landmark year of 1984 starts in October 1983.

During this period, work was being done to organize the first major conference on DID held in Chicago in 1984. This series of conferences, all chaired by Bennett Braun, ran continuously until 1994, and was always held in Chicago. Concurrently, leading figures in the field were preparing for formation of the International Society for the Study of Multiple Personality and Dissociation (ISSMP&D), which was renamed the International Society for the Study of Dissociation (ISSD) in 1994. The annual DID meeting in Chicago and the growth of the ISSD have been major factors in my development, and that of the field. Part of the success of psychoanalysis early in the twentieth century was due to its political organization, with formation of societies and meetings. Janet was politically unsuccessful, which is partly why he fell into obscurity. One cannot overemphasize the importance of the ISSD and the annual Chicago meetings in reestablishing the study of DID.

1984: THE TRANSITION TO A SCIENTIFIC LITERATURE

The other three journals that published special issues on DID were the *International Journal of Clinical and Experimental Hypnosis, Psychiatric Annals,* and *Psychiatric Clinics of North America.* These four issues provided a large body of writing on DID by a number of different people. Diverging and conflicting points of view were represented, in a healthy and alive intellectual atmosphere. The role of iatrogenesis in DID was debated without polarization into pro and con warring factions. The quality of the argument was high.

Virtually all the main contributors to the DID literature in the 1980s had one or more papers in these four special issues. But one observation needs to be made: four men represented in these journals were not involved in the ongoing development of the ISSD, or the annual Chicago meetings. These are Ralph Allison (1984, 1985), John Beahrs (1982), Eugene Bliss (1983, 1984a, 1984b, 1984c, 1985, 1986, 1988; Bliss & Jeppsen, 1985; Bliss & Larson, 1985), and Martin Orne (Orne, Dinges, & Orne, 1984). Why and how this occurred deserves more than a footnote in the history of psychiatry. Ralph Allison and John Beahrs began to speak at ISSD meetings again in 1994 and 1995 respectively, which is a healthy sign.

With the appearance of these four special issues, Richard Kluft (1982, 1983, 1984a, 1984b, 1984c, 1985a, 1985b, 1985c, 1985d, 1985e, 1985f, 1985g, 1986a, 1986b, 1986c, 1986d, 1986e, 1987a, 1987b, 1987c, 1987d,

1987e, 1988a, 1988b, 1988c, 1988d, 1988e; Kluft, Braun, & Sachs, 1984; Kluft, Steinberg, & Spitzer, 1988) and Bennett Braun (1983a, 1983b, 1984, 1985, 1986a, 1986b, 1988a, 1988b; Braun & Sachs, 1985) established themselves as the leaders in the field. They maintained this position throughout the rest of the 1980s by writing, editing, treating patients, consulting, organizing conferences, doing political work, and encouraging the development of young clinicians and researchers. Bennett Braun established the world's first Dissociative Disorders Unit at Rush-Presbyterian-St. Luke's Medical Center in Chicago, and in 1988 the first issue of the first journal devoted exclusively to dissociative disorders appeared, with Richard Kluft as Editor-in-Chief (*Dissociation*, Vol. 1, No. 1, January 1988).

In these four special issues, something new appears in the modern clinical study of DID: *data*. Although many of the papers are summaries of clinical experience, they present several kinds of scientific data. Prior to 1984, only a few scattered studies had contained any scientific information, such as a physiological study by Ludwig, Brandsma, Wilbur, Benfeldt, and Jameson (1972), but none of these were based on large series. In 1984, we begin to hear about the characteristics of series of 30 or more patients, with data about clinical features and treatment response. As well, more elaborate descriptive models of the etiology and maintenance of DID are formulated.

I won't review all the papers in these journals because I will be referring to many of them throughout the rest of this book. One noteworthy article by Bliss (1983) is an outline of a book he published three years later (Bliss, 1986). By 1984, the relationship of DID to childhood abuse had been clearly recognized, as had the severity and chronicity of the abuse (Stern, 1984; Wilbur, 1984). The posttraumatic nature of DID was a given in the field, and discussion of the relationship between DID and other posttraumatic stress disorders had begun (Spiegel, 1984).

A second important relationship, that between DID and borderline personality disorder, is the subject of two papers. One of these, by Clary, Burstin, and Carpenter (1984) is highly metapsychological, but the other contains a detailed analysis of borderline features in 33 cases of DID based on *DSM-III* criteria (Horevitz & Braun, 1984). This paper also provides a discussion of the relevant literature, and thereby stands as the first comprehensive review of a particular subproblem in the DID field. Previous reviews had dealt with the field in a general way.

It is evident from the preceding papers that the relationship of DID to other psychiatric disorders was under serious study by 1984. This was a new development. Another important advance was the recognition and description of childhood DID (Kluft, 1984b). In his paper, Kluft (1984b) states that a review of the literature yielded one childhood case of DID, that of an 11-year-old girl named Estelle, who was treated by Despine Pere from 1836 to 1837 (Ellenberger, 1970; Fine, 1988). Kluft goes on to describe four cases of his own and to give a list of predictors of childhood DID. This is the first sign of the field moving toward its most important objective: the recognition and treatment of childhood DID. Based on clinical experience to date, rapid treatment of childhood DID appears to be possible, with lasting stable integration in the absence of further abuse. This in effect means that primary prevention of adult DID is possible.

Another important set of papers dealt with the Hillside Strangler case (Allison, 1984; Orne, Dinges, & Orne, 1984; Watkins, 1984). In these papers, Ralph Allison, Martin Orne, and John Watkins, all of whom had been expert witnesses in the trial of Kenneth Bianchi, argued their positions in detail. Bianchi was found by the judge to be faking DID and therefore to be ineligible for a defense of "not guilty by reason of insanity." It is of interest that Watkins concluded Bianchi had genuine DID, Allison that he had atypical dissociative disorder caused by the forensic psychiatric examinations, and Orne that he was faking DID. Watkins taught a course every year at the DID meetings in Chicago, and Allison and Orne did not attend.

The four special issues include a number of papers on the use of hypnosis in diagnosis and treatment of DID, as well as several papers on physiological aspects of dissociation, all of which acknowledge the tiny amount of hard data available. Frank Putnam (1984a, 1984b) contributed two papers on research and methodological issues and stated, "The scientific study of multiple personality disorder is just beginning." These papers are characteristic of later workshops, seminars, and conference presentations, and are much expanded and developed two years later (Putnam, 1986a, 1986b).

In these four journals, the leading contemporary writers in the field had begun to make their characteristic contributions. The organizational and editorial skills of Bennett Braun were evident, as was his gift for clinical work; Richard Kluft had expanded his careful observation of a large series of cases (Kluft, 1982), and was leading the field in study of childhood DID; Frank Putnam was defining more rigorous scientific studies; Philip Coons (1984) was writing scholarly, clear papers on diagnosis and phenomenology, characteristic of his large body of work (Coons, 1980, 1984, 1986a, 1986b, 1986c, 1986d, 1988a, 1988b; Coons, Bowman, & Milstein, 1988; Coons & Bradley, 1985; Coons & Milstein, 1984, 1986; Coons, Milstein, & Marley, 1982; Coons & Sterne, 1986) and Eugene Bliss (1984a) was exploring the hypnotic nature of DID and related disorders. These five men published the most work, and generated the bulk of the data on DID in the 1980s. Their contributions are not limited to this highlight of their published work.

Although they have not written as much or contributed as many original observations to the literature, Cornelia Wilbur (1984), who treated Sybil (Schreiber, 1973), and David Caul (1984), who treated Billy Milligan (Keyes, 1981), were present in these journals. They were major contributors to the development of the ISSD, and to the nourishment of young clinicians, as was George Greaves. Finally, as mentioned earlier, David Spiegel (1984) had begun to write on posttraumatic stress disorder and DID, a theme he has pursued since (Spiegel, 1986a, 1986b, 1988; Spiegel, Hunt, &

Dondershine, 1988). Spiegel is a contributor to DID studies who has moved into the area with a preestablished reputation (Spiegel & Rosenfeld, 1984; Spiegel & Spiegel, 1978). As other established investigators move into the field, they will raise standards, guard against insularity and stagnation, and provide credibility for dissociative studies.

The other major events in 1984 were the formation of the ISSD, and the First Annual International Conference on Multiple Personality/Dissociative States in Chicago. The ISSD has grown steadily to a membership of over 3,000 at the time of the 1994 meeting. Among its many functions, the ISSD publishes a newsletter that contains a variety of features and announcements. A future historian will have to record in detail the formation and evolution of this organization, and its impact on psychiatry as a whole. If dissociative disorders obtain a secure position in the mainstream of psychiatry, this will in large part be due to individual and organizational efforts of ISSD members. The ISSD and the annual Chicago meetings, organized by Bennett Braun, are closely interlinked.

In the 1970s, authors submitting papers on DID to journals did not have an easy time. In the 1990s, members of ISSD act as reviewers of many papers on DID submitted to North American journals. This means that a major ideological barrier to publication of DID papers has been removed. The establishment of dissociative disorders as a legitimate field of scientific inquiry has depended on this personal service and behind-the-scenes political work, as is the case in any new area of endeavor. The field of psychiatry as a whole, however, is still highly skeptical about DID.

The annual DID meetings in Chicago provided a forum for in-person contacts, presentation of papers with many different foci, workshops, political organization, and research collaboration. ISSD committee meetings were held concurrently. By the end of 1984, the field had moved from a prescientific stage to an early scientific level of development, with some data, an annual meeting, and a professional organization. Each of these components is essential if DID is to be more than a passing fad, destined to fall into disrepute and obscurity after a decade or two, in repetition of events that occurred 100 years ago.

DEVELOPMENTS FROM 1985 TO 1989

I am not going to review all the developments during this period because most of them will be taken up elsewhere. I diagnosed my third case of DID in September 1985, in consultation to Pam Gahan, who subsequently became a cotherapist and collaborator along with Geri Anderson in the diagnosis and treatment of about 50 cases of DID. In late 1991, I moved to Texas to become the Director of the Dissociative Disorders Unit at Charter Behavioral Health System of Dallas; since my arrival, the Unit has had over 1,000 admissions, and since 1985 I have accumulated an independent series of 236 cases (Ross,

Norton, & Wozney, 1989), 102 cases (Ross, Miller, Reagor, et al., 1990), and 103 cases (Ellason, Ross, & Fuchs, 1995).

This rapidity of personal development gives a measure of the rate of accumulating experience in the field as a whole. The exponential increase in the rate of diagnosis of DID is not an isolated phenomenon; it is a correlate of a great deal of organizational and educational effort.

During the 1980s, Richard Kluft (1985d, 1985f, 1987a) wrote the three major review papers in the field. These were radically different from the reviews published in 1944, 1962, and 1980. The 1987 paper, for example, entitled "An Update on Multiple Personality Disorder," contains 95 references, all but 10 of them from the 1980s and all but 7 of them directly on DID. Greaves's (1980) review, in comparison, contains 85 references, of which 26 are not directly related to DID, and 33 are from before 1970. The volume of literature that a reviewer had to assimilate expanded a lot in seven years. General reviews by a variety of authors appeared in a variety of journals in the 1980s, attesting to the growing interest in DID (Krasad, 1985; O'Brien, 1985; Ross & Fraser, 1987; Ross & Norton, 1987).

Kluft's three review papers contain data on or refer to several large series of cases. He has outcome data to present, can define the general principles of a treatment protocol, references and discusses a variety of treatment techniques, gives a detailed list of primary and secondary diagnostic features, reviews the clinical phenomenology and natural history, and can base his discussion of etiology on data. He is able to make preliminary remarks about the epidemiology. Very little of this was possible for a reviewer less than 10 years earlier. The evolution of review papers on DID gives another measure of the exponential growth of the field.

Two important books on DID were published by the American Psychiatric Press (Kluft, 1985a; Braun 1986b) during the mid-1980s. These continued the rapid development of the field. But now, for me, a potential problem began to appear, one commented on by Margolis (1988), who thought it was apparent in the 1984 special issue on DID of *Psychiatric Clinics of North America*. Contributors to one book are Barkin, Braun, Caul, Kluft, Putnam, Sachs, Spiegel, and Wilbur. Contributors to the other book are Braun, Coons, Frischholt, Goodwin, Hicks, Kluft, Putnam, Sachs, and Wilbur. The contributors cross-reference each other extensively.

On the one hand, this was entirely appropriate and commendable, since the list included the major contributors to the field. On the other, there was a potential danger—formation of an in-club with little tolerance for dissenting opinion. One remedy to this problem was to make a deliberate effort to engage outsiders in serious dialogue. This is a remedy put in place in the form of a debate at the 1988 American Psychiatric Association Annual Meeting, and the remedy has been much expanded and developed in the 1990s. Richard Kluft and David Spiegel supported, and Martin Orne and Fred Frankel opposed, the resolution that "Multiple Personality Is a True Disease Entity."

The APA debate was incorrectly titled because DID is not a true *disease* entity in the biomedical sense. It is a true psychiatric entity and a true disorder, but not a biomedical disease. The debate was nevertheless an important event, and should be ongoing.

To return to the two American Psychiatric Press books of the mid-1980s, one of their main features is the diagnosis and treatment of childhood DID, discussion of the familial incidence of DID, and overall a systemic life-cycle approach to the disorder. This is an important development in dissociative studies; DID must be placed in a social context, taking the life histories of families into account. Still, though, virtually no anthropological or cross-cultural perspective is evident in the two volumes, although such can be found elsewhere in the field (Krippner, 1986; Stevenson & Pasricha, 1979; Varma, Bouri, & Wig, 1981; Villoldo & Krippner, 1986). A cultural analysis is another antidote for insularity. To achieve scientific rigor in our understanding of late twentieth-century North American DID, we must more actively pursue an anthropological viewpoint.

Despite those concerns about the breadth of the two books, they are major contributions. Jean Goodwin's (1985) chapter, "Credibility Problems in Multiple Personality Disorder Patients and Abused Children," is a particularly well-written contribution, which I have found personally helpful. Another chapter worth noting is one on the use of medication in DID by Barkin, Braun, and Kluft (1986). This chapter is important because it highlights the need to conduct controlled, well-designed studies of the use of medication in DID (see Chapter Eleven). To date, one can use medication only on an empirical-trial basis, with little assurance as to the indications or likely response.

Setting aside content, these two books were an important event in the field for several reasons. They showed that mainstream psychiatry was willing to take DID seriously, since the publisher is the American Psychiatric Press. As well; the books demonstrated that a critical mass of contemporary scholars was in communication and able to collaborate on projects. A third consideration that gives a measure of the growth of the field, is that there is enough material to fill 450 pages in two volumes. Two such books would not have been possible 10 years earlier, because there wasn't enough content in the field to support them.

Another important book published in this period was *Multiple Personality, Allied Disorders, and Hypnosis* (1986) by Eugene Bliss. This book is thoroughly reviewed by Gruenewald (1988). I will discuss Bliss's book further in Chapters Three and Seven. *Split Minds Split Brains* (Quen, 1986) provides a broader cultural and historical perspective on the field and is cross-linked with the American Psychiatric Press volumes because it contains a chapter by Frank Putnam. The problem with this book, in terms of linking clinical studies with historical and anthropological work, is that it is not clinical enough. In a sense, that is an irrelevant criticism, since the editor wasn't setting out to bridge contemporary clinical practice and other scholarly studies. However, the problem remains in the field.

The same applies to *The Passion of Ansel Bourne* (Kenny, 1986). A book published in the 1980s, however, that embodies a historical and cultural perspective on clinical dissociation is *Multiple Man: Explorations in Possession and Multiple Personality* by Adam Crabtree (1985). Although this book has been out for 10 years, I don't yet see evidence of its influence on the field as a whole. Crabtree provides a historical review of DID then moves into the most interesting, clinical sections of the book. These contain numerous examples of dissociative disorders he has encountered in practice. Crabtree is able to bring a great deal of scholarship to bear on his clinical work, which is in itself a rare attribute. His thinking challenges preconceptions and stimulates alternate perspectives in a way that is potentially fruitful both for research and other clinicians (Crabtree, 1986).

In the two years 1985 and 1986, then, six scholarly books on DID were published in North America. This is a great deal of work, and it provided further evidence of the maturing of the field. Before closing my commentary on the 1980s, I want to highlight one other development in this period. That is the publication and/or presentation at conferences of the first scientific instruments for the measurement of dissociation, and the making of dissociative diagnoses. Prior to this period, research was hampered by the absence of self-report instruments and structured diagnostic interviews. Both of these are absolute prerequisites for modern scientific study of any psychiatric disorder. Other psychiatric disorders such as schizophrenia, mood disorders, and anxiety disorders have been studied with standardized instruments for some time. The specifics of these instruments are discussed in Chapter Seven.

During the second half of the 1980s, the transition from a prescientific to a scientific body of knowledge was consolidated. The field was now in the stage of early scientific development. This did not mean that there was no further place for case reports, however. An example of a case report that makes an important contribution is a paper by Coons (1988a) that describes the misuse of forensic hypnosis and a false-positive diagnosis of DID. Such reports are required to define problems in the field for further inquiry. They also provide useful clinical instruction. The field was evolving, though, to a point at which the need for single case reports was much less than it had been in the 1970s.

During the 1980s, early signs of preparation for multicenter treatment outcome studies started to become visible. General principles of treatment were defined (Braun, 1986a), an effort to standardize terminology was made (Braun, 1986a), and techniques of treatment were presented by a variety of clinicians (Ross & Gahan, 1988b). Methodological difficulties facing the field were described by Putnam (1986a). The possibility of beginning to prepare for multicenter studies was a topic of conversation among specialists in DID: A few years earlier such talk would have been idle dreaming.

These developments in the last half of the 1980s made it less likely that DID would once again fall into oblivion, after a short period of enthusiasm. The field was creating a database that could bring it into the psychiatric mainstream. One of the most important events in this regard was the launching of the journal *Dissociation* in 1988. With a professional society, a journal, a major specialty meeting, a number of scholarly books, and papers in a variety of journals, the dissociative disorders began to establish themselves in psychiatry, as the anxiety disorders had only a short while earlier. There are many patients with treatable dissociative disorders in North America who could benefit from greater awareness, prompter diagnosis, and more skilled treatment than is often available to them.

The year 1989 saw the publication of the only comprehensive single-author textbooks on the diagnosis and treatment of DID that have appeared to date. These were Frank Putnam's (1989) *Diagnosis and Treatment of Multiple Personality Disorder* and the first edition of this book, *Multiple Personality Disorder: Diagnosis, Clinical Features, and Treatment* (Ross, 1989). With the appearance of these two books, the field had reached a level of maturity that set the stage for the developments of the 1990s.

DEVELOPMENTS FROM 1990 TO 1995

The increase in the size of the dissociative disorders literature in the 1990s has been so rapid that it is now impossible for a single person to read everything that is published. This was not true when I wrote the first edition of this book in 1989, at which time I had a complete grasp of the important current literature. The sociological structure of the dissociative disorders field shifted in important ways in the first half of the 1990s: The membership of the International Society for the Study of Dissociation became much more broadly based, and original research from the Netherlands (Boon & Draijer, 1993), Belgium (Vanderlinden, 1993; Vanderlinden, Van Dyck, Vandereycken, & Vertommen, 1991), France (Darves-Bornoz, Degovianni, & Gaillard, 1995), Norway (Knudsen, Draijer, Haselrud, Boe, & Boon, 1995), Turkey (Tutkun, Yargic, & Sar, 1995; Yargic, Tutkun, & Sar, 1995), Canada (Horen, Leichner, & Lawson, 1995), Japan (Berger et al., 1994), New Zealand (Altrocchi, 1991), Puerto Rico (Martinez-Taboas, 1989, 1991), and India (Lewis-Fernandez, 1994) was published or presented at conferences.

A large number of editors and authors entered the field in the 1990s who were not part of the small inner circle of the 1980s, and the field began to display a divergence of points of view, especially concerning the historical veracity of trauma memories, and the frequency of iatrogenic DID. Also, dissociative data began to appear in papers published by a wide variety of different researchers, none of whom were primarily identified with the dissociative disorders field. Most of this work involved the inclusion of the

Dissociative Experiences Scale (Bernstein & Putnam, 1986) in assessment batteries.

Two journals published special issues on DID in the 1990s, *Psychiatric Clinics of North America,* September 1991, and the *Bulletin of the Menninger Clinic,* Summer 1993. The Menninger Clinic issue was subsequently published as a monograph (Allen & Smith, 1995). The *International Journal of Clinical and Experimental Hypnosis* published two special issues (Hypnosis and Delayed Recall) in October 1994 and April 1995 that contained considerable discussion of DID. Additionally, the journal *Consciousness and Cognition* published a special double issue on The Recovered Memory/False Memory Debate in September/December 1994 which, although it did not mention DID much, was directly relevant to the field. The July 1993 issue of the *American Journal of Psychiatry* was in effect an informal special issue on posttraumatic stress disorder and dissociative disorders, due to the appearance of a large number of papers on those topics. The October 1995 issue of the *Journal of Traumatic Stress* was a special issue on traumatic memory research that mentioned DID repeatedly.

The International Society for the Study of Dissociation issued the *Guidelines for Treating Dissociative Identity Disorder* (1994), the first effort at setting a standard of care for the treatment of DID. The guidelines were produced by the Standards of Practice Committee of the ISSD through an extensive committee process. In the same year, the American Society of Clinical Hypnosis published its monograph entitled *Clinical Hypnosis and Memory: Guidelines for Clinicians and for Forensic Hypnosis* (Hammond et al., 1994). The monograph contained an extensive review of the literature on traumatic memory. Combined with statements about recovered memories of childhood abuse issued by the American Psychiatric Association (1994b) and the American Medical Association (1995), these two sets of guidelines provided much more officially sanctioned information than was available in the 1980s.

A number of edited books appeared or were in press in the first half of the 1990s. These included *Dissociative Disorders: A Clinical Review* (Spiegel, 1993); *Clinical Perspectives on Multiple Personality Disorder* (Kluft & Fine, 1993); *Dissociation: Clinical and Theoretical Perspectives* (Lynn & Rhue, 1994); *Dissociation: Culture, Mind, and Body* (Spiegel, 1994); *Psychological Concepts and Dissociative Disorders* (Klein & Doane, 1994); *Dissociative Identity Disorder: Theoretical and Treatment Controversies* (Cohen, Berzoff, & Elin, 1995); *Treating Dissociative Identity Disorder* (Spira, 1996); and *Handbook of Dissociative Disorders* (Michelson & Ray, 1996). This substantial body of work was evidence that the dissociative disorders field had evolved into a true scientific field. The contributors to these edited volumes represented a wide variety of backgrounds, viewpoints, and interests, and there was a lot of disagreement among contributors. The days of the small group of pioneers were gone.

Several single or multiauthor books on DID and dissociation were published in this same period. These were: *The Osiris Complex: Case Studies in Multiple Personality Disorder* (Ross, 1994b); *Satanic Ritual Abuse: Principles of Treatment* (Ross, 1995a); *Multiple Personality Disorder from the Inside Out* (Cohen, Giller, & Lynn, 1991); *Telling without Talking: Art as a Window into the World of Multiple Personality* (Cohen & Cox, 1995); *Multiple Personality Disorder in the Netherlands* (Boon & Draijer, 1993); *Dissociative Experiences, Trauma and Hypnosis* (Vanderlinden, 1993); *Handbook for the Assessment of Dissociation: A Clinical Guide* (Steinberg, 1995); *From Mesmer to Freud: Magnetic Sleep and the Roots of Psychological Healing* (Crabtree, 1993); *First Person Plural: Multiple Personality and the Philosophy of Mind* (Braude, 1995); *Rewriting the Soul: Multiple Personality and the Sciences of Memory* (Hacking, 1995); *Trance and Possession in Bali: A Window on Western Multiple Personality, Possession Disorder, and Suicide* (Suryani & Jensen, 1993); and *Multiple Personalities, Multiple Disorders* (North, Ryall, Ricci, & Wetzel, 1993).

The authors of these books are from Canada, the United States, Bali, the Netherlands, and Belgium, and their professional backgrounds include psychology, psychiatry, philosophy, art therapy, and theology. It is evident that the dissociative disorders field was neither insular nor isolated to North America by the middle of the decade. I will not attempt to summarize all these books here, but will refer to them in subsequent chapters.

The International Society for the Study of Multiple Personality and Dissociation shortened its name to the International Society for the Study of Dissociation (ISSD) in 1994, which was my Presidency year. The reason for the name change was to conform to the new *DSM-IV* nomenclature, and to broaden the view of the organization to encompass the full range of normal and pathological dissociation. The primary focus of the organization continued to be on DID. The membership of the Society was about 2,600 people in late 1995.

The annual DID meetings in Chicago continued to be held under the chairmanship of Dr. Bennet Braun up until 1994. Beginning with the 1995 annual fall meeting, the Society took full scientific and financial control of the meeting, and it was held outside Chicago for the first time, in Orlando—this was another measure of the maturity of the field. The history of the Chicago meetings, and the great debt the field owes Dr. Braun for running them for a decade, is worthy of a book, and someone should record the history while the principals are still alive, the records intact, and the memories fresh.

The ISSD also held spring meetings in Ottawa, Amsterdam, Vancouver, and Dallas in the 1990s, and the first conferences on DID were held in England under independent sponsorship. Japanese translations of North American books on DID were published, and an original text on DID was published in German (Huber, 1995) and another in Japanese (Hattori, 1995). The Dissociative Disorders Interview Schedule (Ross, 1989), the Structured

Clinical Interview for *DSM-IV* Dissociative Disorders (Steinberg, 1995) and the Dissociative Experiences Scale (Bernstein & Putnam, 1986) were translated into many different languages and used in original research in Asia, Europe, North America, South America, the Middle East, the Caribbean, and Australia.

The *DSM-IV* (1994a) text for DID represented a major advance on *DSM-III-R* (1987), and the diagnostic criteria were improved by addition of an amnesia criterion. All these developments were indicators of the transition out of the early scientific phase of development: A great deal of research was conducted that could be described as *normal science* (Kuhn, 1962) within the trauma-dissociation paradigm. Despite all this work, however, the dissociative disorders were still marginalized within psychiatry and psychology, and did not receive the academic attention or clinical emphasis that was given to the anxiety, mood, psychotic, and substance abuse disorders.

The possibility still existed in 1995 that the dissociative disorders could disappear from professional awareness, repeating the history of the early twentieth century. This seemed unlikely, however, because of the much greater research base, the political organization of the field, and the existence of a dissociative disorders section in *DSM-IV*. The most likely development in the first decade of the twenty-first century is a steady increase in the scientific foundation and international character of the field. As of 1995, the field still awaited the appearance of definitive texts on dissociative disorders in childhood and on dissociative disorder not otherwise specified (DDNOS), although a special issue of *Child and Adolescent Psychiatric Clinics of North America* dealing with dissociation appeared in April 1996.

Diagnosis and Clinical Features of Dissociative Identity Disorder

Part Two reviews the clinical phenomenology, diagnostic criteria, epidemiology, and associated symptoms and diagnoses of dissociative identity disorder. In Chapter Nine, a discussion of nonclinical dissociation is provided to embed the clinical discussion in a broader context. Chapter Nine looks back to the first two chapters in this regard.

DID can be diagnosed with a high degree of reliability and validity. However, it will not be recognized without making a specific inquiry for its signs and symptoms. This inquiry is not part of a standard psychiatric assessment, which is why so many cases are missed. By the end of Part Two, the reader, with the assistance of the Dissociative Disorders Interview Schedule (see Appendix A), will know how to make the diagnosis.

What is DID? DID is a little girl imagining that the abuse is happening to someone else. This is the core of the disorder, to which all other features are secondary. The imagining is so intense, subjectively compelling, and adaptive, that the abused child experiences dissociated aspects of herself as other people. It is this core characteristic of DID that makes it a treatable disorder, because the imagining can be unlearned, and the past confronted and mastered.

DID patients are among the most disturbed people who seek the services of mental health professionals, yet they are often among the most treatable. The treatment must be guided by an understanding of DID and its historical antecedents. The complex details of the personality system can overwhelm the therapist who doesn't have a broad framework within which to conduct therapy.

The process of diagnosing DID leads naturally into the treatment, because the majority of patients have been severely traumatized in childhood. The trauma makes itself known in an array of symptoms and disturbed behaviors that fall into a pattern if the diagnostician knows what pattern to look for. Once the pattern is recognized, specific intensive psychotherapy follows naturally. The symptoms are severe and disabling and do not appear to remit with nonspecific interventions, although definitive data on this point are not available.

DID patients, when studied carefully, reveal many inadequacies in the current diagnostic system in psychiatry, as described in *DSM-IV*. In Part Two, therefore, I discuss a number of different psychiatric disorders from the point of view of dissociation to illuminate the paradigm-threatening potential of DID. The study of DID can yield valuable insight into a variety of issues in both biological and psychosocial psychiatry.

Etiology of Dissociative Identity Disorder

Dissociative identity disorder is a controversial diagnosis. The controversy centers on disagreement about its etiology, from which follows disagreement about its treatment, status as a psychiatric diagnosis, and relationship to other disorders (Atwood, 1978; French & Chodoff, 1987; Kluft, 1986d; Ludolph, 1985; Merskey, 1995; Piper, 1995a; Simpson, 1995). There is more opinion on the etiology of DID than data, a situation that hasn't prevented the expression of extreme views.

Much of the disagreement about the status of DID is purely ideological and occurs without reference to the existing research data. I will critique the skeptics in Chapter Ten. Another characteristic of the controversy is overgeneralization from biased samples, which I will explain in more detail in this chapter.

Before describing four pathways to DID, I will review what I call *the central paradox of DID* (Ross, 1995a). Much of the disagreement about the status of the disorder is based on failure to grasp this clinical logic. I will then explain the lessons to be learned from DID in forensic settings. Then I will review a number of different models of DID in the literature, each of which contributes something to our overall understanding.

THE CENTRAL PARADOX OF DISSOCIATIVE IDENTITY DISORDER

DID is not literally real. It is not possible to have more than one person in the same body. People with DID do not have more than one personality. However, DID is a real disorder that can be treated to stable integration. Untreated, DID often results in high levels of utilization of psychiatric services without significant improvement. In its childhood onset forms, the disorder is an effective strategy for coping with a traumatic environment: It becomes dysfunctional because environmental circumstances have changed by adulthood. The DID adaptation can be unlearned, with a great improvement in function and dramatic reduction in symptoms and need for psychiatric treatment.

Debates about whether or not DID is real are meaningless. The reality of the disorder is that it is both real and not real at the same time. People who say they don't believe in DID fail to grasp the central paradox of the disorder: The reality of DID exists at a metalevel that encompasses the central paradox. Not believing in DID is like not believing in hallucinations. All psychiatrists "believe in" hallucinations and delusions, grasp the fact that hallucinations and delusions are not real, and understand that they are real psychiatric symptoms.

FOUR PATHWAYS TO DISSOCIATIVE IDENTITY DISORDER

Based on my clinical experience, reading, and work as an expert witness, I have devised a scheme for understanding four different pathways by which patients arrive at DID. These are childhood abuse, childhood neglect, factitious, and iatrogenic pathways. Most patients present with a mixture of these different pathways but some occur in relatively pure form.

Prior to crystallizing this scheme, I tended to think of childhood abuse cases as "genuine" and iatrogenic and factitious cases as "phony," and I didn't differentiate iatrogenic and factitious pathways. I then realized that this distinction between real and false cases was based on a cognitive error: It did not follow *DSM-IV* rules. The *DSM* system is phenomenological throughout, and reliance on unproven theory has been removed from the diagnostic criteria sets and the text. This was done to achieve reliability in psychiatric diagnosis, and because psychiatrists tend to be wedded to schools of thought rather than to dispassionate scientific study of psychopathology.

Most of the "debate" about DID takes place at an ideological level and is based on a mistaken distinction between true and false cases. There is nothing in the *DSM-IV* criteria for DID that says anything about age at onset or etiology. This is also true of the diagnostic criteria for schizophrenia, depression, bulimia, panic disorder, and most other disorders. *DSM-IV*

DID exists when the phenomena of switching and amnesia are present—by *DSM-IV* criteria, these do not have to be directly observed by the psychiatrist. This lack of requirement for direct observation of diagnostic criteria also applies to all other disorders. For example, it is commonplace to diagnose bipolar mood disorder when the patient is currently observably depressed, but the mania is confirmed by patient self-report only. Although a collateral history is desirable, it is not essential. A decision to start lithium can be made without conclusive collateral history or direct observation of mania.

Using the rules of the *DSM* system, an iatrogenic case of DID is just as "real" and "genuine" as one with an onset in childhood. This is the reality of psychiatric disorders in the late twentieth century: Mental disorders are real because their diagnostic criteria sets have face validity and diagnostic reliability. The face validity of the different disorders does not have to be universal, only sufficient to permit entry into the system and appearance in *DSM-IV.* By this logic, which is the official logic of the American Psychiatric Association, DID is as real as depression or schizophrenia. None of the anxiety, psychotic, mood, or dissociative disorders can claim any greater form of reality, none has a proven biomedical foundation, and none has a scientifically proven etiology.

Different people could be depressed for purely genetic, purely environmental, or mixed reasons; in the *DSM-IV* system, all are "really" depressed and all receive the same diagnosis. Similarly, the negative symptoms of schizophrenia can be due to medications, depression, the illness itself, or institutionalization, and it is often difficult or impossible to separate out these different pathways to the same common clinical phenomenology. The purpose of the differential diagnosis of negative symptoms of schizophrenia is not to determine which symptoms are "real" but to prescribe differential treatments. This is also true of the analysis of the four pathways to DID.

The four pathways to DID are summarized in Table 3.1. As can be seen in the table, each pathway has a unique pattern that differentiates it from the other three. Some of these differentiating criteria are speculative, and some are supported by published research. It is futile to debate the relative frequency of the four different pathways in the absence of adequate research data, because all parties to the debate are working from biased subsamples, and tend to overgeneralize from their own experience.

A therapist may see predominantly childhood abuse pathway cases that have been treatment failures in conventional psychiatry and may think that iatrogenic cases are rare. A skeptic, on the other hand, will be more likely to see iatrogenic cases that are treatment failures for the dissociative disorders field, and will be prone to the opposite ideologically driven overgeneralization. Neither camp sees the other's treatment successes, and no one has provided empirical data on the frequency of the four subtypes of DID in clinical populations.

Table 3.1A.   **Four Pathways to Dissociative Identity Disorder**

Pathway	Predominant Personality Type	Hypnotizability	DES Score	Type of Therapy	Response of DID to Treatment
Childhood Abuse	Borderline	++	40	DID	Integration
Childhood Neglect	Dependent	+	30	Modified DID	?
Factitious Disorder	Antisocial	?	70	Factitious Disorder	Remission/ Chronic
Iatrogenic	Dependent	+	70	Cult Exit Counseling	Remission

Table 3.1B.   **Four Pathways to Dissociative Identity Disorder**

Pathway	Type of DID	Attachment to Perpetrator	DID Symptoms Prior to Therapy	Elaborate Medical History
Childhood Abuse	Trauma Model	+/−	++	+/−
Childhood Neglect	Trauma Model	−	+/−	−
Factitious Disorder	Factitious Model	−	−	++
Iatrogenic	Destructive Psychotherapy-Cult Model	+	−	−

Childhood Abuse Pathway

The childhood abuse pathway to DID is the one treated most frequently by dissociative disorders therapists, as far as the therapists can tell; this statement is qualified by the fact that iatrogenic cases are rarely recognized as such by the therapists creating them. This subtype is described in detail in the rest of this book and is the target of the techniques described in the treatment section.

The most common etiological theory for this subtype, which I subscribed to in the first edition of this book, is that DID arises during severe, chronic childhood trauma, which in North America is most commonly sexual and/or physical abuse. The little girl being sexually abused by her father at night imagines that the abuse is happening to someone else, as a way to distance herself from the overwhelming emotions she is experiencing. She may float up to the ceiling and watch the abuse in a detached fashion. Now not only is the abuse not happening to her, but she blocks it out of her mind—that other little girl remembers it, not the original self. In this model, DID is an internal divide-and-conquer strategy in which intolerable knowledge and feeling is split up into manageable compartments. These compartments are personified and take on a life of their own.

I have gradually shifted over to a model that differs from the first in subtle but important ways. I now think that the primary driver of the dissociation is not the abusive events themselves, or the feelings they cause, although this mechanism comes into play regularly: I now postulate more of a social-psychological theory.

It seems to me that the fundamental problem in DID is *the problem of attachment to the perpetrator.* This can be so whether the abuse is physical, sexual, or psychological. I arrived at this understanding through thousands of hours of clinical experience, and changed models in a gradual manner. The two theories are not mutually exclusive, and I assume that they co-occur. Barach (1991) and Liotti (1992) have written about attachment in DID.

The abused child cannot escape from the trauma, nor can she control or predict it. The abuse is arbitrary. For example, when I lived in the Canadian Arctic, I observed that childhood trauma and spousal abuse increased dramatically when welfare checks came in, and alcohol was purchased. There is no way that young children could predict this cycle.

The abused child can use dissociation to block out some or all of the actual abusive events, but this strategy does not solve a more pervasive and inescapable problem: The child is overwhelmed, helpless, and powerless. It is this helplessness and powerlessness that is the deepest trauma. The child's developmental problem is that she must attach to her perpetrator in order to survive. The little girl is driven by biological imperatives that have been extensively studied in experimental mammals (van der Kolk, 1987): She must attach to survive biologically, emotionally, and spiritually.

A survival strategy of extreme detachment would be self-destructive and would cause failure to thrive. Therefore the child tries to attach to her perpetrator father and enabler mother, who often is a perpetrator in her own right. To keep her genetically encoded attachment systems up and running, the child must dissociate. The environment, through the abuse, signals the child to shut down her attachment systems, but her genes override this environmental imperative. The two realities do not fit together, and the world does not make sense.

To cope with this fundamental threat to its integrity, and to avoid the paralysis of learned helplessness, the organism, whether a little kitten, duckling, monkey, cat, or child, must dissociate. Because of dissociation, the attachment systems can be kept up and running, given that from their point of view the trauma is not occurring (Freyd, 1993). In a human being, the attachment systems become personified as separate identities who idealize the parents, and are amnesic for most or all of the abuse. The amnesia barriers need not be absolute, as long as they downregulate the traumatic psychophysiology sufficiently to permit attachment.

In this model, an additional drive to the creation of alter personalities is the need to create stable internal persons who are always available for attachment, safety, security, and nurturing. The need for attachment figures drives the narcissistic investment of the alters in separateness, and the delusion of separate physical bodies they often create. In the child with lesser dissociative capacity, this strategy results in the creation of polarized but nonpersonified states that alternate in the taking of executive control. This psychological mechanism is called *borderline splitting*.

It follows from this model that both DID and borderline personality disorder can occur in the absence of overt physical and sexual abuse. The reason that there are very high rates of reported physical and sexual abuse in DID is that the extreme attachment dilemma required to drive the formation of DID usually occurs in families that are also overtly and criminally abusive. The overt acts of abuse are traumatic in and of themselves, but are also markers of inevitable severe attachment conflicts in the family's children.

Additionally, it follows that sexual abuse in less intrusive, violent, threatening, bizarre, and deviant forms occurring in families that are overtly normal and stable, would be less likely to result in DID. In these families, the attachment conflict is not amplified by alcoholic rages, serial live-in boyfriends of the divorced mother, chronic storminess, multiple perpetrators, and other social trauma such as poverty and urban violence. In these less overtly dysfunctional families, simpler forms of dissociation would suffice to maintain attachment, and the incest father would more likely display a range of positive parental behaviors.

Individuals on the childhood abuse pathway have full DID before age 10, and exhibit symptoms of complex dissociation on a chronic basis. These often can be observed in medical records going back for years before the diagnosis. Not uncommonly, family members will describe switching and amnesia prior to diagnosis, and will say that the diagnosis of DID makes complete sense to them. Because of the psychosomatic symptoms that arise from the abuse, childhood abuse pathway patients sometimes will have extensive medical-surgical histories without definitive findings or diagnoses. This need not always be the case, however; therefore, I have rated these individuals as plus or minus on this dimension.

As described in Chapter Seven, childhood onset DID cases are characterized by high scores on standard measures of hypnotizability and average scores in the 40s on the Dissociative Experiences Scale. The predominant personality type is borderline, because of the problem of attachment to the perpetrator, the type of treatment is DID/trauma model, and the response of a successfully treated case is integration. The average duration of therapy is 3 to 5 years.

Childhood Neglect Pathway

I began to become more aware of this pathway in 1993 due to accumulating clinical experience. On our Dissociative Disorders Unit at Charter Behavioral Health System of Dallas, we began to see more and more cases that combined elements of all four pathways, and some in which neglect was the predominant form of trauma. It took me a long time to understand that extreme neglect can be as traumatic as physical or sexual abuse.

Childhood neglect pathway patients describe mothers who were depressed, schizophrenic, alcoholic, or themselves had DID, and who were physically absent and emotionally unavailable. The neglect may have involved being locked in closets and basements or left in a crib for prolonged periods. The pervasive trauma was the absence of a secure attachment figure. These neglected and emotionally deprived children retreated into an internal imaginary world to fill up the emptiness and form internal attachments. They created an elaborate internal landscape populated by characters with histories and complex interactions.

From the starting point of a highly elaborated inner world, the neglect pathway patients seem to take one of three subpathways: In some cases, the person activates inner characters to take executive control to deal with the outside world prior to therapy. Here the diagnostic picture is predominantly one of DDNOS (Dissociative Disorder Not Otherwise Specified) with some preexisting relatively simple DID.

On the second subpathway, the DDNOS is elaborated iatrogenically by therapist error into an artifactual DID. On the third pathway, the patient is DDNOS at entry into therapy and never evolves into DID. Lumping these three subpathways together, the childhood neglect case may show some symptoms of full DID prior to treatment and will not tend to have an elaborate medical history because of the absence of sexual abuse, which I assume to be the main driver of the psychosomatic symptoms.

The neglect cases seem to be highly hypnotizable but are not at the virtuoso level of the childhood abuse pathway. High fantasy proneness and absorptive capacity are required to create the inner world. The predominant personality type appears to be dependent, the treatment modality is modified DID/trauma model, and the response to treatment appears to be favorable overall, with a more rapid remission of the DID into DDNOS than occurs in abuse cases.

The main difference in the therapy, compared with abuse pathway cases, is that the therapist does not enter into the internal system and work at a microlevel within the system. Instead, the therapist pulls out into a more external stance and treats the DID as a single autohypnotic defense. The interpretations, systemic analysis, and correction of cognitive errors are done at a more macrolevel than in abuse cases, and the patient is encouraged to examine the cost-benefit of the dissociation as a monolithic defense.

Factitious Pathway

I have encountered pure factitious pathway cases in my work as an expert witness. In the clinical arena, I have seen cases in which the factitious element predominated but was combined with abuse and neglect elements, and I have made a formal diagnosis of factitious disorder several times. Usually, the factitious elements in combined-pathway cases are discussed in my progress notes but are not highlighted by a separate diagnosis.

In factitious cases, there is no history of dissociative symptoms prior to therapy, but there is usually an elaborate medical-surgical history. This may include self-inflicted infections; anemia; faked withdrawal from substances of abuse; physical injuries; factitious rape reports; multiple investigations, tests, and surgeries without definitive findings; extreme doctor and hospital shopping; prescription drug abuse; and multiple psychiatric diagnoses. The picture is one of factitious disorder as described in the general medical literature (Feldman & Ford, 1994).

The predominant personality type, I suspect, is antisocial—I do not have enough clinical experience with these cases to be confident about that. These people are con artists and are consciously running a scam on the health care system. Somewhere along the line, they get the idea that it would be fun to have DID, and to be in the DID patient role. As is true of medical-surgical factitious disorders, these people can be very hard to spot. Conscientious, ethical, skilled clinicians can get fooled for prolonged periods by the factitious epileptic or the Munchausen's-by-proxy mother.

The factitious pathway cases seem to have low hypnotizability but may have extremely high scores on the DES, up into the 70s or 80s. They are overfaking DID. The treatment for these individuals is a factitious disorder model, and the response to confrontation and redirection can take one of two forms: relatively rapid remission of the DID, or flight to another facility with ongoing factitious DID.

Since the formation of the False Memory Syndrome Foundation in 1992 (Ross, 1995a), factitious patients now have another career option open to them: they can develop *false memory syndrome* and sue the therapists they had previously conned with factitious DID. In the current legal climate, the secondary gain derived from the DID patient role is far outweighed by that of false memory syndrome, which brings pseudo-reconciliation with the family, protection by a lawyer father-substitute, and potentially large sums of money.

In the general medical literature on factitious disorders, no one has been able to accumulate a large series of cases that has stayed in treatment for factitious disorder postconfrontation and diagnosis. The patients simply run away to another doctor and hospital. The medical countertransference toward factitious patients, once they are diagnosed, is usually hostile, rejecting, and blaming, and the professionals who were fooled by the patient are viewed as victims of a clever con artist.

On our Dissociative Disorders Unit, we have been trying to change our countertransference, and the response of factitious DID cases to confrontation. Our goal is to have these cases stay in treatment for real problems, and to save the health care system the costs of prolonged treatment for factitious DID. Our main strategy for accomplishing this is to define factitious disorder as a real, serious, and treatable condition. Factitious DID is a symptom of a more severe psychiatric problem than is abuse pathway DID. So far, with limited experience, we are having some success at treating these cases on our Dissociative Disorders Unit, with frank discussion of the secondary gain in both individual and group therapy. The other patients have by and large been supportive to the factitious pathway patients, without rejecting them as "fakes."

Iatrogenic Pathway

Whereas the factitious pathway arises from conscious deception by the patient, in the absence of significant therapist error, iatrogenic cases are caused by poor therapy techniques. Most cases involve admixtures of all four pathways to varying degrees, but I have seen pure iatrogenic cases in my expert witness work.

In the predominantly iatrogenic case, there is no history of chronic, severe dissociative symptoms prior to therapy, the attachment to parents is more-or-less normal, there is no elaborate medical-surgical history, and the predominant personality type is dependent. This is the pattern I have seen on administering the Structured Clinical Interview for *DSM-III-R*, Axis II Version (Spitzer, Williams, Gibbon, & First, 1990) in six women I have assessed as a plaintiff's expert witness in malpractice cases. In each of these cases, I judged that the plaintiff was an example of iatrogenic pathway DID.

Although some fantasy-proneness and hypnotizability is required to create iatrogenic DID, like the neglect and factitious pathways, these individuals do not seem to have the extreme trance-proneness of childhood abuse cases. During the iatrogenic DID phase, they have high DES scores, but in the retractor phase their scores are normal. In the six cases I have assessed as an expert witness, the DID symptoms remit spontaneously and rapidly once the patient is extricated from her enmeshment with the offending therapist, usually in a matter of a few weeks or months. In clinical assessments totaling up to 12 hours of face-to-face interviewing per case, I have not seen any evidence that the retraction is based on denial or shutting down of the system.

Pure iatrogenic cases, in my limited experience, can arise out of one of three premorbid backgrounds. One group of patients has bipolar mood disorder (Merskey, 1995), which is interpreted by the therapist as switching of alter personalities; the second has complex symptoms of anxiety, mood disorder, eating disorder, personality disorder, and dissociation, but no diagnosable dissociative disorder; and the third has posttraumatic stress disorder but no DDNOS or DID before contact with the therapist.

I have characterized the psychotherapy of iatrogenic DID as cult exit counseling based on my knowledge of the literature on destructive cults (Hassan, 1988; Singer, 1995; West & Martin, 1994), which I review in more detail in my book on Satanic ritual abuse (Ross, 1995a). Margaret Singer, Louis Jolyon West, Robert Lifton (1961), and others belonged to a network of psychologists and psychiatrists who studied coercive persuasion, mind control, brainwashing, and thought reform—all terms for the same process—during the 1950s. West, Lifton and others debriefed U.S. pilots who had been brainwashed by their communist Chinese captors during the

Table 3.2.   Characteristics of a Destructive Psychotherapy Cult

1. Deceptive Recruitment	8. Love Bombing
2. Hierarchical Structure	9. Trance Induction—Meditation,
3. Charismatic Leader	Chanting, Studying Group Doctrine,
4. Alienation from Family—Family	Drugs
Defined as Satanic	10. Questioning of Cult Doctrine
5. Control of Information, Daily	Disallowed
Relationships	11. Creation of a New Cult
6. Sensory Deprivation and Isolation	Personality/Suppression of the
7. Sleep and Food Deprivation	Preexisting Personality

Korean War. These military studies of thought reform were then extended to civilian destructive cults, which use many of the same methods.

Table 3.2 lists the general features of destructive cults, as summarized by Singer (1995). Table 3.3 describes the way in which iatrogenic cases of DID are subjected to the same techniques during prolonged hospitalizations on dissociative disorders units.

The following case study is an example of the creation of iatrogenic DID through coercive persuasion; this case is a composite of the extreme cases I have seen as an expert witness. I suspect from analysis of these extreme cases that the threshold for creation of iatrogenic DID may be higher than many skeptics assume. If one considers the amount of control over a recruit's lifespace required for creation of a new identity by a destructive cult, it seems unlikely that this could be achieved in any significant number

Table 3.3.   A Destructive Psychotherapy Cult—Two Years on a Dissociative Disorders Unit for Iatrogenic Dissociative Identity Disorder

1. Admitting Diagnosis is Not DID	8. Massive Attention and Positive
2. Hospital Clinical and Administrative	Feedback from Staff
Structure	9. Numerous Active Inductions
3. Unit has a Charismatic Director	Prolonged Journalling, Artwork,
4. Family Defined as Multigenerational	Mapping, Guided Imagery
Orthodox Satanic	Multiple Medications and High
5. Mail, Visitors, and Phone Calls	Dosages
Restricted to Minimal or Zero	10. Questioning of Induced Virtual
6. Over 100 Voluntary Restraint	Reality Attributed to Cult
Abreaction Sessions, Two Years	Programming
Physically Inside the Hospital	11. Polyfragmented New Identity Created
Building	Divorce, No Contact with Children
Prolonged Seclusion and PICU	for Years
7. Discharged Biochemically	False Positive Confession to Child
Malnourished, Hospital Food,	Protective Services
Iatrogenic Traumatic Insomnia	

of people through only an hour or two of outpatient psychotherapy a week. G. H. Estabrooks said it took months of special training under military conditions to create artificial DID in selected subjects, so the existing evidence suggests a fairly high threshold for creation of enduring iatrogenic DID.

In the pure iatrogenic cases I have seen, the amount of control and influence by the therapist has been extreme and has involved inpatient admissions as long as two years, or 10 to 15 hours of outpatient contact per week for years. The treatment is provided within a destructive psychotherapy cult, which I will illustrate with a composite inpatient case.

Case Study

Mrs. S. was admitted to the dissociative disorders unit of a hospital far from her home in order to protect her from the Satanic cult to which, according to her therapist, her parents belonged. The specific goal of the admission as stated in the medical record was to work on her cult programming. Mrs. S. had been inducted into DID psychotherapy via deceptive recruitment because her presenting problems were depression and panic disorder, and because she never gave meaningful informed consent to DID therapy.

There was no history of amnesia, auditory hallucinations, flashbacks, other secondary features of DID, or childhood physical or sexual abuse prior to diagnosis. Her medical-surgical history was unremarkable, and there was no history of substance abuse, legal or criminal problems, antisocial behavior, promiscuity, unemployment, or spousal abuse. She functioned well as a mother and professional. Assessed with the SCID I and SCID-II in 1995, she met lifetime criteria for depression, panic disorder, posttraumatic stress disorder related to a rape in adulthood, and dependent personality disorder. Her score on the Dissociative Experiences Scale was under 10, and she did not meet criteria for any dissociative disorders on the Dissociative Disorders Interview Schedule. Her scores and profiles on the Beck Mood Inventory, Hamilton Depression Scale, SCL-90-R, and Millon Clinical Multiaxial Inventory-II were normal.

The hospital had a hierarchical structure both administratively and clinically, and the dissociative disorders unit was run by a charismatic leader to whom all other personnel deferred. During the course of her two years as an inpatient, Mrs. S. was subjected to profound sensory deprivation and isolation simply by virtue of never leaving the hospital. In addition, she had over 200 voluntary restraint sessions for abreactive psychotherapy lasting up to six hours each; over six months of continuous 1:1 nursing observation; prolonged admissions to psychiatric intensive care; and numerous prolonged periods in seclusion rooms, often in involuntary restraints.

Mrs. S. experienced food deprivation through loss of appetite and phobic avoidance of food secondary to iatrogenic memories of cannibalism, and drinking of blood, urine, and semen. She lost weight, experienced fatigue and weakness, and was discharged biochemically malnourished. She experienced severe sleep deprivation due to nightmares and nocturnal abreactions of Satanic ritual abuse. There was no external evidence that she had ever experienced any abuse of any kind, and she had retracted all these allegations within a few months of leaving the hospital.

Trance states were induced countless times by formal hypnotic inductions, and prolonged journaling, artwork, mapping, guided imagery, and internal visualization exercises, as well as high doses of medications. These trance-induction exercises occupied many hours per day for the two years; maps of personality systems were displayed prominently in patients' rooms on the unit, so that they were visible from the hallway, and the maps were so hypercomplex that they often required 20 or more square feet of paper. The problem was not with any one of these techniques used in moderation, but with the massive amount of time and energy devoted to them collectively.

Mrs. S.'s family was explicitly defined as belonging to a multigenerational orthodox Satanic cult, and many staff members repeatedly stated their absolute belief in the reality of the cult to Mrs. S. All mail, visitors, and outside phone calls were cut off for over six months to protect her from cult triggers, and the medical record contained notations that a dentist was brought into the hospital to see her out of concern that another dentist, whom she had previously seen outside the hospital, might be a cult member and might implant a transmitter in her teeth for cult signaling and reprogramming.

All resistance to the treatment plan by Mrs. S. was viewed as evidence of cult programming and this was explicitly noted in the chart. The cult love bombing took the form of massive reinforcement of the beliefs that the patient was safe from the cult in the hospital, that the staff cared for her, and that they would be her new family. The love of the clinical family evaporated when the insurance policy was exhausted.

Instead of creating a single new cult personality, with suppression of the former identity and its connections and allegiances, Mrs. S. created a new polyfragmented cult identity that conformed to the demands, expectations, ideology, and paranoia of the destructive psychotherapy cult. She described in detail asking a copatient questions about how to structure her personality system map to conform with unit expectations, and this copatient similarly taught another patient I assessed. Mrs. S. described being aware that there was something wrong throughout the hospitalization, while simultaneously believing that the induced virtual reality of DID and Satanic ritual abuse was real.

Mrs. S. has not required rehospitalization for three years since discharge, during which time she has not overdosed, abused substances, entered into destructive personal relationships, or acted out in any significant way. She understood and agreed with the rationale for having me as an expert witness, and was fully cooperative with the interview, during which her mental status was unremarkable, and devoid of any hints of psychosis or dissociation.

If all cases of DID occurred exclusively on the iatrogenic pathway, I would have no disagreement with the skeptics discussed in Chapter Ten, and would advocate shutting down the dissociative disorders field with lawsuits, legislation, managed care policing, peer review, and ethical scrutiny. However, my clinical experience tells me that the iatrogenic is only one of four pathways to DID, and not the predominant one.

If I was asked for an informal estimate of the contribution of the four pathways to the caseload of over 1,000 admissions treated on our Dissociative Disorders Unit at Charter Behavioral Health System of Dallas since 1991, I would set the childhood abuse pathway at 50%, and the other three at 16.7% each. I would give the estimated range for the childhood trauma pathway as 25% to 50%, and for the other three 16.7% to 25%. Only a small number of cases have illustrated the nonabuse pathways in relatively pure form. I mean by these estimates that this is the contribution of the four pathways in our patients up to the first time they are admitted to our Unit.

False positive diagnoses of DID were not a significant problem when I was writing the first edition of this book in 1988 because few clinicians were making the diagnosis: At that time, the problem of false negatives far outweighed the problem of false positives. Now with thousands of clinicians making the diagnosis of DID, many of whom were never formally trained in differential diagnosis and have never worked directly with a broad range of psychopathology, a significant amount of iatrogenic DID exists.

There is still a major problem with false negative diagnoses, however. The shift from the 1980s to the mid 1990s is in the quantity of DID cases diagnosed: If a quarter of the current DID diagnoses in North America are false positives, this would not likely be any higher than the rate of false positive diagnoses of schizophrenia, given the interrater reliability of the diagnosis of schizophrenia on structured interview, as I will discuss in Chapter Seven.

The field needs to move from polarized ideological pseudodebates about the validity of DID to scientific studies and collection of data concerning the four pathways.

DISSOCIATIVE IDENTITY DISORDER IN FORENSIC PSYCHIATRY

In this section, I am going to review selected aspects of forensic DID. I'm not a forensic psychiatrist and can't make detailed recommendations about how to do assessments of criminals with DID. My focus will be on nonforensic DID, and what we can learn about it by considering criminal cases, especially what we can learn about the four pathways described earlier. An inventory of civil and criminal cases involving DID is given in Goettmean, Greaves, and Coons (1992).

Coons (1988a) has published a case that illustrates the harmful effects of the abuse of forensic hypnosis. In his case, a woman lost her job and children because of incorrect interviewing, misused hypnosis, and a false positive diagnosis of DID. The patient appeared to be innocent and to have no interest in simulating DID. The supposed DID was never used as a defense because she was not brought to trial. Nor was she detained on psychiatric grounds. The negative consequences ensued because of events set in motion by the false diagnosis and included losing her children in custody disputes.

Those concerned that criminals might fake DID for secondary gain should be aware that factitious DID may create more loss than gain. The difficulties of establishing whether a criminal does or doesn't have "real" DID are illustrated by the debate about the Hillside Strangler (Allison, 1984; Orne, Dinges, & Orne, 1984; Watkins, 1984). I was persuaded by Martin Orne's argument that Kenneth Bianchi was faking, but it was a complicated case. Perhaps both factitious and childhood trauma DID were coexistent in Kenneth Bianchi. Whatever the truth is about that one case, no test or battery of tests can establish scientifically, beyond doubt, whether a given criminal does or does not have genuine DID. This means that expert testimony is based on clinical judgment, and is inexact and imperfect. It is therefore necessary to be cautious about the relevance of DID in criminal proceedings.

Many professionals think that DID is always iatrogenic. What does forensic DID teach us about the possibility that clinical DID is an artifact caused by the doctor? Faked DID in the forensic context is an artifact not of the doctor-patient relationship, it seems to me, but of the legal system. It makes sense to fake DID, when charged with crimes, only if that is a good legal strategy. If the legal system was structured such that criminals with DID received jail sentences that were twice as long as those received by criminals without DID, we would not encounter malingered DID in forensic psychiatry. In fact, we would expect malingered false negative diagnoses of DID to occur. In this scenario, criminals would not manifest either factitious or iatrogenic DID no matter how many leading or suggestive questions the psychiatrist asked.

In forensic settings, neither iatrogenic nor factitious DID are caused solely by the doctor, or by the relationship between doctor and criminal. The causality is systemic in nature, and both doctor and criminal are players in a systemic game. The cause of the DID is the rules of the system, which make it "smart" to have DID. Both criminal and doctor are playing according to rules that reward criminals for displaying mental illness.

The problem, in forensic assessment of DID, is a systemic rule that says criminals can be found not guilty by reason of insanity (Ross, 1986b). Not guilty by reason of insanity is bad therapy for DID patients.

Today we have a legal system in which a defendant who killed a child while driving drunk can claim that it was the bartender's fault for serving him too much alcohol. This can actually result in a lighter sentence and the possibility of a suit against the bar owner. Even without that added twist, criminals may get lighter sentences for murder if they were drunk at the time. Rapists get lighter sentences if they express remorse, seek counseling, or go to church. There are currently court challenges in the United States based on the claim that some murderers on death row are not mentally competent to be executed. In my view, using DID as a tactic on this perverse playing field that we call the legal system may be good legal strategy, but it does not teach patients how to take ownership of their lives, or responsibility for their actions. Therapists are misguided if they try to "help" their

DID patients by telling the judge that the patient wasn't responsible, on the grounds that an alter personality committed the crime.

I am not saying that forensic psychiatry is a waste of time. Quite the opposite: It is an extremely important branch of medicine. What I am talking about is shutting down the rewards for artifactual DID. A few highly publicized cases in which DID has been used as a defense illustrate the perversity of "not guilty by reason of insanity." In the case of Billy Milligan, for example (Keyes, 1981), the patient might have spent less time locked in institutions, and received less harassment after discharge, if he had been found guilty and served his time as a regular criminal. A psychiatric defense is not always in the defendant's best interest, even as a strategy for getting a lighter sentence.

There is a simple solution to the artifactual creation of DID in criminal cases. Mental state and psychiatric history should be irrelevant to a determination of guilt. If you did it, you are guilty. If you didn't do it, you are innocent. And, you are innocent until proven guilty. Those simple principles would immediately eliminate all secondary gain for having a psychiatric diagnosis. But should mentally ill criminals be treated the same as other criminals? No, of course not. They need psychiatric treatment if they have treatable psychiatric disorders. Such treatment is in the best interests of both the criminal and society.

Criminal trials should be held in two stages. In the first stage, no testimony about mental state or psychiatric history should be allowed. If the person is found innocent, proceedings stop. If he is found guilty, then the defending lawyer has the option of asking for psychiatric testimony to be heard in determination of sentencing. This would only delay courtroom manipulation and secondary gain, however, if a psychiatric diagnosis could result in a lighter sentence. Therefore, the length of sentence should be set at the end of the first stage, and the defending lawyer should only be able to request psychiatric testimony after that.

What would be the point of psychiatric testimony, then? To determine whether the prisoner should serve his time in regular prison, the psychiatric wing of a prison, or the forensic ward of a psychiatric hospital. If the sentence does not involve a jail term, there is no need for psychiatric testimony. Whatever flaws it might have, such a system would eliminate motivation to fake or unconsciously simulate DID, and for genuine DID patients charged with crimes to augment, exacerbate, or perpetuate their disorder for secondary gain.

The point I am making, in a book about clinical DID, is that it is possible to shut down secondary gain, to minimize faked or artifactual dissociation, and to keep a focus on recovery and improved function. This is what I try to do in the clinic. The second point is this: If artifactual clinical DID does occur, it is not necessarily caused by the doctor in a simple linear manner. Like forensic DID, clinical DID must be analyzed in a systemic context. In a health care system in which psychotherapy for depression was paid for but psychotherapy for DID was not, there would be a strong drive toward false positive diagnoses of depression, and false negative diagnoses of DID. Reverse the billing procedure, and the "incidence" of DID would increase. In either case, both patient and doctor are players in a systemic game, and the features of DID are influenced by systemic rules.

Iatrogenic DID is the product of a wide social context, not just of the doctor-patient relationship as an isolated entity, as illustrated by the case history given earlier. Analyzing the causes of artifactual DID must involve a much wider focus than the doctor-patient relationship. Blaming the doctor for DID is like blaming him for the sore back of a carpenter on compensation. In factitious cases, the doctor doesn't *cause* the sore back. He is a participant in a social ritual with defined rules, structure, and outcomes. The doctor assesses some genuine sore backs and some fake ones, and has trouble differentiating the two.

In assessing an artifactual case of DID, it is essential to determine whether the case is primarily factitious or primarily iatrogenic. The skeptics have not made this distinction and assume that all cases are iatrogenic.

The defense of not guilty by reason of insanity is bad therapy for DID patients. Two of the foundations of DID treatment are defining the patient as not crazy, and expecting the patient to be and to become responsible for her life and actions. These are essential principles of therapy. The treatment of trauma pathway DID involves defining the disorder as a good survival strategy, based on talent and ability, not on defect or incapacity. The patient did not develop DID because there was something wrong with her brain, her ego, or any other aspect of her. The DID was a creative and adaptive strategy for surviving a traumatic childhood. Treatment is required in adulthood because the strategy has becoming self-defeating.

If treatment is based on this essential principle, how can the DID patient who commits a crime be not guilty by reason of insanity? You can't have it both ways at once, except in an inconsistent, contradictory, and double-binding world, such as the one DID patients grow up in. It is also essential, especially in working with severely disturbed multiples, who are prone to theatrical, manipulative, and double-binding behavior, to insist that the patient is responsible for the behavior of all alters. To "let her off" because it was an alter that broke a window, molested a child, or broke the treatment contract, is to reinforce secondary gains for dissociation.

Many DID patients have been molested by parents who themselves have DID (Braun, 1985). The fact that the parent had an abusive alter, hidden behind an amnesia barrier, does not excuse the abuse. It does not make the abuse less wrong, less criminal, or less destructive. Nor does the fact that the parent had DID mean that the child's dissociated anger is less legitimate. If the abusive DID parent is not let off, in an emotional sense, within the therapy of his child, why should the child be let off for criminal behavior of her own? Why should the child be let off for abusive, manipulative, or destructive behavior directed at the therapist, office furniture, or other staff?

As I see it, sane therapy requires clear, consistent rules. Therefore I am opposed to the defense of not guilty by reason of insanity, for DID and other dissociative disorders.

THE IATROGENIC MODEL OF DISSOCIATIVE IDENTITY DISORDER

Serious students of dissociation have thought about the artifactual aspects of DID since the nineteenth century (Binet, 1890/1977b). There is irrefutable evidence that features of DID can be created in experimental subjects (Estabrooks, 1971; Harriman, 1942a, 1942b, 1943; Kampman, 1976; Leavitt, 1947; Spanos, Weekes, & Bertrand, 1985; Spanos et al., 1986). This fact is established beyond doubt, and is an important facet of the understanding of DID. The question is, what is the significance of these experiments?

First, one must understand that none of these experiments result in the creation of trauma pathway DID. DID is not a transient phenomenon existing only in cross-section. Nor does it exist in isolation from a wide range of signs and symptoms that accompany it. There is no doubt that one can get college students to act as if they have alter personalities quite easily. But these students don't have a history of childhood abuse, numerous psychiatric symptoms, extensive involvement with the mental health system with limited benefit, and specific primary and secondary features of DID stretching back for decades (see Chapter Six). None of the experiments with normal college students have resulted in the creation of anything even remotely approaching full clinical DID.

Imagine that there was a controversy about the iatrogenesis of osteoarthritis. Imagine that Spanos took a group of normal college students and, in an experimental setting, got them to limp and complain of hip pain. Would that prove, or even suggest, that osteoarthritis is an artifact of the doctor-patient relationship? Obviously not. But Spanos is arguing, by analogy, that because he can get college students to limp, patients who are diagnosed by doctors as having osteoarthritis are manifesting an artifact created by the doctor's questions, expectations, and rewarding of the patient for having artifactual osteoarthritis by prescribing medications, physiotherapy with attractive young women, home support, disability pension, and further appointments.

There is a catch. Osteoarthritis can be demonstrated on X-ray. We don't have the equivalent of an X-ray for any psychiatric disorder, other than a few specific intoxication states or organic brain syndromes. Lack of a DID "X-ray" does not explain why DID is singled out among all psychiatric disorders for the charge of iatrogenic artifact. Why not borderline personality disorder or panic disorder? Because of ideology and bias, not because of data or science.

Compare DID with panic disorder, for example. Panic disorder was rarely diagnosed by psychiatrists 20 years ago, but now it is recognized to be common, has specific effective treatments, and is the subject of a great deal of research (Walker, Norton, & Ross, 1991). Few if any North American psychiatrists worry that panic disorder is artifactual. It is a clinical commonplace that coming to the doctor's office for appointments often causes the patient to panic. Some patients are so housebound that home visits are necessary.

Does anyone argue that because panic patients get anxious coming for their appointments, the disorder is artifactual? The treatment for panic involves exposure, a procedure deliberately designed to evoke symptoms. In the initial stages of treatment, the patient may have more anxiety due to the exposure exercises than she had while avoiding the supermarket before treatment. This increase in symptoms is an unavoidable consequence of exposure treatments for panic. The increase in panic symptoms that can occur as a by-product of treatment has never been used to argue against the validity of either the diagnosis or treatment.

The same logic should apply to DID. In treatment, as the patient is exposed to her traumatic memories, which had been hidden behind amnesia barriers, dissociative symptoms transiently increase. Since DID is a more complex and severe disorder than panic disorder, the increased symptoms have longer duration and greater complexity. The DID patient has been using dissociation to avoid an internal phobic stimulus (the abuse memories), whereas the panic patient has been using restriction of her physical movement to avoid an external stimulus. Any increase in symptoms during the initial stages of treatment is a perfectly comprehensible consequence of the disorder, for both panic disorder and DID.

Now let me compare DID with paranoid schizophrenia. A paranoid schizophrenic comes to emergency complaining that the FBI and his mother have been conspiring since his birth to control his thoughts. His mother, the patient says, signed a consent to have a device implanted in his brain at age two days. The FBI uses this device to control his thoughts and actions because they know that he has state secrets to give to the KGB, and they are trying to prevent him from completing his education. The FBI is afraid that if he completes his education, he may be able to move to Russia.

The patient is admitted. Two weeks later, he has incorporated the psychiatric staff into his delusional system. The patient now states that all the rooms on the ward are bugged by the FBI, that the nurse is actually his mother who has undergone plastic surgery, the doctor is an FBI agent, and the medication is a substance given to reprogram the device in his brain. Does it make sense to blame the doctor for the schizophrenia, or for the inclusion of the staff in the patient's delusional system? No. It is the nature of the patient's disorder that anyone in contact with him becomes incorporated into his delusional system. The same logic should apply to DID.

When paranoid schizophrenics see psychiatrists, they may create delusions about the psychiatrist. Panic patients may get anxious coming to see their doctors. DID patients may display more dissociative symptoms. In each case, this is a comprehensible consequence of the patient's disorder. There is no sound reason to classify DID as more iatrogenic than other psychiatric disorders based on experiments with college students, or an increase in dissociative symptoms in the early phases of treatment. As I will discuss in Chapter Six, much of the increase in dissociative symptoms during the early and middle phases of treatment is probably due to the uncovering of preexisting alters, rather than the creation of new ones in treatment. In this case, the analogy is with exploratory surgery that identifies unsuspected metastases in a cancer patient.

It would be bad medicine for the paranoid schizophrenic's psychiatrist to introduce himself as an FBI agent. It would be bad practice to prescribe exposure for agoraphobia if there was no benefit to the patient. Likewise in DID, the practitioner must be careful not to amplify the patient's symptoms unnecessarily and must be aware of potential secondary gains the patient may get from displaying symptoms. The treatment needs to be structured to control and minimize artifactual amplification of the illness. As I said earlier, however, this does not imply that all cases of DID are artifactual, any more than sciatica is invalidated as a diagnosis by fraudulent compensation cases.

The experiments on creation of analogs of isolated features of DID are valuable for a number of reasons. Rather than undermining the status of DID as a legitimate psychiatric disorder, these experiments help us to understand the iatrogenic pathway to DID. DID is often thought to be an extravagant deviation from normal experience, a rare curiosity with little connection to everyday psychology or reality. Probably the main reason it has been considered to be rare is the perception of DID as fantastic and improbable. Experiments by Spanos and others previously cited help to correct this misperception, and lead to a different guess as to how common the disorder is in North America.

The ability to create analogs of alter personalities is a capacity of the normal mind. Many college students can easily create such analogs when the right demands are made of them by a psychology professor. One thing it is important to recognize is that these experiments involve intensive signaling and shaping by the experimenters. Besides the possibility of course credit, approval for providing data the experimenter can publish, the enjoyment of playacting DID, and self-approval for participating in science, there were numerous instructions to behave in an unusual way. The environment of the experiments was highly structured to elicit certain behaviors, and these behaviors were reinforced in many ways.

What does that tell us about DID? It tells us that normal people can easily create alter personalities in the right environment. The ability to create alters, as I see it, is a specialized development of the normal ability to become intensely involved in childhood play, books, or movies. Creating imaginary identities is a normal aspect of child development, as any parent knows. DID patients have drawn on this ability demonstrated in normal childhood play, in Spanos's experiments, and in G. H. Estabrooks's military work, to cope with trauma. What better way to survive incestuous abuse than to imagine that it is happening to someone else?

It is an ability of the normal highly hypnotizable mind to be able to erect amnesia barriers. The DID patient has used this ability to create amnesia barriers between her imaginary "people." As the abuse goes on year after year, the amnesia and the illusion that the alters are really different people are reinforced and entrenched. What is surprising or difficult to understand about this process? In my view, DID is a commonsense disorder that draws on capacities of the normal mind. The evidence that iatrogenesis theorists draw on to invalidate DID, actually points to its essential nature, and helps us to understand why DID is treatable.

If "DID" patients created in Spanos-like experiments and actual abuse-pathway DID patients were interviewed by me under blind conditions, I could assign them to their two respective groups with 100% accuracy after diagnostic interviews lasting less than five minutes.

DID is not a fantastic curiosity in which there is more than one person in the same body. There is only one person, an abuse victim who has imagined that there are other people inside her in order to survive. This is an adaptive use of the human imagination which, at least in its rudiments, appears to be available to a large segment of the population. Since childhood sexual and physical abuse are common, and the ability to create alters is common, DID should be far from rare, in both its full classical form and in partial forms.

I think that DID is singled out for the accusation of iatrogenic artifact because of the link between DID and childhood physical and sexual abuse. Not long ago, incest was thought to be as rare in North America as one in a million families (Weinberg, 1955). We now know that that estimate was out by four orders of magnitude. Memories of childhood incest are still assumed to be fantasies by many North American psychiatrists, however. It is not surprising, in this social and ideological context, that DID is singled out for dismissal as an iatrogenic artifact. The charge of artifact, when massively overextended, is a defense against dealing with the reality of childhood abuse in North America. We have a popular superstition in North America that our children are our most valued resource and that the intact nuclear family is a good place to grow up. For many children this is a lie. The intact family, for many North American children, has been a war zone of physical and sexual abuse, a private Vietnam. It is not acceptable to dismiss the psychic scars and amputations resulting from this childhood trauma as artifact.

Properly understood and used, the experiments about creation of analogs of DID are important and valuable. They point to social factors in the creation and maintenance of DID that tend to be underemphasized by therapists. They provide a reminder of the need for careful diagnostic assessment, and monitoring of the effects of treatment interventions. There is no doubt that treatments can go wrong, and that patient and therapist can get stuck, with harmful amplification of dissociative symptoms. The same applies to bad surgical technique, which can make cancer spread more rapidly or an aneurysm rupture prematurely.

We have gathered data that argue against the theory that DID is primarily an iatrogenic artifact. In a series of 236 cases (Ross, Norton, & Fraser, 1989), we identified 44 cases reported by 40 Canadian psychiatrists, and 48 cases reported by 44 American psychiatrists. The Canadian psychiatrists were generalists who had seen an average of 2.2 cases of DID, while the Americans were subspecialist members of the ISSMP&D who had seen an average of 16.0 cases of DID.

We then went on to gather data on 22 of my cases and 23 cases seen by George Fraser, another Canadian psychiatrist specializing in DID (Ross & Fraser, 1987). This resulted in four groups of DID cases, two seen by single Canadian psychiatrists specializing in DID, one seen by 44 different American psychiatrists specializing in DID, and one seen by 40 Canadian general psychiatrists. The data on my and George Fraser's cases were gathered by research assistants blind to the results in the series of 236 cases, as described in the paper reporting these data (Ross, Norton, & Fraser, 1989).

We reasoned that if DID is an iatrogenic artifact, the following would be observed:

1. Cases seen by Canadian general psychiatrists will have fewer personalities.
2. Cases seen by Canadian general psychiatrists will not differ in features of DID known to the general public. These will include histories of physical and sexual abuse.
3. Cases seen by Canadian general psychiatrists will have fewer features known only to specialists, because only specialists will cue their patients to report these features. These will include a history of numerous previous psychiatric diagnoses.
4. Cases seen by Canadian psychiatrists will have been in the mental health system longer prior to diagnosis, because the Canadians will not be so quick to create DID in their patients.
5. If hypnosis is one means by which the iatrogenic artifact of DID is created, specialists will have used hypnosis more both before and after diagnosis.
6. The patients reported by DID specialists will meet the NIMH diagnostic criteria more often, because specialists are more familiar with these criteria, and more likely to cue their patients to report them.

7. The DID specialists will report DID as occurring more frequently in the first-degree relatives of their patients, compared with the frequency of DID in the first-degree relatives of patients diagnosed by Canadian general psychiatrists.

The data refuted all these predictions of the iatrogenic theory. The four groups did not differ in age, sex, marital status, or number of children. There were no differences between the four groups in the percentages that met each of the five NIMH diagnostic criteria for DID, the number of personalities at the time of diagnosis, or the number of personalities at the time of reporting. Of the four groups, it was the Canadian psychiatrists who diagnosed DID in first-degree relatives most frequently, and this difference was statistically significant. The fact that the specialists in DID diagnosed less DID in first-degree relatives suggests that they are not diagnostically "trigger-happy." Nor do they influence patients to act as if they have DID in an indiscriminate fashion.

An important finding of the study was that there was wide variation between the groups in the use of hypnosis, at statistically significant levels. The data showed that wide variations in the use of hypnosis do not produce differences in the specific features of DID. This is important to establish because DID is widely thought to be an artifact of hypnosis. The creation of DID through hypnosis is a corollary of the general theory of iatrogenesis.

Although the study with Fraser provided strong evidence against the iatrogenesis of DID, we wanted to examine the effects of hypnosis on the clinical features of cases in the overall series of 236 cases. We found that information on the use of hypnosis was provided by the respondents for 214 cases. Of these, 176 (82.2%) had been hypnotized. This meant that 17.8% had never been hypnotized. Of the 176 cases that had been hypnotized, 85 (48.3%) had been hypnotized only after diagnosis, whereas 56 (31.8%) had been hypnotized both before and after diagnosis. If hypnosis has an effect on the clinical features of DID, comparison of these three groups (never hypnotized, hypnotized only after diagnosis, hypnotized both before and after diagnosis) would demonstrate it. The statistical power of the analysis was sufficient for quite small differences between groups to be significant at $p < .05$.

The results showed no differences between the three groups on frequencies with which cases met each of the five NIMH diagnostic criteria for DID, the number of personalities identified at diagnosis, or the number of personalities identified at the time of reporting (Ross & Norton, 1989c). DID patients who are hypnotized before and/or after diagnosis are no different from those who have never been hypnotized, at least not in the specific features of DID. The three groups did not differ in age, sex, marital status, or number of children. These data argue against the hypothesis that DID is exclusively an artifact of hypnosis, or that its features are influenced by hypnosis. Taken together, these two studies provide evidence that DID is not solely an iatrogenic artifact. Although there are methodological limitations to the research, as for any questionnaire study, the questionnaire method is as likely to amplify observer bias, making it easier to detect, as to conceal it. Therefore reservations about the unreliability of the diagnoses actually make the data stronger, because such unreliability would be expected to result in greater variation between cases than actually exists, or to magnify idiosyncrasies of the respondents.

These two studies provide the only empirical evidence on the iatrogenesis of DID available to date. Anyone who wishes to establish that all cases of DID follow the iatrogenic pathway must provide very strong data on clinical DID to overcome our evidence against iatrogenesis. The main problem with the iatrogenic theory is that it is founded on the classical cognitive error of dichotomization, or all-or-nothing thinking. In reality, DID is far too complex a phenomenon to be entirely noniatrogenic, or purely artifactual.

Discussion and research should focus on the role of demand characteristics, secondary gain, and the ideology of the diagnostician, on the presentation and treatment of DID, without making dichotomous assumptions or overgeneralizing the results of studies of normal college students. Otherwise, an unproductive and polarized confrontation ensues, accompanied by behind-the-scenes political machinations to have the "enemy" discredited, or at least not published.

PSYCHOANALYTIC MODELS OF DISSOCIATIVE IDENTITY DISORDER

I am not an advocate of purely psychoanalytic models of DID for several reasons:

1. Such models cannot be tested, or even modified by data.
2. They are too closely linked to Freud's repudiation of the seduction theory.
3. They overemphasize the Oedipus complex, and underemphasize the Osiris complex.
4. They reify a semantic distinction between splitting and dissociation.
5. Only a tiny proportion of DID patients could make use of classical analysis.
6. DID occurs in a systemic context, and cannot be adequately understood by an exclusively intrapsychic school of thought.
7. The vocabulary of psychoanalytic theory is obscurantist.
8. Psychoanalytic theory has too many tautological qualities, which make it difficult to integrate with other schools of thought.

Instead of discussing classical psychoanalytic theories of DID, I will do what I do in practice, which is to blend certain Freudian ideas into my thinking throughout. For example, practitioners need to be aware of transference and countertransference in the treatment of DID. This doesn't mean that a classical analysis of transference is required. DID therapy, in my hands, involves long short-term dynamic psychotherapy. By this, I mean that the treatment resembles the active short-term dynamic psychotherapies in style, more than classical analysis, but it takes a few years.

Analytical papers on DID, for the interested reader, include ones by Clary, Burstin, and Carpenter (1984); Ganaway (1995); Gruenewald (1977, 1984); Lasky (1978); Marmer (1980); and Wilbur (1986). This is an incomplete list. Since Richard Kluft and Cornelia Wilbur have both advocated the psychoanalysis of selected cases of DID, and the use of psychoanalytic principles in all cases, and since I respect these two DID specialists, there is probably more apparent than real difference between the approach defined in this book and psychoanalytical treatment of DID. Probably the differences are more important in the written theory and would be less visible in videotapes of therapy sessions.

DISSOCIATIVE IDENTITY DISORDER AS AUTOHYPNOSIS

There is a strong connection between DID and hypnosis, in etiology, phenomenology, and treatment (Carlson & Putnam, 1989). Clinical experience and research evidence to date support the belief that DID patients are highly hypnotizable. They frequently enter trance states, and Bliss has shown that they have high scores on standard scales of hypnotizability. Bliss's work appears in a series of papers; these papers are further developed in his book (Bliss, 1986). Since Eugene Bliss has done most of the work on the autohypnotic etiology of DID, I will refer to him.

The special issue of the *American Journal of Clinical Hypnosis* on DID in October 1983 contained a number of articles on hypnosis. Other papers by Braun (1984), Kline (1984), and Miller (1984) in the special issue of the *International Journal of Clinical and Experimental Hypnosis* on DID address the relationship between DID and hypnosis as well. Hypnosis is generally referred to throughout the DID literature, and is discussed at length by Ellenberger (1970), Hilgard (1977), and Carlson and Putnam (1989). These references will lead any interested reader into the literature.

Autohypnotic models of DID basically state that DID is created by self-hypnosis. The data in support of the model are the high hypnotizability scores of DID patients; the numerous phenomena of hypnosis displayed by DID patients; the usefulness of hypnosis in treatment; the ease with which transient analogs of DID can be created in normal subjects using hypnosis; the historical link between interest in hypnosis and interest in DID, which suggests the two are related; and the close relationship between DID and other disorders that seem to be autohypnotic in nature.

There is a major problem with the autohypnotic model of DID. It is basically tautological. As enunciated by Bliss, it takes the following logical form:

1. DID patients are good hypnotic subjects.
2. DID patients display phenomena of hypnosis.
3. All DID phenomena must be autohypnotic.
4. The etiology of DID must be autohypnotic.

This is equivalent to stating that pneumonia is caused by fever. Just because fever is a phenomenon of pneumonia doesn't mean it is the cause. Also, Bliss arbitrarily describes DID patients as entering trance when they switch from the presenting personality to any other personality. This is arbitrary, because it could just as easily be the presenting personality who is in trance, and other alters with more complete memories who are not.

Empirically, it will be difficult, if not impossible, to demonstrate whether DID is autohypnotic when it arises in childhood. If one discovers a child in whom DID is forming, it immediately becomes necessary to stop the abuse, which interrupts the natural experiment. Conceptually, as Kluft (1987a) has pointed out, it is possible that DID patients are born highly hypnotizable and that only people with high dissociative capacity can form DID in the face of severe trauma. On the other hand, DID patients may be born with an average dissociative ability, which is environmentally reinforced, whereas that of nonabused children is not. This seems possible because it is known that hypnotizability scores decline through childhood and adolescence in the overall population. As usual in nature versus nurture arguments, reality probably combines the two possibilities in ratios that vary from case to case.

In either event, it is tautological to label DID phenomena as autohypnotic, then classify DID as an autohypnotic disorder. Such a classification is an artifact of the initial labeling. The autohypnotic model is based on inferring etiology from phenomenology, a common error in psychiatry. A similar error is made by biological psychiatrists who assume that a positive dexamethasone suppression test implies that the patient's depression is a biomedical illness (Ross, 1986a; Ross & Pam, 1995).

The autohypnotic model of DID isn't really a model. It is more a comment that DID patients display many phenomena of hypnosis. In fact, the field lacks an adequate theory or model. Nevertheless, Bliss has done a great deal of original work. There is no doubt that dissociation and hypnosis are closely related in DID patients. From a medical school teaching point of view, DID patients are superb subjects for teaching medical students about hypnosis. A comprehensive model of DID needs to take into account much more than autohypnosis, however.

A final, and fatal, problem with the autohypnosis model is that the correlation's between scores on the Dissociative Experiences Scale and standardized measures of hypnotizability are quite weak in samples other than DID patients (Carlson & Putnam, 1989).

ROLE-PLAYING AND SOCIAL LEARNING MODELS

The idea that DID is an artifact of the doctor-patient relationship, based on role demands, cues by the doctor, mutual reinforcement of role performance by doctor and patient, and similar mechanisms, is most developed in the work of Spanos (Spanos, Weekes, & Bertrand, 1985; Spanos et al., 1986; Spanos, Burgess, & Burgess, 1995). I have discussed this model at length earlier in this chapter.

Role theory provides insight from a blind man examining a small portion of the total elephant. Such theories, models, and schools make valuable contributions, except that they tend to be grossly overextended by their advocates. This is especially the case for armchair-quarterback "explanations" of DID based on experiments with normal college students, conducted by professors who have never met a patient with DID. The findings from such studies should be generalized to DID patients with caution. As data relevant to the understanding of clinical DID, Spanos's work is equivalent to a small number of experiments with rats in a single laboratory. No matter how interesting, such rat data could never "explain" a complex, heterogeneous phenomenon like human cancer, or DID.

The real value of social role theory will be its contribution to our understanding of the interactions in abusive families, during the time that DID is forming in the children. The social cues, reinforcements, and role demands coming from the sexually abusive father, and the mother who does nothing, are important etiological factors. Spiegel (1986b) has written about the role of double binds in the creation of DID: His analysis points to a line of empirical research. Social psychologists should make detailed maps of the interactions in families of children with DID. Combined with a mapping of the cognitions that accompany these interactions (Ross & Gahan, 1988a), a data-based cognitive-social psychological treatment package could be developed.

In the meantime, in the absence of such studies, social role theorists have made a minor contribution to the understanding of clinical DID, other than the predominantly iatrogenic pathway cases.

NEUROLOGICAL CAUSES OF DISSOCIATIVE IDENTITY DISORDER

Since the time of Charcot in the nineteenth century, there has been a suspicion that DID might, at least in some cases, be a neurological disorder. It was thought that DID might be the psychological and behavioral manifestation of epileptic discharges in the temporal lobes. Since 1980, a number of reports have appeared in the literature describing small series of patients with concurrent DID and temporal lobe epilepsy (Benson, Miller, & Signer, 1986; Mesulam, 1981; Schenk & Bear, 1981). These cases were interpreted by the authors as suggesting that DID might be a form of seizure disorder. Another issue is whether DID might be an interictal disorder secondary to epilepsy (Benson, 1986).

In Chapter Eight, I will discuss the relationship between DID and temporal lobe epilepsy at length and will present data which demonstrate that DID and temporal lobe epilepsy are separate disorders with little phenomenological overlap.

A second possible neurological cause of DID that has been proposed is a disconnection of the left and right hemispheres (Benner & Evans, 1984). Sidtis (1986) has provided the definitive analysis of this possibility, and discounted it. The main problem with hemispheric disconnection theories is that they were devised to explain dual personality, but cannot possibly account for complex DID. In any case, it is hard to see how a neurologically caused disorder could be cured by psychotherapy. Dual personality, which is the form of DID that most lends itself to explanation by disconnection theories, is probably the easiest form of DID to treat with psychotherapy. This does not make sense if dual personality is the form of DID most likely to have a cause in the hardware of the brain.

There is no evidence that DID is a neurological disease. Conversely, there is substantial evidence that it is a psychosocial disorder. In a computer analogy, DID is a disorder of software, occurring in patients whose brain hardware is intact. Since structure and function are interwoven in a complex way in the human mind and brain, however, the computer analogy is a gross oversimplification. The physiological study of brain function in DID may yield important insights into mind-body interaction and the psychophysiology of trauma (Larmore, Ludwig, & Cain, 1977; Mathew, Jack, & West, 1985), and physiological techniques may prove to be useful in the study of DID (Loewenstein, Hamilton, Alagna, Reid, & de Vries, 1987). None of these will imply that the etiology of DID is endogenous and biological, though. That is all there is to say about neurological models of DID.

THE FEMINIST ANALYSIS OF DISSOCIATIVE IDENTITY DISORDER

When I speak of the feminist analysis of DID, I am referring to the writing of Margo Rivera (1987, 1988, 1989, 1991), who has done extensive work on this aspect of the disorder. Chapters by Ellen Borges (1995) and David Sackheim and Susan Devine (1995) in my book *Pseudoscience in Biological Psychiatry* (Ross & Pam, 1995) are also directly relevant. As pointed out by Rivera, DID occurs in a broad social context that includes the division of power between the sexes, sex role socialization of men and women in North America, and institutionalized sexual exploitation of women and children. It is an error to view the sexual abuse of children as an isolated phenomenon. Such abuse, according to the feminist analysis (Rush, 1980), is an extreme expression of the patriarchal power structure that dominates our society.

Women are sexually exploited in advertising, films, locker room jokes, the workplace, the home, and the massage parlor (a short list) in North America. Sexual abuse of girls by men is the earliest and most extreme aspect of the socialization of women into subservient roles. The patriarchal role for women, at least in our society, is a combination of sex object, property, doormat, and punching bag. DID, then, is caused primarily by a sick social structure. The sexually abusive father is an embodiment of patriarchal corruption. Although officially abhorred, his behavior is consistent with societal norms. That is why incest and child pornography are so widespread: They are inevitable consequences of the power structure.

There is a lot of truth in this analysis. There are also some problems. Although girls are abused more often than boys in our society, boys too are victims of a billion-dollar pornography industry, homosexual prostitution, physical abuse by their fathers, and pathological socialization. Their development is warped and scarred by perverted sexuality in North America.

The female:male ratio in clinical series of DID is 9:1 (Ross, Norton, & Wozney, 1989). However, many males with DID are probably in prison, or do not go to see doctors, so the ratio in the overall population is probably lower. As I will discuss in Chapter Six, there is no difference between DID in males and DID in females (Ross & Norton, 1989a). Males with DID have as much abuse, as many personalities, as many suicide attempts, and many other features in common with females.

A second problem with the feminist thesis is that many of the incestuous fathers probably have DID themselves. They are themselves victims of abuse by DID parents, both fathers and mothers. Over the next 10 years, we may gain insight into an extremely intricate multigenerational transmission of incest involving amnesia, abusive paternal alters having intercourse with alters in their children, and DID mothers amnesic for their own direct contributions to the cycle.

There is no doubt that orthodox psychiatry is mistaken if it resists the feminist analysis. In the future, the task for the feminists is to translate their theory into the gathering of scientific data. In the absence of such data, social and political action is still imperative, as the feminists insist (Rush, 1980).

HILGARD'S NEODISSOCIATION THEORY OF DIVIDED CONSCIOUSNESS

Hilgard (1977) has provided an extensive discussion of dissociation that places it in a broad and general context. He reviews the history, experimental data of his own and others, clinical cases, related literature, and theory. His book single handedly revived the serious study of dissociation. Hilgard reconnects us with the nineteenth century while taking into account modern discoveries about information processing (Andorfer, 1985), divided attention, and brain processing.

His focus is not on DID, however, and he does not appear to have seen a case himself. Hilgard does not provide us with a synthesized understanding of DID itself, rather he organizes a great deal of background information and allows us to see the disorder in the context of modern experimental psychology. His theory is called neodissociation theory partly because it takes nineteenth-century understanding into account without making an ideological commitment to any one of the nineteenth-century schools.

One of the most helpful ideas in the book for a clinician treating DID is Hilgard's distinction between vertical and horizontal splitting. Vertical splitting results in dissociation, while horizontal splitting results in repression, as shown in Figure 3.1. In my view, splitting and dissociation are synonyms. I believe that repression is a form of dissociation (Jorn, 1982), dissociation being a general term. It isn't essential which terms are used in which way, but we need to arrive at consistent use of terms in the field.

Following a vertical split, psychic material is pushed to the side, or to the back of the mind. The dissociated material is not "unconscious," however, it is merely dissociated. It is available for direct transaction with the external world. This is very different from unconscious, repressed material, which can only be recovered using "deep" techniques. DID teaches us that dissociated material, in the form of alter personalities, can be rational, organized, and coherent. Contacting the material hidden behind a vertical split is usually fairly easy from a technical point of view.

The "depth" psychology's and psychotherapies are based on an assumption that horizontal splitting is the more important defense. This is repression in Freud's sense. DID teaches us that much of what was thought to be repressed id material, governed by primary process and available only using free association, or dream analysis, is in fact not far away, and is easy

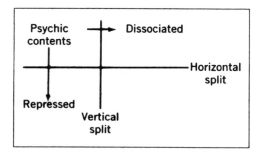

Figure 3.1. Vertical and Horizontal Splitting

to get at. Much of what was thought to be the unconscious is actually dissociated ego. In this sense, DID teaches us that the unconscious is not unconscious. Hilgard's diagram helps us to understand this, and connects us back
to Estabrooks, Myers, Binet, and Janet.

An example will clarify what I mean. A patient presents with a conversion paralysis of the left arm. If this is due to an unconscious conflict hidden behind a horizontal split, understanding why the patient's arm can't
move will require deep exploration of the unconscious. Considerable time
and a great deal of complicated, untestable theory will be required to analyze and treat the problem. If the cause of the paralysis is hidden behind a
vertical split, however, the clinician simply calls out the alter personality
who is causing the paralysis and asks the alter why she is doing that. The
clinician receives an explanation, negotiates a different solution to the
problem, and contracts for cure of the symptom. This may take a while if
the alter is hostile, but the process is one of rational negotiation and discussion. There is nothing deep or hidden.

Hilgard's book is important because it sets the treatment of DID in a
modern scientific context. I will discuss the difference between repression
and dissociation at greater length in Chapter Ten.

STATE-DEPENDENT AND STATE-OF-CONSCIOUSNESS MODELS OF DISSOCIATIVE IDENTITY DISORDER

The state-dependent line of thinking about DID has a number of important features. For one, it leads directly to experimental work on dissociation (Silberman, Putnam, Weingartner, Braun, & Post, 1985). It is linked to
a large empirical literature on mood and state-dependent learning, and it
has immediate implications for many other psychiatric disorders. For example, Putnam is interested in what the switching process in DID might
teach us about the onset of panic attacks, switches from depression to
mania in bipolar affective disorder, rapid changes of state in borderline
personality disorder, and a host of other phenomena (Putnam, 1988). These
models work against the view that DID is an isolated curiosity.

An intriguing aspect of Putnam's thinking is the observation that infants
switch rapidly from one state to another, and that their states tend to be
discontinuous. There is apparently a large literature on this aspect of normal development. It is possible that the switching of alters in DID draws on
this normal ability. DID may represent a trauma-driven developmental
delay in the maturation of the ability to integrate experience. If this is so,
DID may teach us something about normal child development.

It is possible to study DID using metaphors and principles from physics,
within the framework of state-dependent models. Physicists have studied
boundary phenomena extensively, and the transmission of signals across
boundaries. Their discoveries might shed light on the boundaries between

alters. In turn, physicists might learn something from DID. These models have no specific limitations because they are abstract and systemic.

Like DID patients, the field is greater than the sum of its parts. Although state-dependent theories and models are only one part of the field of dissociative studies, they are a potentially important part.

DESCRIPTIVE CLINICAL MODELS OF DISSOCIATIVE IDENTITY DISORDER

When descriptive clinical models of DID are called "descriptive clinical models," it seems to imply that they are low powered. Other models sound more prestigious and scientific. Actually, descriptive clinical models aren't even "models." They are clinical descriptions. There is a widespread misconception that to be worth anything, one's understanding must be puffed up into "a model." Since I am a clinician and have never done an experiment on dissociation, my contribution is a clinical one. I don't feel a strong need to erect a model. Clinical practice is the most important source of data, understanding, and treatment techniques: Clinical practice is the touchstone, the guide, and the focus.

It is important that the clinical treatment of DID be guided by science, data, and rigorous thought. But it is the treatment of patients that provides meaning and purpose for the science. Without patients who can benefit from treatment, the science becomes a hobby for academics who have no serious work to do in the world.

The best clinical formulations of the traumatic etiology of DID come from Richard Kluft (1984c) and Bennett Braun (1986a, 1986b; Braun & Sachs, 1985). Obviously, these two men have not worked in isolation, and have borrowed a great deal from others. Braun and Sachs propose a 3-P model of DID derived from the standard predisposing, perpetuating, and precipitating factors used in clinical psychiatry. Kluft has proposed a four-factor theory of DID.

Both these clinical accounts of the etiology of DID emphasize two points:

1. Patients with DID are extremely good at dissociation.
2. Patients with DID have used dissociation to cope with severe childhood trauma.

In a nutshell, that is all that needs to be said about the etiology of childhood trauma pathway DID. Since this is a book, not a nutshell, I will say a bit more.

I will refer only to Kluft's four-factor theory because it encompasses the 3-P model of Braun and Sachs. Although Kluft lists a number of examples illustrating each of the four factors in his theory, these are really only lists and have not been woven together into what could properly be called a theory. The first two factors are the two items already stated—dissociative ability and trauma.

The third factor in the etiology of DID is "shaping influences and substrates that determine the form taken by the dissociative defense." Kluft lists, among other things, multiple systems of cognition and memory, libidinal developmental lines, and imaginary companionship as relevant to this factor. Actually integrating all of these into a theory, rather than simply listing them, would be a major intellectual feat (the contents of the list should be modified because there is an unintended pun on "multiple"). Kluft's fourth factor is "inadequate provision of stimulus barriers and restorative experiences by significant others, for example, insufficient 'soothing.'"

Restated, the third and fourth factors in the etiology of DID are:

3. The form and structure of DID vary depending on the person's temperament and nonabuse experience.
4. The abuse didn't stop, and the victim did not receive enough consistent love and care to heal her wounds.

The third factor encompasses social and cultural factors that contribute to the creation of DID. The fourth factor points to the power of the reinforcers for dissociation, and the huge number of times they were applied throughout childhood and adolescence, in complex cases of DID.

The clinical descriptive model of DID is the best one. It was arrived at by therapists who had spent thousands of hours working directly with DID patients. The model is simple, and that is one of its best properties. As a general outline it accounts for all the major features of childhood-onset DID, provides a rationale for treatment, and is consistent with the response to treatment. Confirmation of the model is given by alter personalities in response to open-ended questions: The alters state the four factors directly to the therapist, in response to questions such as "Why were you created?"

CONCLUSION

What is DID? DID is a little girl imagining that the abuse is happening to someone else. Since the human mind and human culture are complicated, the disorder is not a simple one. We should not lose sight of the basic simplicity of this etiological model of DID, nor should we cloak it in too much jargon or fancy language.

A great deal of data support the descriptive clinical model of DID. Rather than reviewing it here as evidence in support of the model, I will discuss the abuse histories and other features of DID patients in detail in Chapter Six. A comprehensive account of the etiology of DID must take into account all the schools, viewpoints, and pathways I have outlined in this chapter. It isn't necessary to produce a complicated diagram with arrows and boxes, showing supposed relationships between all of these; as more data accumulate, everything will fall into place. For now all that is required is an acknowledgment that DID is a complex biopsychosocial disorder with numerous determinants. DID is a strategy for surviving a traumatic childhood. It can also be factitious or an artifact of bad therapy.

In the absence of adequate data, dogmatic opinions about the frequency of the four pathways to DID among diagnosed cases are meaningless.

Diagnostic Criteria for Dissociative Identity Disorder

Until 1980, dissociative identity disorder (DID) did not have defined diagnostic criteria. With the publication of the third edition of the *Diagnostic and Statistical Manual of Mental Disorders* (*DSM-III*; American Psychiatric Association, 1980), the disorder first attained official recognition as a legitimate psychiatric entity. This was an important political event, and undoubtedly contributed to the exponential increase in the diagnosis of DID in North America in the 1980s. Outside North America, where *DSM-IV* is used less, DID is still rarely diagnosed. My sense of the situation is that DID is still underdiagnosed even in North America, despite the problem of false positive diagnoses and iatrogenic pathway cases.

In this chapter, I am going to review the *DSM-IV* (American Psychiatric Association, 1994a) criteria for DID. As well, I will discuss the status of DID in *ICD-10* (World Health Organization, 1992). Also, I will discuss DID in the context of a spectrum of dissociative disorders, a concept not adequately elaborated in *DSM-III, DSM-III-R,* or *DSM-IV* (Ross, 1985). In Chapter Eight, I will set the dissociative disorders in a broader context of what I call trauma disorders and propose a revised classification. First, though, some discussion of the function of diagnostic criteria is required.

THE FUNCTION OF DIAGNOSTIC CRITERIA AND THE ORGANIZATION OF *DSM-IV*

The function of diagnostic criteria might seem obvious: It is to define illnesses in a valid and reliable way, in order to guide treatment and provide a prognosis. The first problem is that few disorders in *DSM-IV* are biomedical illnesses. Some have no known effective treatment, and for many the natural history and prognosis are uncertain. The disorders in *DSM-IV* vary widely in presumed etiology and treatment. Alcohol withdrawal has a single specific cause, while bulimia probably has numerous contributing causes that vary widely from patient to patient. The management of alcohol withdrawal probably does not vary much throughout North America, whereas bulimia might be treated with antidepressants, short-term cognitive therapy, psychoanalysis, self-help groups, or any one of numerous different approaches. The natural history of alcohol withdrawal is short-term resolution or death, whereas bulimia lasts for years in most cases.

According to *DSM-IV*, mental retardation, premature ejaculation, schizophrenia, narcissistic personality disorder, and stuttering are all "mental disorders." No category can meaningfully encompass so many disparate phenomena, and no organizational rules can adequately account for all of them. In fact, *DSM-IV* has many different principles of organization within its different sections, as did *DSM-III* (Ross, 1985). To understand the diagnostic status of DID, it is necessary to have some idea of how *DSM-IV* is organized. It is also important to realize that *DSM-IV* is a resting point en route to *DSM-V* and later destinations.

DSM-IV is organized into a number of major sections that bear no stated logical relation to each other. These include substance-related disorders, schizophrenia and other psychotic disorders, mood disorders, anxiety disorders, and personality disorders. The dissociative disorders have a section of their own. Within each of these sections, there are a number of diagnoses that may or may not have a specified relationship to each other.

The principles of organization of the different sections of *DSM-IV*, and even different diagnoses within one section, vary widely. The concept of a continuum is a frequently used organizing principle, of which I will give some examples.

Schizophrenia

DSM-IV takes into account that psychoses must be diagnosed on a "temporal continuum." This continuum has therapeutic and prognostic implications, and it impels the clinician to be more careful in diagnosing schizophrenia (its purpose is to reduce premature false positive diagnoses of schizophrenia). A schizophrenia-like illness lasting more than one day but less than month is called a brief psychotic disorder. If a patient has a schizophrenia-like illness for more than one month but less than six months, the diagnosis is schizophreniform disorder. After six months, the diagnosis is schizophrenia.

Depression

A somewhat analogous temporal continuum is combined with a poorly operationalized "continuum of severity" in the *DSM-IV* diagnosis of depressions. Here the analog of brief psychotic disorder is adjustment disorder with depressed mood (there is no adjustment disorder with psychotic features). On a continuum of severity, there are different diagnoses for depression: adjustment disorder with depressed mood; dysthymic disorder; major depressive disorder (MDD), mild; and MDD, severe with mood-incongruent psychotic features, which represents the severe end of the continuum.

Bipolar Mood Disorder

Here an organizing principle is "polarity of symptoms," resulting in a diagnosis of bipolar mood disorder, subtyped as most recent episode mixed, manic, or depressed. Additionally, a continuum of severity results in bipolar mood disorder being divided into hypomanic (Type II) and manic (Type I) subtypes.

Phobic Disorders

In the anxiety disorders, there is a continuum of severity based on the number of stimuli that generate a phobic response. This is in effect a "continuum of pervasiveness of pathological response." At one end of the continuum lies the specific phobia. In the middle lies social phobia, in which numerous situations sharing a common social element provoke a phobic response. When the phobic response is generalized to the largest number of stimuli, the most severe diagnosis—panic disorder with agoraphobia—is made.

Pervasive Developmental Disorders

The pervasive developmental disorders of childhood are diagnosed according to age of onset, with prognosis thought to improve with later onset. This is a "continuum of age of onset." In *DSM-IV,* Rett's disorder has an onset between 5 and 30 months, autistic disorder has an onset before the age of 3 years, while childhood disintegrative disorder begins before age 10.

Mental Retardation

Mental retardation may be diagnosed as mild, moderate, severe, or profound according to the IQ. This particular form of continuum is worth noting because it is the only *DSM-IV* diagnostic continuum that is based on valid and reliable psychological testing. It is a "continuum of test scores."

Alcohol Intoxication and Withdrawal

Withdrawal from alcohol or any other substance of abuse or addiction must be preceded by long-term use, and the two diagnoses follow each other according to a "continuum of physiological response," in which the withdrawal state is preceded by the intoxication. A physiological continuum exists for sexual dysfunctions also, in which arrest at any one stage causes inhibition of the following stages. In *DSM-IV*, the stages are called hypoactive sexual disorder, female sexual arousal disorder or male erectile disorder, and female orgasmic disorder or male orgasmic disorder.

Delusional Disorders

In the schizophrenia and other psychotic disorders section, *DSM-IV* gives recognition to the possibility of "contagion of symptoms" as a way to conceptually relate two diagnoses: delusional disorder and shared psychotic disorder. This is one of the few areas of *DSM-IV* where a systems approach is implied, and with it a "gradient of psychopathology" from the primary partner to the less severely disturbed and secondarily involved partner.

Personality Disorders

DSM-IV recognizes that the personality disorders are not a randomly assorted group of independent entities. They fall into three clusters: (a) paranoid, schizoid, schizotypal; (b) histrionic, narcissistic, borderline, antisocial; and (c) avoidant, dependent, obsessive-compulsive. The principle inherent in this grouping of personality disorders is an overlapping sets or "Venn diagram" system of organizing a diagnostic section of *DSM-IV*.

There are numerous principles of organization within the different sections of *DSM-IV*. How are the dissociative disorders organized? The answer is that they aren't. The dissociative disorders are simply listed in *DSM-IV*, without a statement as to how they are related to each other.

Any one of many possible principles of organization could, in theory, bring conceptual order to the dissociative disorders section of *DSM-IV*. Bennett Braun (1986a, 1988a) and I (Ross, 1985) have proposed independently that the dissociative disorders be organized on a continuum of increasing severity, with DID at the far end. I have not heard a specialist in dissociative disorders object to this scheme. I have concluded since 1985, based on research data and clinical experience, that DID should be reclassified in the context of trauma disorders (see Chapter Eight). Within the trauma disorders, however, the relationship of the different dissociative disorders remains the same as that proposed by Braun and myself. In this chapter, I will discuss only the dissociative disorders, without setting in them in the larger context.

DISSOCIATIVE DISORDERS ON A CONTINUUM OF INCREASING SEVERITY AND COMPLEXITY

The dissociative disorders could be classified on a continuum of increasingly large amounts of psychic material dissociated. This is a simple organizational principle that fits with clinical experience. There is insufficient research evidence to date to support or refute this or any other organizational principle for the dissociative disorders. We have to go with what seems to make sense.

The simplest dissociative phenomenon is a normal dissociative state such as absorption in a movie. The simplest dissociative *disorder* is dissociative amnesia. Dissociative amnesia is defined in *DSM-IV* as "one or more episodes of inability to recall important personal information, usually of a traumatic or stressful nature, that is too extensive to be explained by ordinary forgetfulness." The disorder cannot be due to a known organic cause, such as blackouts during alcohol intoxication (I will propose that alcohol blackouts are often actually psychogenic dissociative phenomena, and not necessarily organic in nature, in Chapter Eight), or better understood as part of another disorder. DID is an exclusion criterion for the diagnosis of dissociative amnesia disorder. In other words, if one has DID, one cannot also have dissociative amnesia, since such amnesia is a facet of the more complex dissociative disorder.

Moving further along the spectrum, as illustrated in Figure 4.1, one encounters dissociative fugue and dissociative disorder not otherwise specified (DDNOS). DDNOS currently encompasses partial forms of DID which in fact are not at all atypical, and are probably more common than

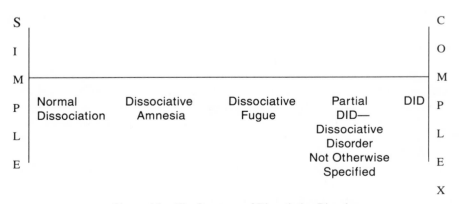

Figure 4.1.   The Spectrum of Dissociative Disorders

full DID. Fugue and partial DID are more complex dissociative disorders than simple amnesia, and therefore are placed further out the spectrum. The best reviews of dissociative amnesia and fugue are by Coons (1992) and Loewenstein (1993a, 1993b).

Depersonalization disorder is the only diagnosis in the Dissociative Disorders Interview Schedule with a low interrater reliability ($r = .56$). It is the only dissociative disorder that does not occur more frequently in DID than in panic disorder or eating disorders (Ross et al., 1989a). Further, it is the only dissociative disorder that occurs more commonly in partial complex seizures than in controls (Ross et al., 1989b). The best review of depersonalization disorder is by Steinberg (1994). It may occur as a feature of DID, in complex partial seizures, as a limited symptom panic attack, or as a feature of other psychiatric disorders. I won't discuss depersonalization disorder further.

At the extreme end of the continuum is DID. DID is not subtyped in *DSM-IV,* but clinical experience indicates that it could be divided into at least four pathways, as reviewed in the previous chapter. It appears that the simpler forms of DID are probably associated with less severe trauma, and are easier to treat, but data are lacking. Kluft (1991a) has offered a clinical typology of different subtypes of DID that needs to be investigated systematically.

Even in complex DID, there are usually not more than seven or eight major personalities that have handled the bulk of the life experience, and do most of the work in therapy. Then there tend to be a number of fragments with each of which the therapist may spend minutes or a few hours throughout the therapy. Braun (1986a) proposes that fragments be subtyped as special purpose fragments and memory trace fragments, but I don't see the clinical utility of these differentiations. In complex DID, the therapist will usually contact most or all of the major named alters and fragments at least once, even if only for a brief conversation prior to an integration ritual.

In polyfragmented DID, there may be hundreds of states with separate names and ages. It is logistically impossible and therapeutically unnecessary to contact all these states directly, although the patient may have them all recorded in a chart. Patients with polyfragmented DID have taken the process of dissociation to its extreme. Hundreds of experiences are split into separate pieces and given names and ages. When there are hundreds of fragments, the process may not be the same as the formation of alters: The person may name memories in a "labeling" manner, without dissociation as such occurring. It is important not to fall victim to the illusion that there are "hundreds of personalities inside one person" in such cases. Such claims discredit DID as a serious disorder, and stretch the meaning of the word "personality" far beyond any meaningful limit. There is no sound reason for subtyping DID according to characteristics and number of alter personalities. My clinical experience tells me that polyfragmentation is often factitious or iatrogenic and may occur on a foundation of simpler DID, DDNOS, or no dissociative disorder at all.

What are the *DSM-IV* criteria for DID? There are four of them (American Psychiatric Association, 1994a):

A. The presence of two or more distinct identities or personality states (each with its own relatively enduring pattern of perceiving, relating to, and thinking about the environment and self).

B. At least two of these identities or personality states recurrently take control of the person's behavior.

C. Inability to recall important personal information that is too extensive to be explained by ordinary forgetfulness.

D. The disturbance is not due to the direct physiological effects of a substance (e.g., blackouts or chaotic behavior during Alcohol Intoxication) or a general medical condition (e.g., complex partial seizures). *Note:* In children, the symptoms are not attributable to imaginary playmates or other fantasy play.

One argument in favor of more elaborate diagnostic criteria is that DID is insufficiently operationalized and that the *DSM-IV* criteria will result in too many false positive diagnoses. This is an argument I advanced myself about the *DSM-III* criteria (Ross & Fraser, 1987). The argument applied even more to the *DSM-III-R* criteria, which were simplified from the three *DSM-III* criteria to two in number.

In our series of 236 cases (Ross, Norton, & Wozney, 1989), we excluded any cases reported to us that did not meet the first two of the five NIMH criteria proposed by Frank Putnam (personal communication, 1986), which are more rigorous than the *DSM-IV* criteria, so by definition all 236 cases met NIMH criteria A and B. For the remaining three NIMH criteria, 94.4% met criterion C, 95.7% met D, and 94.9% met E. What does that tell us? It means that, consistent with my own experience, most cases of DID meet all five NIMH research criteria. What would be the point of using all five criteria, then? There would be little point. By using more rigorous criteria, one would exclude only a small number of cases as false positives.

Because there were too few cases for statistical analysis in our series of 236 cases, our data did not tell us whether cases that did not meet criteria C, D, and E, were simpler cases, had experienced less trauma, were easier to treat, or differed in any other meaningful way. I will discuss the question of the vagueness of *DSM-IV* criteria for DID at greater length in Chapter Ten.

What data exist to support the concept of a continuum of dissociative disorders? Three studies by Boon and Draijer (1993), Coons (1992), and Ross, Anderson, Fraser, et al. (1992) compared DID and DDNOS cases, and in all three studies, DID patients had higher DES scores, displayed more dissociative symptomatology, and reported more comorbidity. The Boon and Draijer studies involved the SCID-D and my study the DDIS.

In my study (Ross, Anderson, Fraser, et al., 1992), 166 subjects with a clinical diagnosis of DID had an average DES score of 39.7 (*SD* 18.3), while 57 subjects with a clinical diagnosis of DDNOS had an average DES score of 21.7 (*SD* 17.0), (t(193) = 6.106, p < .00001). The DID subjects also reported more symptoms on all the major symptom clusters of the DDIS and more severe childhood trauma. The mere presence or absence of amnesia did not differentiate the two groups, but the degree and complexity of amnesia did. The existing evidence indicates that the *DSM-IV* amnesia criterion for DID do not differentiate DID from DDNOS by themselves. However, a discriminant function analysis using the subsections of the DDIS, resulted in the DDIS being able to correctly assign 91.4% of the DID subjects to the DID group. Much of the power of this discrimination came from the secondary features of the disorder, rather than from the diagnostic criteria alone.

SECONDARY FEATURES OF DISSOCIATIVE IDENTITY DISORDER

The primary diagnostic criteria for DID, which are the *DSM-IV* criteria, are straightforward, as they should be. Anyone can look them up. It is the secondary features of DID that are most valuable to the clinician, however. Usually, DID does not present in an obvious overt fashion. In most cases, patients will not walk into the office announcing that they have DID and spontaneously exhibiting named alters. Kluft (1985e) found that in a clinical series, 5% of cases presented as self-diagnosed but were generally disbelieved by their psychiatrists, 15% openly dissociated during assessment or treatment, 40% presented with signs that could alert a clinician with a high index of suspicion for DID, while 40% of cases were highly disguised and were discovered while he was testing a special diagnostic protocol.

DID often presents in a highly covert fashion even when the patient is being assessed by Richard Kluft, who has made a more detailed clinical analysis of more patients than anyone in the world. The longest I have personally worked with a patient before eventually contacting an alter personality is two years; this was a case of DDNOS, not DID, and the entity was not a *DSM-IV* identity state or alter personality (Ross, 1994b).

Clinicians who say that they have been in practice 10 or 20 years, and never seen a case of DID, are really saying that they have never seen a case that falls into Kluft's 5%, the self-diagnosed group. In my experience, clinicians who do not seriously consider DID in their differential diagnoses can observe florid dissociation without seeing it as a diagnostic clue for DID. They therefore do not pursue the diagnosis with detailed and specific inquiry, and never "see" cases.

During a period of a year (July 1, 1985–June 30, 1986), I diagnosed DID in 3 of 68 (4.4%) general adult inpatients assigned to me (Ross, 1987). These were cases that had come to emergency and been assigned to me on the ward. There was no strong selection bias, and my overall caseload was similar to that of any general inpatient psychiatrist in North America. Yet no other inpatient psychiatrists at my hospital made a diagnosis of DID during this period, out of a total of nearly 500 admissions. The three patients I diagnosed had between 1 and 13 previous admissions for borderline personality disorder under other psychiatrists.

All three patients had exhibited numerous secondary features of DID for years. Of the three, two have since been treated to integration. Does this mean that I was the only competent inpatient psychiatrist at my hospital? No. It means that I was the only psychiatrist who seriously considered DID in his differential diagnoses and made a specific inquiry for its signs and symptoms. If the other psychiatrists had done the same, they too would have diagnosed cases on a regular basis.

In a study done at St. Boniface Hospital in Winnipeg (Ross & Clark, 1992), my research nurse, Patti Clark, reviewed 774 written emergency room psychiatric consultations from July 1, 1985 through June 30, 1991. We found that in 96.1% of the written consultations, there was no comment on whether amnesia was present or absent in the case, indicating that this symptom is simply not asked about. Similarly, auditory hallucinations were not commented on in 61.2% of cases, suicidal ideation in 26.6%, and depressed mood in 29.3%. Additionally, there was no comment on whether there was or wasn't a reported history of childhood sexual abuse in 87.6% of cases, and of childhood physical abuse in 89.7% of cases.

Unless the secondary features of DID are inquired about routinely and systematically, cases of DID will be missed, as they were at my teaching hospital in Canada. I will discuss the secondary features of DID in detail in subsequent chapters.

DISSOCIATIVE IDENTITY DISORDER IN *ICD-10*

The dissociative disorders are handled very differently in *ICD-10* (World Health Organization, 1992), compared with *DSM-IV*. They are found in a general section entitled "Neurotic, stress-related and somatoform disorders," which includes seven subsections: phobic anxiety disorders; other anxiety disorders; obsessive-compulsive disorder; reaction to severe stress, and adjustment disorders; dissociative [conversion] disorders; somatoform disorders; and other neurotic disorders.

Overall, the *ICD-10* scheme for classifying dissociative disorders is more like the scheme I proposed in the first edition of this book than is the *DSM-IV* system (see Chapter Eight of this edition). In *ICD-10,* dissociation is considered to occur in all areas of the cortex, giving rise, in *ICD-10* vocabulary, to disorders of memory (dissociative amnesia), state of consciousness (dissociative stupor), motor function (dissociative motor disorders), sensation (dissociative anesthesia and sensory loss), and identity (multiple personality disorder). In *ICD-10*, dissociation and conversion are treated as synonyms, whereas in *DSM-IV* they belong to separate categories of mental illness.

In *DSM-IV*, dissociative disorders of memory are classified as dissociative disorders (dissociative amnesia), of state of consciousness as anxiety disorders (acute stress disorder), of motor function as somatoform disorders (conversion disorder), of sensation as somatoform disorders (undifferentiated somatoform disorder or pain disorder), and of identity as a dissociative disorder (DID). Obviously, both systems cannot be scientifically correct. The differences between *ICD-10* and *DSM-IV* are ideological and political, and are not based on definitive research data.

In *ICD-10*, DID is still called multiple personality disorder. More importantly, it is categorized as a subtype of "Other dissociative [conversion] disorders," along with Ganser's syndrome, transient dissociative (conversion) disorders occurring in childhood and adolescence, and other specified dissociative (conversion) disorders. In the text (p. 152), it is stated, "All types of dissociative state tend to remit after a few weeks or months, particularly if their onset was associated with a traumatic life event." The conceptualization of DID in *ICD-10* is radically different from that in *DSM-IV*: in *ICD-10*, DID is a transient form of conversion disorder that remits spontaneously in a short period. This is the position taken by many skeptics in North America and Europe. Stated in *DSM-IV* vocabulary, in *ICD-10*, DID is a form of DDNOS, whereas in *DSM-IV*, DID is an exclusion criterion for DDNOS.

These differences between *ICD-10* and *DSM-IV* illustrate that there is radical disagreement about the nosological status of DID throughout the world.

In subsequent chapters, I will review the relationship between dissociation and conversion, the relationship between dissociation and other mental disorders, the secondary features of DID, the difference between vertical and horizontal splitting, and subtypes of DID in more detail. The primary purpose of this chapter has been to present the *DSM-IV* criteria for DID and discuss some of the controversies about them.

Epidemiology of Dissociative Identity Disorder and Dissociation

A great deal has been learned about the epidemiology of dissociative identity disorder (DID) and dissociation in the past 10 years, but this area of study is still in its infancy. None of the research I will review in this chapter takes the four pathways to DID into account. The epidemiology of DID is at the core of the controversy about the disorder, as I will describe in Chapter Ten.

In this chapter, I will discuss of the epidemiology of dissociation in general then focus on DID. For discussion of the clinical literature on amnesia, depersonalization, and fugue, I refer the reader to Hammond et al. (1994), Loewenstein (1993a, 1993b), and Steinberg (1993).

DISSOCIATION IN THE GENERAL POPULATION

One study of dissociation has been conducted in the general population in North America (Ross, 1991a; Ross, Joshi, & Currie, 1990; Ross, Joshi, & Currie, 1991), and one in Europe (Vanderlinden, 1993). A stratified cluster sample of 1,055 adults in the city of Winnipeg, Canada, completed the Dissociative Experiences Scale (DES) and provided demographic information. Details about the procedure and sample are given in the main paper arising from the study (Ross, Joshi, & Currie, 1990). The sample was representative of the city as a whole when compared with census data, and there were no methodological problems with the sampling procedure.

The distribution of DES scores among the 1,055 respondents is shown in Figure 5.1. The curve is highly left-skewed. It shows that most people in the general population have very few dissociative experiences, while a small number have a lot: The vast majority of individuals in the general population report never experiencing the most pathological DES items. A reanalysis of the data done by Neils Waller (Waller & Ross, unpublished data, 1995), showed that, based on a statistical method called the HIT-MAX, 3.3% of the 1,055 subjects were *in the taxon*. This is a technical term meaning that 3.3% of the respondents appeared to have pathological dissociative experiences, and therefore presumptively had a dissociative disorder. Subjects were clearly either in the taxon or out of it, with few or no intermediate or grey-zone cases.

A principal components analysis of the 1,055 DES responses (Ross, Joshi, & Currie, 1991) showed that the DES has three factors. These three factors have been found in most DES studies involving college students and are called *absorption/imaginative involvement, amnesia,* and *depersonalization/derealization.* In our paper, I called the amnesia factor *activities of dissociated states,* but this term is too cumbersome.

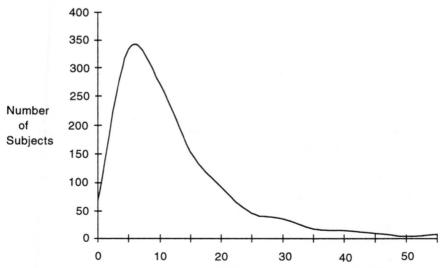

Figure 5.1. Distribution of Dissociative Experience Scale Scores in the General Population (*N* = 1055)

All DES factor studies show that the absorption/imaginative involvement items are much more common than those in the other two factors. All investigators are agreed that the absorption items are not inherently pathological, even when an individual item score is high. It appears from reanalysis of DES data gathered by Frank Putnam and Eve Carlson (Waller, unpublished data, 1995) that the three DES factors are a statistical artifact of frequency of item endorsement. When one controls statistically for how common the different experiences are, then a single DES factor emerges. I include this information to show that current research on the epidemiology of dissociation involves sophisticated statistical analyses.

The main point remains valid, that most of the items on the DES are not inherently pathological, and that clinical interest should be focused on the average score for the critical items. I will discuss the details of all of this in Chapter Seven. The scores on the 28 different DES items in the sample of 1,055 people from the general population are shown in Table 5.1.

The items in Table 5.1 are ranked from the highest to the lowest average score: The possible score for each item ranges from 0 to 100, depending on how frequently one has the given experience. The overall DES score is the sum of the 28-item scores divided by 28, and therefore also ranges from 0 to 100. The second column in Table 5.1 is the frequency of endorsement of each item, or the prevalence: This is the percentage of respondents scoring above zero for that item. The third column is the percentage of respondents who experience this item more than 30% of the time: I chose 30 because it is regarded as a cutoff score for the pathological range by many investigators.

Among the 1,055 respondents, there were no differences in overall DES scores due to any demographic factors, including gender, income, family composition, religion, and ethnic background. The only exception was a slight decline in scores with age: this decline was statistically significant but of doubtful clinical or theoretical significance, since it involved a drop in average score from 15.2 in the 18–29 age range to 5.9 in the 60–69 age range. Differences this small within the normal range of DES scores are of unknown if any significance.

Vanderlinden (1993) found a similar distribution of dissociative experiences in the Netherlands and Belgium using his Dissociation Questionnaire (DIS-Q). Based on DIS-Q scores, he predicted that the prevalence of dissociative disorders in his sample was 2.1%. The number of subjects scoring in the range for DID was 0.52%.

A number of DES studies have been done in college students in a variety of countries, and the findings are highly consistent. The average DES score usually lies between 10.0 and 20.0 and the distribution is highly left-skewed. I have summarized these findings elsewhere (Ross, 1996b). These studies have been conducted in Japan (Hattori & Ross, unpublished data, 1995); Canada (Ross, Ryan, Voigt, & Edie, 1991), and the United States (Frischholz et al., 1990; Ray & Faith, 1995); other related studies are reviewed by Ray (1996).

Table 5.1. *Dissociative Experience Scale Scores in the General Population in the City of Winnipeg, Canada (N = 1,055)*

Item	Mean Score	Prevalence (%)	Subjects Scoring > 30 (%)
Able to ignore pain	25.6	74.7	33.4
Missing part of a conversation	24.3	83.0	29.0
Usually difficult things can be done with ease and spontaneity	22.8	73.1	28.4
Not sure whether one has done something or only thought about it	21.2	73.1	24.7
Absorption in television program or movie	20.2	63.9	24.2
Remembering past so vividly one seems to be reliving it	17.4	60.4	19.2
Staring into space	15.3	62.6	25.7
Talking out loud to oneself when alone	15.2	55.6	17.7
Finding evidence of having done things one can't remember doing	13.5	58.4	14.3
Not sure if remembered event happened or was a dream	12.6	54.6	12.5
Being approached by people one doesn't know who call one by a different name	12.4	52.4	4.1
Feeling as though one were two different people	11.5	47.0	11.8
So involved in fantasy that it seems real	10.0	44.5	10.9
Driving a car and realizing one doesn't remember part of the trip	9.0	47.8	7.5
Not remembering important events in one's life	8.8	37.9	9.5
Being in a familiar place but finding it unfamiliar	8.6	40.0	8.2
Being accused of lying when one is telling the truth	7.3	40.8	6.0
Finding notes or drawings that one must have done but doesn't remember doing	6.7	34.0	6.3
Seeing oneself as if looking at another person	5.3	28.6	4.3
Hearing voices inside one's head	5.3	26.0	7.3
Not recognizing friends or family members	5.1	25.8	4.6
Other people and objects do not seem real	4.9	26.3	4.1

(continued)

Table 5.1.   (Continued)

Item	Mean Score	Prevalence (%)	Subjects Scoring > 30 (%)
Looking at the world through a fog	4.7	26.3	4.0
Finding unfamiliar things among one's belongings	4.5	22.1	4.1
Feeling as though one's body is not one's own	3.9	22.7	3.6
Finding oneself in a place but unaware of how one got there	2.8	18.8	2.0
Finding oneself dressed in clothes one doesn't remember putting on	1.9	14.6	1.4
Not recognizing one's reflection in a mirror	1.8	13.6	1.2

I haven't gone into this literature in a comprehensive fashion because it is too technical. The overall conclusions are clear, however: The distribution of dissociative experiences in the general population closely resembles that in college students, except that students are younger and do not manifest the slight decline in DES scores that occurs with age; the findings are consistent across many studies and in a variety of different cultures and languages; most people do not report any pathological dissociative experiences; many dissociative experiences are normal and benign; and extrapolations from self-report data set the lifetime prevalence of dissociative disorders in the general population in the range of 2% to 11%.

DISSOCIATIVE DISORDERS IN THE GENERAL POPULATION

To date, only one study has attempted to determine the lifetime prevalence of the dissociative disorders in the general population (Ross, 1991a). An attempt was made to reinterview the 1,055 respondents in Winnipeg who completed the DES using the DDIS: the structured interviews were administered by trained undergraduates who were blind to the DES scores. We were able to find and interview 502 of the 1,055 respondents: Comparison of the 502 subjects who participated in the structured interview with the 553 who did not revealed no differences in demographics or DES scores.

The paper reporting these findings (Ross, 1991a) presents an analysis of only the first 454 respondents, since data collection was not completed in time for publication in the special issue of *Psychiatric Clinics of North America.*

There are a number of serious methodological limitations to the DDIS portion of this study: No validating clinical interviews were conducted; the validity of the DDIS in nonclinical populations is unknown; the sample size is too small; the data come from only one city; and no other standardized interview was administered. Because of these limitations, the data from the study, shown in Table 5.2, must be regarded only as first approximations.

The 1% prevalence of DID is a conservative interpretation of the data, because over 3% of respondents endorsed *DSM-III-R* criteria for multiple personality disorder. I excluded most of these people as false positives because they reported neither trauma histories nor the rest of the DDIS symptom profile for DID. It is clear that the DID cases detected in this study are far milder in symptom severity than clinically diagnosed cases, including their DES scores.

Several other interpretations of the data are possible. First, the prevalence of severe DID may be less than 0.2% because no such cases were detected in a sample of 502 respondents. Second, these data provide the strongest existing scientifically based (as opposed to ideologically based) argument in favor of the iatrogenic amplification of DID. If cases existing in the general population are mild, and those diagnosed clinically are severe, it is possible that symptom levels get amplified during recruitment into the mental health system in a substantial proportion of cases.

Much more research and more advanced methodology are required before any firm conclusion can be reached about the epidemiology of DID in the general population.

However, two additional studies with the DDIS have been done in college student populations, and these yield roughly the same findings as the general population study. Ross, Ryan, Voigt, and Edie (1991) administered the DES to 345 college students in Winnipeg, then gave a battery of further measures including the DDIS to 22 students scoring under 5 on the DES and 20 scoring above 22.6. The high scorers were selected by starting with the highest DES score in the sample of 345 students, and working downward until 20 subjects had consented to complete the follow-up battery.

Table 5.2. The Prevalence of Dissociative Disorders in the General Population of Winnipeg, Canada (N = 502)

Disorder	Percent
Dissociative amnesia	6.0
Dissociative fugue	0.0
Depersonalization disorder	2.8
Dissociative identity disorder	3.0
Dissociative disorder NOS	0.2
A dissociative disorder of some kind	12.2

High and low DES scorers differed at very high levels of significance on all measures: Of the 20 subjects scoring above 22.6 on the DES, 14 (70%) met DDIS criteria for a dissociative disorder including 8 with DID. None of the low scorers had a DDIS dissociative disorder. Extrapolations from the data based on simple arithmetic yielded a lifetime prevalence for DID of 6.3% and for the dissociative disorders overall of 11.0%. I don't believe that 6.3% is the true prevalence of DID in college students, but the data do lead to this conclusion. The limitations of the study are the same as for the general population study. It is impossible to say whether the consistent figure of about 11% for the lifetime prevalence of dissociative disorders in the general population is an artifact or an accurate finding.

In the other college student study, in which I also participated, Pat Murphy (1994) administered the DES to 415 college students in Idaho, then gave the DDIS to a follow-up sample. She found a mean DES score of 14.7 (*SD* 10.8), with 8.9% of the sample scoring above 30, which is similar to all other studies. She administered the DDIS to a subsample of 18 students scoring above 30 on the DES and 9 who scored below 30: Of the 18 students scoring above 30, 16 met criteria for a dissociative disorder including 4 with DID. This sets the conservative prevalence of DID on the DDIS among Idaho college students at 1%. Murphy's conclusion was that the lifetime prevalence of dissociative disorders in the general population may be in the range of 5% to 10%.

My role in the Murphy study was to review 8 of the DDISs to render an opinion as to whether I agreed with the diagnostic conclusions of the trained college students who administered the DDIS. I agreed in 7 cases, but in one disagreed because I did not think there was enough symptomotology to warrant a diagnosis of DDNOS.

So far, no studies have disconfirmed the finding that about 10% of people in the general population will suffer from a dissociative disorder at some time in their lives. More conservative estimates based on sophisticated statistical analyses of DES scores set the figure closer to 3%—even 3%, however, means about 10 million cases in North America. If we set the prevalence of full clinical DID at about 0.1%, this means hundreds of thousands of current cases in North America.

A reasonable conclusion from the existing data is that DID and the other dissociative disorders are unlikely to be rare in the general population. DID could be about as common as schizophrenia and bipolar mood disorder, but also might prove to be only one tenth as frequent.

DISSOCIATIVE DISORDERS IN CLINICAL POPULATIONS

Much more work has been done on DID in clinical populations, and the work has been replicated in a number of different countries and institutional settings. All existing studies show that most clinically diagnosed

DID patients score in the top few percent of the general population distribution of DES scores; that is, they are *in the taxon.* Findings from Canada, the United States, the Netherlands, Turkey, and Puerto Rico (four languages on three continents) are shown in Table 5.3.

These data do not tell us the relative contributions of the four pathways to DID, but they do indicate that DID patients report far more pathological dissociation than anyone else. They endorse the rare DES items at high levels. This is why the DES functions as a screening tool for DID—high scores on the critical items increase the odds that the person has DID or another dissociative disorder.

A number of different studies including one of ours (Chu & Dill, 1990; Ross, Anderson, Fleisher, & Norton, 1992) have shown that the distribution of DES scores is shifted right in clinical compared with nonclinical populations, but the difference is not dramatic. The prevalence of DID has been studied in two clinical populations: general adult psychiatric inpatients and chemical dependency patients, with consistent results, as shown in Tables 5.4 and 5.5.

I won't go into all the methodological details of these studies, but they all involve screening with the DES and interviewing follow-up subjects with a structured interview, either the DDIS or Marlene Steinberg's (1995) Structured Clinical Interview for *DSM-IV* Dissociative Disorders (SCID-D). In our study in Winnipeg, we also did validating clinical interviews on subjects positive for DID on the DDIS and matched controls, conducted by an interviewer blind to the DES and DDIS results. The other studies did not involve screening as large a sample or as rigorous a

Table 5.3.   Dissociative Experiences Scale Scores in Dissociative Identity Disorder

Study	N	Average DES Score
United States		
Fink	16	48.6
Loewenstein	9	47.5
Frischholz	33	55.0
Canada/United States		
Ross	82	41.4
Carlson	228	42.8
Netherlands		
Ensink	7	49.3
Turkey		
Tutkin	20	47.2
Puerto Rico		
Martinez-Taboas	16	60.3

Table 5.4.   Prevalence of Dissociative Identity Disorder and
the Dissociative Disorders among General Adult Psychiatric
Inpatients

Study	DID (%)	Dissociative Disorder (%)
Canada		
Ross	5.4	20.7
Horen	6.0	17.0
USA		
Saxe	4.0	15.0
Latz	12.0	46.0
Norway		
Knudsen	4.7	8.2

methodology for clinical validation (Horen, Leichner, & Lawson, 1995; Knudsen, Draijer, Haselrud, Boe, & Boon, 1995; Latz, Kramer, & Hughes, 1995; Saxe et al., 1993). Except for the higher figures obtained by Latz and colleagues, the prevalence of undiagnosed DID among general adult psychiatric inpatients is very consistent in the range of 4% to 6%. I consider this prevalence rate to be accurate and conservative, and I predict that it will be confirmed by systematic replications throughout the world. Confirming data should emerge from Turkey, Australia, England, France, Japan, and other countries within the next decade.

The prevalence of DID and the other dissociative disorders varies more widely in chemical dependency populations. In my opinion, this is more likely due to an actual greater variability in psychopathology across the different clinical settings, compared with the inpatient samples, than to imprecision of measurement.

Our sample of 100 subjects came from a teaching hospital setting in Winnipeg (Ross, Kronson, Koensgen, Barkman, Clark, & Rockman, 1992), whereas our sample of 102 subjects was from Charter Behavioral Health System of Dallas, a freestanding private for-profit psychiatric hospital (Ellason, Ross, Sainton, & Mayran, 1996). The two other studies involve Veterans Administration samples in the United States (Dunn, Paolo, & Ryan, 1993; Leeper, Page, & Hendricks, 1992).

Table 5.5.   Prevalence of Dissociative Identity Disorder and the
Dissociative Disorders among Chemical Dependency Patients

Study	DID (%)	Dissociative Disorder (%)
Ross ($N = 100$)	14.0	39.0
Leeper ($N = 99$)	5.1	15.4
Ross ($N = 102$)	18.6	56.9
Dunn ($N = 100$)	7.0	15.0

A realistic conclusion concerning the prevalence of DID in chemical dependency populations is that it is at least as common as among general adult inpatients, possibly affecting as many as 15% of patients in treatment for drug and alcohol problems. The existing data suggest that dissociative disorders are at least as common a form of comorbidity as mood and anxiety disorders in chemical dependency populations, and are vastly underdiagnosed clinically.

When we administered the Structured Clinical Interview for *DSM-III-R* (SCID) (Spitzer, Williams, Gibbons, & First, 1990) to 85 chemical dependency subjects who also completed the DDIS, out of our overall Dallas sample of 102 patients, we found that mood disorders had occurred in 40.0% and anxiety disorders in 36.5%, which is typical of the findings from a large number of other comorbidity studies, none of which assessed for dissociative disorders. It appears that our Dallas sample is representative of chemical dependency patients in terms of overall comorbidity, therefore the findings for dissociative disorders may be accurate.

DISSOCIATIVE DISORDERS IN CHILDREN AND ADOLESCENTS

The epidemiology of dissociation and dissociative disorders in children and adolescents is even less understood than in adults. I review the existing literature elsewhere (Ross, 1996b). The key study to date is one by Marcia Waterbury (1991) involving 231 children admitted to a facility in Baltimore for treatment of children who are difficult to manage in foster care. Careful assessment of these children, including review of extensive records and extensive interviewing of collateral sources, resulted in a finding that 23% met criteria for multiple personality disorder, 33% met criteria for DDNOS, and 17% met criteria for dissociative identity disorder of childhood, a diagnosis proposed for *DSM-IV* but not adopted (Putnam & Peterson, 1994). The trauma histories of these children were extreme and often well documented.

Waterbury commented that many of the DID children had personality systems that were complex, crystallized, and very similar to adult DID systems. If these diagnostic and clinical findings are replicated, and supported by the use of standardized measures, it will be accepted that dissociative disorders are common in severely traumatized children.

In an unpublished study, my research team in Winnipeg interviewed 45 adolescents in treatment at a teaching hospital inpatient facility with the DDIS, and found that 44.5% met criteria for a dissociative disorder, including 15.6% with DID. In another unpublished study, we compared 11 adolescents with clinically diagnosed DID to 166 adults with clinically diagnosed DID on their DDIS profiles, and found only two differences at $p < .05$: The adolescents reported fewer somatic symptoms and fewer positive amnesia items. Otherwise the adolescent profile was identical to that of adults.

These are the only systematic screening studies in children and adolescents of which I am aware; the remaining literature on dissociative disorders in children consists of small case series, single case reports, and studies of measures of dissociation, but not epidemiological studies. In my review (Ross, 1996b) I conclude that the existing data on children, adolescents, and adults, supports a tentative estimate that 5% to 10% of children in North America will develop a dissociative disorder prior to age 18.

The same cautions concerning the estimated prevalence of dissociative disorders in adults apply to children and adolescents, except that the data are much sparser in children.

CONCLUSION

All existing research consistently points to the conclusion that undiagnosed dissociative disorders are common in clinical settings. No scientific study has been published disconfirming this conclusion. The lifetime prevalence of the dissociative disorders in the general population is uncertain but likely lies in the range of 3% to 11%, based on research conducted to date. The distribution of dissociative experiences in the general population, as measured by the DES and DIS-Q is well studied, and future research is unlikely to shift the findings to any significant extent. The quest now is to find cultures that show markedly different patterns, then to understand what is different about them. The epidemiology of dissociation is a scientific field with a substantial database, although much work remains to be done. Only 10 years ago, no systematic data of any kind existed: The field has advanced steadily at a good pace, given the modest amount of research funding for studies of dissociation.

Clinical Features of Dissociative Identity Disorder

The clinical features of dissociative identity disorder (DID) consist of two main subsets: generic or nonspecific symptoms, and symptoms specific for DID. The clinician, to reach an accurate diagnosis and guide treatment effectively, must be familiar with both. With this in mind, I am first going to describe a general scheme for thinking about dissociation, which I will expand on in Chapter Eight. Then I will discuss the diagnostically nonspecific features of DID and will conclude with those aspects of the disorder that do not occur in other psychiatric illnesses. The specific aspects of DID are subdivided into phenomena most important in diagnosis, and those most relevant in treatment.

A GENERAL SCHEME OF DISSOCIATION

DID is a dissociative disorder and, by definition, is based on the defense mechanism of dissociation. We do not, however, have a good definition of dissociation. Dissociation is defined in *DSM-IV* as "a disruption in the usually integrated functions of consciousness, memory, identity, or perception of the environment." This is a rough-and-ready clinical definition of dissociation that does not have a lot of empirical support. It arbitrarily limits dissociation to those areas of the brain concerned with identity, memory, perception, and consciousness. There is an overlap between a number of related concepts including fantasy proneness, hypnotizability, absorption, and dissociation (Lynn & Rhue, 1988); trying to sort these out into meaningfully distinct terms is a difficult research problem.

As well, there is a problem about the difference between splitting and dissociation (Clary, Burstin, & Carpenter, 1984; Gruenewald, 1977; Horevitz & Braun, 1984; Ross, 1985; Young, 1988). I consider splitting and dissociation to be synonyms, and I consider borderline personality disorder, which is based on splitting, to be an Axis I dissociative disorder. Because there is a great deal of ideological investment in the term "splitting," it is difficult to enter into an empirically grounded dialogue with colleagues who hold that multiples are "really just borderlines." The relationship between DID and borderline personality disorder, which is based on splitting, will be discussed in detail in Chapter Eight.

I favor a simple definition of dissociation. Dissociation is the opposite of association. It is not a coincidence that in the nineteenth century academic psychologists were preoccupied with theories of mental association, and studied clinical dissociation. For definitional purposes, the psyche may be reduced to a collection of elements in complex relationships with each other. Psychic elements include thoughts, memories, feelings, motor commands, impulses, sensations, and all the other constituents of psychic life. Any two psychic elements may be in a dynamic relationship with each other, which is to be associated, or relatively isolated and separate, which is to be dissociated.

The normal mind carries out an infinite number of associations and dissociations as part of its everyday function. On one day, for example, the smell of a perfume, a memory of a romantic dinner, and a calculation about next year's foreign travel budget may be closely linked in conscious awareness. The next day, these three elements will have been dissociated, to be recombined later with the same or other elements. Dissociation is an ongoing dynamic process in the normal psyche, subject to modulation and control by numerous other psychic contents.

Since dissociation is a pervasive aspect of normal mental function, one would expect disordered dissociation to be a feature of many, if not all, psychiatric illnesses. Logically, pathological dissociation may arise in two ways: as a failure of normal association, or as abnormal dissociation. A person with a psychogenic anesthesia of the right hand would not be able to associate the visual image of a hot object with a sensation of pain (unless this association had been learned prior to the onset of the anesthesia). This could be viewed as a failure of normal association, or as a dissociative disorder in the sensory sphere. Association and dissociation are opposite sides of the same coin.

Dissociation can occur in several forms. Two elements that are normally linked may be split apart and separated. A common example of this in DID is the patient's feelings about her father, and her memory of incest. The host personality may enter treatment with unconflicted positive feelings for her father and complete amnesia for the incest. Dissociation can occur when normally dissociated elements are held in rigid separation from each other. This would be a failure in the fluidity and reversibility of normal dissociation. Or there may be a dysregulation of dissociation/association such that two psychic elements are abruptly reassociated, and then equally as abruptly redissociated. One could imagine and classify numerous permutations of dissociation along such lines.

Psychodynamically, dissociation is the basic defense mechanism that precedes and underlies the other defense mechanisms. Before conflicted psychic material can be projected onto the environment, or displaced from one location in the environment to another, it must first be dissociated from its normal psychic connections. If this did not occur, projection either would not work or would result in complete emptying of the mind. Reaction formation necessarily involves a dissociation between the surface attitude, feelings, and cognitions and the underlying equivalents against which it is a defense. Likewise, before two psychic elements can be abnormally associated, as in symbolic and paralogical thinking, they must be dissociated from their normal connections. Any psychiatric disorder characterized by abnormal defense mechanisms therefore exhibits abnormal dissociation.

Dissociation can be subdivided into four main quadrants, as illustrated in Figure 6.1. Dissociation can be normal or abnormal, and it can be biologically or psychosocially driven. These distinctions are in practice impossible

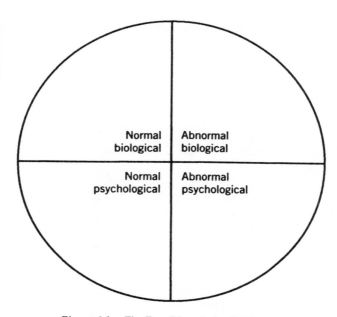

Figure 6.1.   The Four Dissociative Quadrants

to make much of the time: This is simply a general scheme for organizing one's thinking. There is an arbitrary tendency in psychiatry to assume that dissociation is by definition a psychologically driven process. This is not true. For example, an alcoholic may have to get drunk to remember where he hid a bottle the last time he was drinking. Sober, he can't remember. This is an example of state-dependent learning, in which a memory is organically dissociated from the sober consciousness. Organically driven dissociation may be reversible by hypnosis, and psychologically driven dissociation may be reversible by sodium amytal.

There is no sound reason to assume two separate spheres, one of biologically caused and treated dissociation, another of psychological etiology and treatment. I will suggest some possible examples in each of the four quadrants:

1. *Normal psychosocial dissociation.* Daydreaming during a boring lecture.
2. *Normal biological dissociation.* Forgetting that you got up in the night to go to the bathroom.
3. *Abnormal psychosocial dissociation.* Amnesia for incest.
4. *Abnormal biological dissociation.* Amnesia following a concussion.

These examples illustrate that dissociation may involve the trivial or the traumatic. Some forms of dissociation would be hard to classify as biological or psychological. For example, anesthesia for battleground wounds must be based on an ancient evolutionary skill, built into the central nervous system. On the other hand, the same degree of injury in a civilian car accident is likely to require more morphine because of the different meaning, social context, and consequences of the tissue damage. Psychological and biological causation may coexist. This is probably true in DID, which draws on primitive skills and properties of the brain, but in a highly complex social context.

This scheme for classifying dissociation, which is unchanged from the first edition of this book, was restated by Cardena (1994), and is consistent with neodissociation theory (Hilgard, 1994), and the views of Kilhstrom (1994) and others.

Dissociative disorders are arbitrarily limited to disorders of memory and identity in *DSM-IV*. Dissociation can presumably occur throughout the brain, including all regions of the limbic system, cortex, and reticular activating system. DID is a complex dissociative disorder, in which dissociation occurs in virtually all psychic functions, including sensation, memory, motor function, feeling, and cognition. It makes sense that there should be simpler examples of dissociative disorders limited to one or two psychic functions. *DSM-IV* allows only one of these: dissociative amnesia, which is a simple dissociation of memory.

What about a simple dissociation of motor function? This is a conversion disorder. Or a simple dissociation of enraged behavior? This is an impulse-control disorder. A simple dissociation of the ability to have an orgasm? This is a sexual dysfunction. Dissociative disorders are scattered throughout *DSM-IV,* and are grouped with other disorders in an inconsistent fashion (see Chapter Eight). As mentioned in the previous chapter, *ICD-10* organizes its dissociative diagnoses according to the principles I favor, and it does a better job at this than does *DSM-IV.* At the same time, *ICD-10* conceptualizes DID as a simple, spontaneously remitting disorder on the same level as a pure conversion disorder; this conceptualization of DID is inconsistent with a large body of clinical and research literature.

The purpose of this general scheme of dissociation is to lay the groundwork for a comprehensive clinical description of DID, which includes its relationship with other psychiatric disorders. DID almost always coexists with other *DSM-IV* psychiatric disorders, some of which could be thought of as independent concurrent entities, but many of which are actually further examples of pathological dissociation.

Braun (1988a, 1988b) has proposed a BASK model of dissociation that incorporates the principles I have just reviewed. In his scheme, dissociation can occur in various permutations and combinations of four continua: behavior, affect, sensation, and knowledge. A pure dissociation of behavior is a motor conversion disorder, a dissociation of knowledge is an amnesia, and so on. Braun understands clearly that DID involves many types and combinations of dissociations in all four dimensions. His scheme, in my experience as a teacher, consultant, and clinician, is well accepted by therapists and clients, and is helpful in organizing clinical interventions. It should be part of the basic reading for any training course on dissociative disorders.

NONSPECIFIC FEATURES OF DISSOCIATIVE IDENTITY DISORDER

DID patients rarely come for treatment with obvious or overt multiplicity. It is curious that in the nineteenth century syphilis was regarded as "the great imitator" in medicine. It could present with the signs and symptoms of almost any other medical illness. The task of the clinician was to perceive the underlying unity in the phenomenology, in order to make the diagnosis and provide treatment (which became specific and effective in the twentieth century). Syphilis is directly linked to sexuality, often to disordered or deviant sexuality. In the twentieth century, DID is the great imitator in psychiatry, and it too is directly linked to sexuality.

Childhood Trauma Histories

The relationship between DID and childhood trauma is described throughout the literature, and is prominent in all clinical reports and large series of cases. In almost all of this literature, the childhood abuse is reported retrospectively in adulthood and has not been confirmed by outside corroboration. However, in the two studies in which efforts were made to confirm the childhood trauma in series of dissociative cases, Coons (1986d) was able to get outside corroboration in 17 out of 20 adult cases of DID, and 18 out of 19 cases of adolescent DID and DDNOS (Coons, 1994). There are no empirical studies demonstrating the rate of confabulation of childhood trauma in DID.

Clinically, and in research series, at least 88% of DID patients report childhood physical and/or sexual abuse at first assessment for DID, and describe continuous memory for some of the abuse throughout their lives. Almost all patients recall further details during therapy, which can be explained by increased effort at recall and situational cuing of memories, without appeal to metapsychological constructs. The stereotype of the patient with no trauma memories at all prior to diagnosis of DID applies only to a small minority of cases, and in my experience mostly to iatrogenic and factitious pathway cases.

Table 6.1 shows the rates of reported childhood trauma in five large North American series of DID cases (Coons, Bowman, & Milstein, 1988; Putnam, Guroff, Silberman, Barban, & Post, 1986; Ross, Miller, Reagor, et al., 1990; Ross, Norton, & Wozney, 1989; Schultz, Braun, & Kluft, 1989). Similar patterns have been observed in Europe (Boon & Draijer, 1993) and Turkey (Tutkun, Yargic, & Sar, 1995). In round figures, it appears that 5% to 10% of DID patients fail to report childhood physical and/or sexual abuse at first assessment for DID. Logically, this group could include patients who were never abused, patients who remember their abuse but don't want to talk about it, and ones who are completely amnesic for their trauma. The proportions of these subgroups in the 5% to 10% not reporting abuse are unknown. If each represents one third of the 5% to 10%, then about only 2% to 3% of DID patients are completely amnesic for their abuse at the time of diagnosis. This is a rough figure that establishes the *maximum* rate of complete traumatic amnesia at diagnosis: It illustrates that the *tabula rasa* subgroup of DID is very small, if it exists at all.

The abuse histories are severe, begin early, and last a long time. In our series of 102 cases, we reported the types of acts described by these

Table 6.1. Reported Childhood Abuse Histories of Dissociative Identity Disorder Patients in Five Large Series

Type of Abuse	Putnam (N = 100) (%)	Ross (N = 236) (%)	Coons (N = 50) (%)	Schultz (N = 355) (%)	Ross (N = 102) (%)
Sexual	83.0	79.2	68.0	86.0	90.2
Physical	75.0	74.9	60.0	82.0	82.4
Physical or Sexual or Both	—	88.5	96.0	—	95.1

Table 6.2.   Types of Childhood Sexual Abuse Reported by 102 Dissociative Identity Disorder Patients

Type of Sexual Abuse	Subjects Reporting This Type (%)
Hand-genital contact	77.5
Other types of fondling	76.5
Intercourse	54.9
Performing oral sex on a male	52.9
Oral sex performed on patient by a male	52.9
Passive anal intercourse	37.3
Simulated intercourse with a female*	24.5
Performing oral sex on a female	20.6
Pornographic photography	20.6
Oral sex performed on patient by a female	19.6
Forced sex with animals	13.7

* Female patients only (N = 92).

patients, as shown in Table 6.2, and the identities of the perpetrators, as shown in Table 6.3 (Ross, Miller, et al., 1991). These findings are typical of my clinical experience with over 1,000 admissions to our Dissociative Disorders Unit.

In adult DID, sexual dysfunction is usually present (Coons & Milstein, 1986), and conflicts about gender identity and sexual orientation are frequent as well (Ross, 1994b). Like syphilis, DID is often highly treatable and could be prevented by a modification of sexual behavior in society at large, although this is unlikely to happen.

In our 236 cases, 19.1% had worked as prostitutes. In another study, we found DID in 1 out of 20 prostitutes and 7 out of 20 exotic dancers using the DDIS (Ross, Anderson, Heber, & Norton, 1990). This means that there is a

Table 6.3.   Childhood Sexual Abuse Perpetrators Reported by 102 Dissociative Identity Disorder Patients

Perpetrator	Subjects Reporting This Type of Perpetrator	
	Physical Abuse (%)	Sexual Abuse (%)
Father	45.1	39.2
Mother	45.1	15.7
Stepfather	10.8	15.7
Stepmother	4.9	2.9
Sibling	28.4	24.5
Male relative	29.4	46.1
Female relative	16.7	10.8
Other male	46.1	62.7
Other female	20.6	21.6

concrete connection between DID and syphilis. More importantly, there is probably a large number of AIDS-positive male and female prostitutes with DID in North America. Many of these people would potentially stop prostituting if they were diagnosed and treated for their DID. The probable connection between DID, childhood sexual abuse, prostitution, sexual promiscuity, and venereal diseases including AIDS, makes DID a major unrecognized public health problem in North America. I expand on this testable hypothesis elsewhere (Ross, 1994a). These potential connections between childhood sexual abuse and sexually transmitted diseases are only one of the many research hypotheses that flow from the study of DID.

In a prospective study described in Chapter Eleven, Joan Ellason and I observed that 12 DID patients treated to stable integration did not retract any elements of their childhood trauma (Ellason & Ross, 1995b). These 12 integrated individuals were part of a cohort of 54 patients followed prospectively, the rest of whom had not yet reached integration; there were no retractors among the other 42 patients. However, we have treated a number of full retractors on our Dissociative Disorders Unit at Charter Behavioral Health System of Dallas. These individuals presented a mixture of factitious and iatrogenic pathways and retracted their DID and much of their child abuse in a clinically plausible fashion. The more time goes by since the peak of the Satanic ritual abuse hysteria in the late 1980s and early 1990s (Ross, 1995a), the more individuals we see retracting their cult memories; these people usually do not retract their domestic physical, sexual, and emotional abuse histories, however.

The final word on the amount of historically accurate recall of childhood trauma occurring in DID is not available yet. However, my clinical experience and the existing research data tell me that the majority of DID patients have experienced serious chronic trauma in their childhoods.

Prediagnosis Mental Health Treatment

There are many striking findings in the two large series of 100 and 236 cases from the 1980s; one of these is the long period DID patients spend in the mental health system from first presentation for symptoms of DID to diagnosis. In Putnam's series, the average length of time was 6.8 years, and in ours 6.7 years. Since our figure was actually 6.74 years, I quote the average for the two series as being 6.8 years. In Putnam's series, the average number of previous psychiatric diagnoses was 3.6 and in ours it was 2.7.

Most DID patients will come for treatment with a long history of involvement in the mental health system. The picture in old charts, discharge summaries, consultation notes, and agency reports will likely be inconsistent and confusing. Table 6.4 shows the percentage of patients in our series of 236 and 102 cases who had received various psychiatric diagnoses prior to diagnosis of their DID, and Table 6.5 shows the types of treatment they reported.

Table 6.4.   *Prior Diagnoses of Dissociative Identity Disorder Patients in Two Large Series*

Diagnosis	Ross (N = 236) (%)	Ross (N = 102) (%)
Mood disorder	63.7	72.5
Personality disorder	57.4	—
Anxiety disorder	44.3	46.1
Schizophrenia	40.8	26.5
Substance abuse	31.4	—
Adjustment disorder	26.1	—
Dissociative identity disorder	19.7	35.3
Somatization disorder	18.8	—
Eating disorder	16.3	—
Organic mental disorder	12.8	—

As well as long histories of involvement in the mental health system, DID patients have often been extensively involved with legal, welfare, and other social systems. They may have complicated nonpsychiatric medical histories, even to the extent of having Munchausen's syndrome (Goodwin, 1988). In our series of 236 cases, 11.9% of patients had been convicted of a crime, and 12.3% had been in jail. Two published studies (Rivera, 1991; Ross & Dua, 1993) document the high costs of DID patients to the Canadian social service system prior to diagnosis: In a sample of 15 DID cases treated by me as inpatients in Winnipeg, Canada, from 1986 to 1991, the total tabulated lifetime psychiatric health care costs for the 15 women were 4.1 million dollars, most of which had been spent prior to diagnosis of the DID.

Most DID patients are female and in their 20s or 30s at the time of diagnosis. When the large series are added together, the female/male ratio is almost exactly 9:1, and the mean age is in the 30s. This means that the

Table 6.5.   *Prior Treatments Reported by Dissociative Identity Disorder Patients in Two Large Series*

Type of Treatment	Ross (N = 236) (%)	Ross (N = 102) (%)
Psychotherapy	89.7	94.0
Antidepressant	68.9	72.5
Inpatient	74.6	—
Benzodiazepine	60.3	—
Nonbenzodiazepine sedative	59.5	—
Antipsychotic	54.5	55.9
Lithium	21.9	29.4
Electroconvulsive therapy	12.1	16.7

clinician's index of suspicion should be raised whenever he is assessing a young woman with a long inconsistent psychiatric history.

At this point, a caution is in order. The large clinical series I have been describing represent a highly biased sample of DID patients. As described in the previous chapter, there may be a large number of people in the general population with DID who are high-functioning, relatively free of overt psychopathology, and no more in need of treatment than most of their peers. They may not have abuse histories and may have evolved a creative and adaptive multiplicity. If these people exist, virtually nothing is known about them. On the other hand, the clinical research samples probably fail to describe the most severely disturbed multiples, who are dead, in jail, or living on skid row.

I think it's safe to say that the large published series are reasonably representative of cases currently in treatment in North America. In our series of 236 cases, we had 28 males, which allowed for statistical comparisons of males and females with DID. We found no difference in the specific features of DID, and little difference in their general psychopathology (Ross & Norton, 1989a). The differences we did find were those we expected to observe: Males were convicted of crimes and had been in jail more often; females received a diagnosis of depression more often, were prescribed antidepressants, benzodiazepines, and hypnotic-sedatives more often, and overdosed more often. These are differences between males and females one would expect to see in the general population. The net conclusion is that the diagnostic clues and features of DID are basically the same in men and women. Loewenstein and Putnam (1990) described 21 males with DID and similarly concluded that the basic features of DID are consistent in men and women.

A diagnostic clue for DID mentioned by Kluft (1985d) is the failure of the patient to respond to adequate trials of conventional treatment, which is borne out by subsequent research. A good place to look for undiagnosed DID is among treatment nonresponders in drug trials. If these people could be screened out, the active medication response rate might improve while the placebo response rate declined. As well, exclusion of previously unrecognized DID cases from biological research studies in psychiatry might increase the sensitivity of biological markers for mental illness, and reduce the amount of noise in many different psychopharmacological and biological studies (Ross, 1992; Ross & Anderson, 1988; Ross & Pam, 1995).

Self-Destructive Behavior

Self-destructive behavior is very common in DID and is the main reason for inpatient admission. The rates of different forms of self-destructive behavior in our series of 236 and 102 cases are shown in Table 6.6. In our clinical experience in Dallas, we are aware of four patients completing suicide postdischarge out of over 500 individuals admitted in a four-year period. This compares with a long-term rate of completed suicide of about

Table 6.6.   Self-Destructive Behavior Reported by Dissociative Identity Disorder Patients in Two Large Series

Type of Behavior	Ross (N = 236) (%)	Ross (N = 102) (%)
Recurrent suicidal thoughts	—	92.0
Suicide attempt (overall)	72.0	72.5
Overdose	68.0	56.9
Self-inflicted burns or other injuries	56.6	23.5
Wrist slashing	49.3	40.2
Gun, knife, or other weapon	—	26.5
Attempted hanging	—	12.7
Completed suicide	2.1	—

10% for individuals diagnosed with major depressive disorder, schizophrenia, or borderline personality disorder. Since our follow-up period is still short, we cannot conclude whether the rate of completed suicide is lower in diagnosed DID than in individuals with other disorders, but it appears that it may be.

DID patients may be amnesic for their suicide attempts, or may report that they felt depersonalized while harming themselves: This is because of the copresence of another alter personality who was responsible for the behavior (copresence can be confirmed in conversation with the alter at some point in treatment). The self-destructive behavior is not usually primarily a "cry for help" or "attention-seeking," and is most often a sign of internal dispute, cognitive errors, and hostility in the personality system.

We divided our series of 236 cases into those who had attempted suicide (N = 167) and those who had not (N = 48), in an attempt to identify risk factors for self-destruction (Ross & Norton, 1989b). We found that the parasuicidal group had more physical and sexual abuse, and rape. They also had more severe psychopathology. This was evidenced by higher rates of affective disorder diagnoses, which would be expected. However, the parasuicidal group also had a higher frequency of past diagnoses of schizophrenia, substance abuse, adjustment disorder, somatization disorder, and organic mental disorder. They had more frequently been treated with antidepressants, nonbenzodiazepine sedatives, benzodiazepines, antipsychotics, and lithium. As well, they more frequently experienced seven of the Schneiderian first-rank symptoms of schizophrenia: voices arguing, voices commenting, made impulses, audible thoughts, delusions, made feelings, and thought withdrawal.

We took these findings to be evidence both of the more severe general psychopathology of the parasuicidal group, and of greater diagnostic and therapeutic confusion on the part of clinicians faced with these patients. The findings strike one optimistic note. Since the self-destructive behavior occurs partly during a seven-year period in which the DID is not diagnosed, it is possible that earlier diagnosis might reduce the suicide attempts. The parasuicidal group had spent twice as long in the mental health system prior to diagnosis as those who had not harmed themselves. I plan to redistribute the same questionnaire in the next few years to see if this and other characteristics of DID have changed with greater awareness of the disorder.

An interesting finding in our parasuicide study was a clinical triad of made impulses, voices in the head, and suicide attempts. This triad should alert the clinician to the possibility of DID, especially if the made impulse is self-destructive, and the voice is commanding suicide, or is hostile and critical. The triad is indicative of the activity of a dangerous persecutor personality, and has a differential diagnosis that includes schizophrenia.

The self-destructive DID patients also differed in the specific features of DID. They had manifested twice as many personalities by the time of reporting (an average of 18.0 personalities, compared with an average of 7.4 for nonsuicidal patients). They had more of four out of nine types of alter personality inquired about. These were: protector personality, personality of opposite sex, demon personality, and personality identified as a dead relative. The self-destructive DID patient tends to have a more complex personality system and a more severe abuse history. The inner logic and meaning of the different personality types will be discussed later in this chapter.

The figure of 12.1% to 16.7% of DID patients having received electroconvulsive therapy (ECT) shown in Table 6.5 is an indicator of the levels of suicidal ideation in this population. This ECT may be politically costly to psychiatry, since misdiagnosed and mistreated DID patients are likely to be among the most vocal members of the antipsychiatry movement. Within a decade, failure to diagnose DID, combined with treatment with ECT or antipsychotic medications, will likely be grounds for a malpractice suit. The first test case I am aware of concerning failure to diagnose and treat DID was reported in the September 2, 1988, issue of *Psychiatric News* (Vol. 23, No. 17, pp. 20, 27).

Chronic self-destructive behavior in a woman with a long psychiatric history and childhood trauma should always prompt a thorough diagnostic evaluation for DID.

COMORBIDITY

The other psychiatric diagnoses given to these patients before diagnosis of their DID raise a question: Are the other diagnoses errors or correct concurrent diagnoses? The answer is, they may be either. Many DID patients experience classical panic attacks (Fraser & Lapierre, 1986) and clinical depressions. In 20 DID subjects we interviewed in our initial study with the DDIS, 17 (85%) had met the *DSM-III* criteria for major depressive episode at some time in their life. We found that 7 (35%) met the criteria for somatization disorder (Ross, Heber, Norton, & Anderson, 1989b). This compares with 18.8% in the series of 236 cases who had received a diagnosis of somatization disorder in the past.

In the late 1980s, our structured interview findings and clinical experience suggested to us that the rates of other psychiatric disorders in the series of 236 cases were conservative estimates of the actual rates. This was true for mood disorder, personality disorder, anxiety disorder, substance abuse, somatization disorder, and eating disorder. DID patients can often meet *DSM-IV* criteria for 10 or more diagnoses simultaneously. Clinicians who have made these diagnoses in the past are therefore not mistaken. Their error is not to have diagnosed the DID.

In this section, I will review the comorbidity of DID based on a study we did with the Structured Clinical Interview for *DSM-III-R* (SCID-I and SCID-II) (Spitzer et al., 1990). The SCID is a structured interview widely used in psychiatry that makes a broad range of Axis I diagnoses and all the Axis II diagnoses. We administered it to a series of 103 DID patients admitted to our Dissociative Disorders Unit in Dallas in 1992 and 1993. The results are shown in Tables 6.7 and 6.8.

Because the version of the SCID we used does not diagnose posttraumatic stress disorder (PTSD), we administered the PTSD section of the Diagnostic Interview Schedule (Robins, Helzer, Croughan, & Ratcliff, 1981) as well.

Dissociation Mistaken for Psychosis

In our series of 236 cases, 40.8% had a previous diagnosis of schizophrenia, and in the series of 102 cases 26.5% had received this diagnosis, while the figure in Putnam's series of 100 cases was just under 50%. As can be seen in Table 6.7, 68.2% of DID patients receive a SCID diagnosis of schizophrenia or schizoaffective disorder, and 74.3% receive some type of psychotic diagnosis on structured interview. On clinical and research grounds, I believe these to be almost all false positive diagnoses of psychosis. We have had only a handful of cases referred to our Dissociative Disorders Unit in which we concluded that the correct diagnosis was schizophrenia rather than DID. But I have met a DID patient who has received between 8 and 10 courses of electroconvulsive therapy for schizophrenia "when the voices get bad" (Ross, 1994b). Anyone with a diagnosis of schizophrenia who does not seem to have blunted affect, a thought disorder, or the empty, deteriorated air of chronic schizophrenia, should be suspected of having DID. The differential diagnosis can be complicated when the DID patient reports that the injections he has been getting every two weeks for 10 years "calm my nerves."

I participated in an interrater reliability training session for use of the Brief Psychiatric Rating Scale in a multicenter study of a new medication for schizophrenia. There were three videotaped vignettes of schizophrenics

Table 6.7.   Lifetime Axis I Diagnoses in 103 Dissociative Identity Disorder Patients on the Structured Clinical Interview for DSM-III-R (SCID)

Diagnosis	Percent
Mood Disorder	
Some type of mood disorder	98.1
Major depressive episode	97.2
Bipolar I	9.3
Bipolar II	7.5
Dysthymia	0.9
Anxiety Disorder	
Some type of anxiety disorder	91.4
Panic disorder	69.2
Obsessive-compulsive disorder	63.6
Social phobia	45.8
Simple phobia	28.0
Agoraphobia	15.9
Generalized anxiety disorder	1.0
Psychotic Disorder	
Some type of psychotic disorder	74.3
Schizoaffective disorder	49.5
Schizophrenia	18.7
Psychotic disorder NOS	2.8
Delusional disorder	1.9
Substance Abuse/Dependence	
Some type of substance abuse/dependence	65.4
Drug dependence	58.9
Alcohol dependence	50.5
Both drug and alcohol	42.1
Somatoform Disorder	
Some type of somatoform disorder	43.9
Somatization disorder	41.1
Pain disorder	28.0
Hypochondriasis	2.8
Somatoform disorder NOS	1.9
Eating Disorder	
Some type of eating disorder	38.3
Bulimia nervosa	27.1
Nonamenorrheic anorexia	15.0
Anorexia nervosa	8.4

Table 6.8.   Lifetime Axis II Disorders in 103 Dissociative
Identity Disorder Patients on the Structured Clinical
Interview for DSM-III-R (SCID-II)

Diagnosis	Percent
Borderline	56.3
Avoidant	48.5
Self-defeating	46.6
Paranoid	43.7
Dependent	39.8
Compulsive	35.9
Schizotypal	27.2
Antisocial	23.3
Passive-aggressive	12.6
Narcissistic	12.6
Histrionic	8.7
Personality disorder NOS	8.7
Schizoid	5.8

being interviewed by research psychiatrists. One of the patients was a suicidal middle-aged man who heard voices in his head, and thought he was
going crazy, but who displayed no illogical thinking. He reported blank
spells lasting half a day in which he had a vague intimation that he did
things very out of character. He was a drinker. Although a possible diagnosis was alcohol hallucinosis, this man probably has DID. The diagnosis
could probably be established in less than half an hour if the right questions
were asked.

I mention this vignette to illustrate that well-trained, research-oriented
psychiatrists miss cases of DID on a regular basis. This is not because they
are stupid or incompetent. It is because they have been trained to think that
DID is rare and have not trained to ask the necessary questions to establish
the diagnosis. Similarly, the most rigorous application of *DSM-III-R* diagnostic rules for psychosis, using the SCID, results in a false-positive diagnosis in three quarters of DID patients. Of all the diagnostic errors in
psychiatry, a false positive diagnosis of schizophrenia is probably the most
dangerous, and the most difficult to reverse. It can lead to a self-fulfilling
prophecy of lifetime medication, and deteriorating function in the absence
of correct treatment.

I used to think that it was the DID patient's voices that lead to a false
positive diagnosis of schizophrenia, and stated this in print (Ross & Fraser,
1987). I was wrong, at least according to the available data. In our series of
236 cases, we compared cases with and without a past diagnosis of schizophrenia (Ross & Norton, 1988). The cases did not differ in the frequency
with which they experienced auditory hallucinations or thoughts out loud. It
is the other Schneiderian first-rank symptoms of schizophrenia that are

leading clinicians astray. Schneiderian symptoms are very common in DID, and are another diagnostic clue for the disorder (Kluft, 1987b).

In the 236 cases, the average number of Schneiderian symptoms per patient was 4.5. This is similar to an average of 3.4 in a series of 34 DID patients reported by Kluft (1987b). In our 20 cases assessed by structured interview, the average number of Schneiderian symptoms per DID patient was 6.6. This was not significantly different from the average of 4.4 Schneiderian symptoms endorsed by 20 schizophrenics interviewed in the same study (Ross et al., 1989a). I will discuss Schneiderian symptoms and the relationship between DID and schizophrenia further in Chapter Eight.

The quality of the DID patient's auditory hallucinations should be touched on here, though. It is a general rule of thumb that DID voices tend to come from inside the head, while schizophrenics experience their voices as coming from outside. The voices may be commanding and persecutory, and may order the patient to harm herself or others. Alternatively, they may be soothing and reassuring. The two types of voices may discuss the patient, referring to her in the third person. Usually the DID patient does not have a thought disorder, and describes the voices in a lucid manner. The content of the voices' statements is usually not bizarre and "crazy," though it may be.

It is often possible to engage DID voices in an indirect conversation. To do this, the clinician explains to the patient that he wants to try to talk to the voice. The clinician then asks the voice a question, the voice answers, and the patient reports what the voice said. It may be necessary to identify the voice being addressed in the following way: "I want to ask the voice that Mary says sounds like a little girl a couple of questions. I want the voice to answer, and Mary will tell me what the voice said. First I want to know if the voice that sounds like a little girl can hear me." If the patient answers that the voice said, "Yes," the clinician then proceeds with further questions.

Practitioners should always remember that what looks like psychosis could be dissociation. An established psychotic diagnosis should raise the index of suspicion for DID when the patient has had unusual non-*DSM-IV* diagnoses such as "hysterical psychosis" or "hysterical psychotic reaction" or when the diagnosis has shifted back and forth from schizophrenia to schizoaffective disorder, to bipolar mood disorder (especially rapid-cycling bipolar mood disorder), to mood or psychotic disorder not otherwise specified. The shifting clinical picture cannot be captured within one of these diagnostic categories on a stable basis because the true diagnosis is DID, with comorbid depression, unstable mood, auditory hallucinations, and other Schneiderian symptoms.

Mood Disorders

Almost all DID patients (98.1%) meet lifetime criteria for a mood disorder, and most inpatients with DID are currently depressed. This is true comorbidity and will appear as such clinically and on all self-report and physician-administered measures of depression. The only false-positive diagnoses are some of the bipolar diagnoses, which resolve on successful psychotherapeutic treatment of the DID, and are due to switching-related mood instability.

There are no systematic drug trials of any kind in DID, but the newer serotonin reuptake blocker antidepressants are very useful in DID. They work as antidepressants and can also help the anxiety, PTSD, and compulsive and addictive symptoms. Depression in DID can get incorrectly subtyped as psychotic due to the voices and other Schneiderian symptoms but a careful history will show that the voices persist for long periods in the absence of active mood symptoms. This persistence of voices can then push the diagnosis over to schizoaffective disorder: The clue that schizoaffective disorder is also incorrect is the lack of negative symptoms and thought disorder.

A frequent error of nonmedical therapists is to persist with "memory work" and abreaction when the patient is deteriorating—very often the patient is clinically depressed by the time an admission occurs. Our inpatient treatment then involves both an antidepressant and a restructuring of the psychotherapy.

Anxiety Disorders

PTSD occurred in 79.2% of 72 DID patients who completed the Diagnostic Interview Schedule in our study. As discussed in Chapter Eight, I do not consider PTSD to be an anxiety disorder, so I will not discuss it further here. The other anxiety disorders occur in 91.4% of DID patients. Clinically, they occur in two overlapping clusters: a panic-generalized anxiety-phobic cluster, and an obsessive-compulsive cluster. Virtually all DID patients suffer from severe anxiety symptoms in the first cluster during the initial phase of therapy.

The obsessive-compulsive symptoms experienced by DID patients are nearly always dissociative in nature and due to the intrusions of alter personalities into the awareness and motor control of the host personality. Therefore they respond to psychotherapy. However, they may also respond partially to serotonin reuptake blockers and/or buspirone.

Substance Abuse

Substance abuse is a big problem in DID, occurring in 65.4% of cases on the SCID. This is consistent with clinical experience. Reciprocally, dissociative disorders are frequent in chemical dependency populations, as outlined in the previous chapter. A large subgroup of DID substance abusers are consciously using substances to dampen down their psychological pain. They are self-medicating their trauma histories and comorbidity, and reinforcing their dissociation. Often there will be specific alter personalities that abuse substances, but it is also common for the host personality to be psychologically addicted.

As in other populations, withdrawal states can be misunderstood as psychotic, anxiety, or dissociative symptoms. Also, substance-driven symptoms can be misinterpreted as dissociative. It is common to have inpatients on our Unit who have been clean and sober for years, and who are active in Alcoholics Anonymous, others who have never abused substances, and others who are current active users, so generalizations to the whole population are not possible. Treatment of the current active abuser involves a chicken-and-egg analysis of whether the dissociative disorder or the substance abuse should be the primary target, so usually the two are addressed concurrently. As shown in Chapter Eleven, the treatment outcome of DID in terms of substance abuse is excellent.

Somatic Symptoms

In our series of 102 DID cases, patients reported an average of 15.2 (*SD* 7.3) *DSM-III-R* somatic symptoms, and 60.8% met criteria for somatization disorder. In our series of 103 patients, 41.1% met criteria for somatization disorder, while in our series of 236 cases, 18.8% had received a prior diagnosis of somatization disorder. Although the figures vary from series to series depending on the method of assessment and the population, it is established that DID patients are highly somatizing. These are the "body memories" referred to by therapists.

When we compared 50 DID patients and 50 patients with confirmed multiple sclerosis on the DDIS (Ross, Fast, Anderson, Auty, & Todd, 1990), we found that the DID patients had significantly more abdominal pain, nausea, palpitations, amnesia, intolerance of foods, vomiting, bloating, chest pain, pain during intercourse, and pain in the genitals. The multiple sclerosis patients reported significantly more trouble walking and paralysis or muscle weakness.

The findings in the multiple sclerosis study made sense and were consistent with all other research and clinical writing in the field, which I reviewed elsewhere (Ross, 1994a). DID patients report somatic symptoms primarily in the gastrointestinal and genitourinary systems, plus anxiety-related somatic symptoms. This makes sense because the gastrointestinal and genitourinary are the two body systems that bore the brunt of the sexual trauma. Clinically, the psychosomatic symptoms appear to be the ones most directly linked to the childhood sexual abuse.

In another study (Siemens & Ross, 1991), we compared patients in treatment for three different groups of disorders: (a) irritable bowel syndrome (b) Crohn's disease and ulcerative colitis, and (c) other gastrointestinal disorders. The irritable bowel group reported three times the frequency of childhood sexual abuse as the other two groups (37.9% compared with

9.1% and 11.6%). The rates of somatization disorder in the three groups were (a) 20.7%, (b) 3.0%, and (c) 2.3%. Although this study needs to be replicated and extended, it appears that psychosomatic symptoms are related to childhood sexual abuse. It is also clear from the data that childhood sexual abuse is only one pathway to somatization.

In the only study I am aware of evaluating women with a primary diagnosis of somatization for childhood sexual abuse, Morrison (1989) found a reported history of sexual abuse in 60% of 60 subjects. Overall, then, clinical experience and the existing data indicate that somatic symptoms are related to childhood sexual abuse both inside and outside DID, and that DID patients illustrate this relationship because of their extensive trauma histories.

Eating Disorders

The SCID data on eating disorder comorbidity in DID are deceptive, and underestimate the scope of the problem. I think this is true for several reasons. Although 38.3% of DID cases meet formal criteria for an eating disorder, the vast majority have seriously unhealthy eating patterns. They eat junk food excessively, cannot socialize normally at restaurants or dinners, binge occasionally, have trauma-related phobic responses to certain foods, and are often obese. If one included pathological overeating and these other disordered eating behaviors, I would guess that at least 80% of DID patients have serious problems with food. As is true of eating disorders in general, I think that DID patients hide their *DSM-IV* eating disorders more often than any other form of comorbidity. The frequency of frank observable anorexia nervosa of 8.4% seems about right to me, since excessive weight loss cannot be hidden.

The eating disorders are almost always directly related to trauma-driven cognitive errors, a common one being *If I am fat (or thin) perpetrators will not come after me*. Based on clinical experience, I suspect that the eating disorders respond less well to treatment focused on the DID than does the substance abuse, mainly because the eating disorders are much more reinforced by the culture.

Personality Disorders

The average person admitted to our inpatient unit meets lifetime SCID criteria for 3.6 (*SD* = 2.5) different personality disorders, in addition to 7.3 (*SD* = 2.5) Axis I disorders. This average of 10.9 lifetime psychiatric disorders on the SCID does not include PTSD, dissociative, sleep, or sexual and gender identity disorders, none of which are diagnosed by the SCID. The literature on the difficulty of dual diagnosis patients is amusing to me, since we never see such simple cases on our Dissociative Disorders Unit.

Among the anxiety disorders, Cluster C diagnoses are the most common, Cluster B intermediate, and Cluster A most uncommon: 39.7% of our patients meet criteria for a diagnosis from each of the three clusters. These data obviously don't make sense, since a patient cannot in reality suffer from three or four different personality disorders at the same time, given that even DID patients have only one personality. The *DSM-IV* Axis II conceptual system obviously doesn't make sense, if the personality disorders are supposed to be separate entities. My solution to this problem is proposed in Chapter Eight.

I will also discuss the relationship between DID and borderline personality disorder in Chapter Eight.

Clinically, DID patients fall into one of three Axis II groups: (a) no serious character pathology or management problems, only occasional or no inpatient care required preintegration and none postintegration, (b) an intermediate group with more severe Axis I and II pathology early in treatment but a good prognosis, and (c) a group in which character pathology and treatment-resistant Axis I symptoms predominate, resource utilization is high, and prognosis poorer. This pattern can be seen in all Axis I sections of *DSM-IV.*

An important consequence of the DID diagnosis is that many people regarded as high-character pathology/poor prognosis cases by other psychiatrists prove to have a good prognosis when the DID and the childhood trauma are addressed systematically by a skilled treatment team.

Sexual and Sleep Disorders

I do not have any systematic data on sexual and sleep disorders in DID, but both are extremely common. The sleep disorders include trouble going to sleep and staying asleep, early wakening, and excessive sleep, as well as trauma-driven phobic avoidance of sleep and nightmares. Deciding whether to attribute the sleep problems to anxiety, depression, dissociation, PTSD, or surreptitious substance abuse can be impossible, but fortunately serotonin reuptake blockers cover most of the bases.

Disorders of desire, arousal, and orgasm are virtually universal in DID, and often respond dramatically and fully to DID treatment. At the same time, good sexual adjustment can be maintained by certain alters and preserved through dissociation in many cases. DID patients often need a great deal of basic education about normal sexuality. In many cases, inhibited sexuality and promiscuous acting out can coexist, with different alters responsible for each.

Amnesia

The final nonspecific diagnostic clue is blank spells. Like childhood trauma, blank spells occur in virtually all cases of complex childhood-onset DID. Some patients do not remember having had blank spells and are "amnesic for their amnesia," as Kluft puts it. Others may fill the blank spells with confabulation, or be so afraid to acknowledge them that they will deny amnesia. Besides voices in the head, the blank spells are often the symptom that most frightens patients. The blank spells and the voices make patients think they are going crazy. I always begin my inquiry about blank spells with open-ended, general questions about "trouble with your memory," and then make my questions more and more detailed and specific.

Classical DID blank spells have a discrete onset and ending. They may vary from seconds or minutes to hours or days. Some patients have amnesic episodes of years, periods when other alters were continuously in control. Since the blank spells are really specific features of DID, once the differential diagnosis has been pursued, I will discuss them in more detail.

Headache

A final common feature of DID is headache, occurring in 78.7% of cases. The headache is often associated with switching, so that headache followed by a blank spell is a strong clue for DID.

DID headaches are complicated, like much else about the disorder. They may be migraine, tension, or mixed (Packard & Brown, 1986). I have seen DID migraine respond to prophylactic ergotamine, and tension headache unaffected by huge amounts of aspirin or acetaminophen. The switching headache may be distinct from the migraine, and the headache may dramatically resolve on integration. Alternatively, one kind of headache may resolve at integration, while another persists.

There are a number of nonspecific diagnostic clues for DID, then, which, when they occur together, make DID by far the most likely diagnosis. In fact, I would say that nearly 100% of the patients who present with these features have classical DID:

1. History of childhood sexual and/or physical abuse.
2. Female sex.
3. Age 20–40.
4. Blank spells.
5. Voices in the head or other Schneiderian symptoms.
6. Meets or nearly meets *DSM-IV* criteria for borderline personality.
7. Previous unsuccessful treatment.
8. Self-destructive behavior.
9. No thought disorder.

This list summarizes the main features of DID that are not specific for the disorder. Most complex multiples exhibit most of these features, whether male or female. The list, like DID patients, touches on most of the content of a general textbook of psychiatry.

FEATURES SPECIFIC FOR DISSOCIATIVE IDENTITY DISORDER

DID is an unusual disorder in that it can almost be diagnosed from a constellation of nonspecific signs and symptoms. The important word is *almost*. You don't have a case of DID until you have talked to the alters. There is an exception to this rule when clear, reliable collateral observation of alter personalities is available. Certainly, from a research point of view, no subjects should be included in studies as having DID if alters have not been observed directly by a reliable professional.

Strictly speaking, the only specific features of DID are the *DSM-IV* criteria. Once these are met, DID is the only possibility, other than malingering. A group of secondary features are specific for the disorder, though, and need to be inquired about. These are the secondary features of DID listed in the DDIS (see Appendix A). These features are evidence of the existence, activity, and influence of the alters. They all follow logically from the existence of alter personalities that take control of the body, and for which the presenting personality is amnesic.

The frequency of the secondary features of DID in our series of 102 cases is shown in Table 6.9. Bearing in mind the need for replication in other samples, these figures are the frequencies at which the secondary symptoms are endorsed at the time of diagnosis of the DID.

I will describe some of the secondary features of DID in more detail.

Amnesia

As previously stated, the patient will describe blank spells. These may have a pattern, or may appear to be random. For example, a patient may state that she always seems to blank out whenever a male approaches her sexually. Later, one can learn about the life history and motivation of the sexually promiscuous personality responsible for these spells. Alternatively, the responsible personality may be assaultive and hostile to men. The triggers for blank spells are the triggers for switching.

Examples of triggers for switching include a color, touch, sexual arousal, the need to perform a specific function, the company of certain people, a specific emotion such as fear or anger, looking in the mirror, hearing a baby cry, a phone call from a past abuser, physical pain, having a bath, and a psychotherapy appointment. Alters hostile to therapy may take control shortly before an appointment, and relinquish it after the hour is up. This may result in confused phone calls from the patient inquiring about whether she was at her appointment.

As one can see from the list, the triggers for blank spells are infinite in number, and often related to specific details of the childhood trauma. In behavioral terms, the treatment can be thought of as a desensitization to these triggers, combined with exposure to the avoided internal stimuli, which are memories and feelings. Whether or not the therapist identifies

Table 6.9.   Secondary Features of Dissociative Identity Disorder in a Series of 102 Cases

Secondary Feature	Percent
Another person existing inside	90.2
Voices talking	87.3
Voices coming from inside	82.4
Another person taking control	81.4
Amnesia for childhood	81.4
Referring to self as "we" or "us"	73.5
Person inside has a different name	70.6
Blank spells	67.7
Flashbacks	66.7
Being told by others of disremembered events	62.8
Feelings of unreality	56.9
Strangers know the patient	44.1
Noticing that objects are missing	42.2
Coming out of a blank spell in a strange place	36.3
Objects are present that cannot be accounted for	31.4
Different handwriting styles	27.5

himself as a behaviorist, a thorough analysis of the triggers for switching is part of the treatment.

When sustained, organized behavior in an alert state is reported by observers, during a period for which the patient is amnesic, DID is really the only possibility. Only those desperate for an organic explanation for everything will cling to epilepsy as a possible diagnosis. A related misdiagnosis is the fiction of murder committed by a somnambulist. In a case in Ontario (Sneiderman, 1988), a man got out of bed in the night, drove 23 kilometers (about 14 miles), crossing nine traffic lights, and killed his mother-in-law. He was examined by five psychiatrists and let off on the grounds that he was sleepwalking. This seems to me a more serious clinical and legal error than any defense related to DID.

The five psychiatric witnesses were reported to have ruled out fabrication because of the consistency of the man's reports of amnesia. One psychiatrist was quoted as saying that the sleepwalker's brain is "effectively in a coma," and another that the killing was "unconscious activity, uncontrolled, and unpremeditated." Since I have access only to a newspaper editorial by a law professor describing the case, I cannot challenge these five expert witnesses. Let me tell a story, though.

I was referred a patient who had been treated for epilepsy with medication for 20 years, as described in more detail in *The Osiris Complex*. She was referred to me for an opinion as to whether her seizures might be panic attacks. The "seizures" consisted of her waking up in the night terrified and disoriented. She spoke only French, did not recognize her family, and tried to run away. She was amnesic for these spells. She also had short memory blanks during the day, and would sometimes come to with bruises, lying on the floor, or in another room. Epilepsy? Sleepwalking? If she killed someone in this state, would that mean her behavior was unconscious, uncontrolled, and unpremeditated? You wouldn't know until you examined the altered state.

In this case, the "seizure" state was a child alter personality who could easily be called out. She was unaware of the passage of time since the sexual abuse in her childhood, was frightened that the abuse was about to begin again, and spoke rationally with us. The child alter remembered us immediately when called out in a second session. She spoke only French because the woman had not learned English until chronologically older than the age of the alter. The amnesia barrier between the child personality and the adult was easily lowered, and an explanation was given that this was a special kind of dreaming. A more complete explanation would have been given, but the patient declined psychotherapy.

I find it very doubtful that anyone could drive 14 miles and murder his mother-in-law while asleep, in a coma, or sleepwalking. The amnesia barrier should be breached in the Ontario case. The most likely diagnosis is a dissociative disorder, although not necessarily full DID. The behavior may recur if the man is not treated, or alternatively, this may not be the first murder. These are the possible consequences of mental health professionals not learning about DID. Apparently, sleepwalking has been used as a successful defense against homicide in 50 cases in legal history. Subjects diagnosed as suffering from somnambulism (or sleepwalking disorder, as it is called in *DSM-IV*) should be carefully screened for dissociative disorders (Kales et al., 1980).

The blank spells may not be complete. Instead they may consist of "fuzzy" periods of partial recall. This represents the memory component of the presence of an alter, just as depersonalization may represent the identity component, and made impulses the behavior. Such fuzzy periods should not be dismissed as due to drugs or alcohol, even when a patient abuses both. DID blank spells may be mistaken for alcohol blackouts (see Chapter Eight) and may occur *prior* to alcohol ingestion in a carefully taken history. This was the case for the man I watched being interviewed on videotape by a research psychiatrist.

Another variation of the blank spell is one that is contracted for during treatment, which by definition does not occur on a spontaneous basis prior to diagnosis. An example of this is the "playback" of a memory. During treatment, one may contract with an alter to allow the amnesic host personality to remember the conversation, or a specific memory, or all memories held by the alter. One switches back to the host, and waits while she gets the memory back as an internal videotape.

The blank spells have usually occurred over an extended period but there may be spans of years in the past when the alters were quiescent. A variation on this is the patient who reports a period of years during which she experienced frequent depersonalization but no amnesia: During this time the alters were copresent without amnesia. Or the DID may simply have gone into remission (Kluft, 1985e). A general rule in DID phenomenology is that all possibilities have happened to some patient somewhere.

The periods of missing time may be of any length from minutes to years, but usually are for a few hours at a time, up to a couple of days. The clinician wants to clarify if possible whether the blank spell had a clear onset and offset, like someone throwing a switch. Some patients describe a much fuzzier dawning of awareness that several hours appear to have gone by that cannot be accounted for. When the blank spells are vague and short and there is no change of location, it can be impossible to differentiate them from lack of concentration, or unstructured "spacing out." The main point about all the secondary features is that in a fully active DID case they will occur in both vague and sharply crystallized forms. The interviewer must focus on the sharply defined symptoms to diagnose full DID. There are no data on the relative frequencies of the secondary features on the four different pathways to DID.

The discrete blank spells are often accompanied by a massive, general amnesia for childhood that cannot be attributed to the presence of any one personality. This is a form of amnesia similar to the amnesia for childhood in patients who do not have complex dissociative disorders, but who were abused as children. Here, again, the differentiation of a diagnosable dissociative disorder from normal childhood amnesia can be difficult or impossible. In a clear case, the patient will describe a complete absence of all memory prior to age 12, and a sudden onset of memory at a specific time; a period of amnesia from age 9 to 12, with normal memory before and after; inability to recall major family events recalled by both younger and older siblings; or other patterns of amnesia clearly out of the range of normal in the absence of any discernible organic cognitive problems.

An individual personality can have amnesia for her own experience: I had to hypnotize an alter to recover memories of repeatedly entering her parents' bedroom in a trance, as an adolescent, with a knife, in the middle of the night. The sexual abuse by these parents continued into the patient's 20s by her report and, she alleged, included being raped by a man her father hired for the purpose. If this girl had killed her father, would that have been sleepwalking, insanity, or justifiable homicide? Murder or self-defense? This alter had blank spells that coconscious alters also experienced. In this case, I have not been able to decide how many false memories occurred and how much was accurately reported trauma, and the patient has been lost to long-term follow-up. Sometimes an alter may simply repress a memory in the usual psychodynamic fashion.

One consequence of these complex distortions of memory is that the integrated multiple has trouble understanding what normal forgetting should be like. She may ask whether it is normal not to remember minute details from early childhood, or all of last week's daily activities. Other distortions of memory besides amnesia also occur. One of these is hypermnesia, which is unusually complete memory. The DID patient has an incredible volume of detailed childhood memories stored in her alter personalities.

The quantity of memory presents a problem: how much is accurate recall, and how much is elaboration? This problem should be solvable with the techniques of cognitive psychology. Often the details of abreacted abuse are confirmed by sisters who witnessed or were victims of the same abuse (to witness is to be abused). DID patients provide a rich field for investigation by the cognitive psychologist interested in normal and/or abnormal mental function.

The way in which traumatic and normal memory are processed in the DID patient is analogous to the processing and repair of DNA: There can be inversions, deletions, insertions, repair errors, reading errors, replication errors, virtually any type of error one can imagine. The mind of the DID patient is like a laboratory in which all the properties of human memory are demonstrated in extreme detail and complexity, including accurate recall.

When the patient is fully amnesic for times when other personalities are in control, several associated phenomena occur. These are probably highly culture-bound. Let me give an example from the anxiety disorders that will illustrate this point: I flew to a native community in northern Manitoba on a regular basis from 1983 to 1991 to do consultations. I saw quite a few native people with classical panic attacks that were indistinguishable from those that affect urban whites. But I didn't see the same kind of agoraphobia. That was because there were no buses, elevators, traffic lights, huge crowds, or other agoraphobic stimuli to avoid in the isolated northern community. There is a parallel with DID.

DID patients often report that they come out of a blank spell in another location, for example in a bar in the company of strangers. They report that strangers claim to know them, or call them by a different name. This couldn't happen in an isolated native community in which there were no strangers. Friends tell them about things they have done, which they don't remember. All of this is evidence of the activity of alter personalities in a complex urban society.

The patient may state that objects are frequently missing, including money. Alternatively, objects may be present in her environment that she can't account for. Again, these symptoms could not occur in a culture without bank accounts, stores, and the acquisition of consumer goods. Kluft (1985b) has pointed out that these features are likely to be muted or absent in urban childhood DID because children do not have the independence and mobility of adults. Similarly, a DID patient in a wheelchair in a nursing home would have fewer secondary features than in earlier years.

The secondary features of DID all occur at a very low baseline frequency in the general population; for example, everyone forgets where they put something, or may occasionally be recognized by a stranger. In the DID patient, these symptoms occur far more frequently and in much more elaborate detail than in anyone else. For example, a patient described being in line to buy a ticket at a movie theater when the woman ahead of her turned around, greeted her, and talked about the two-hour luncheon they had had together the previous week. The stranger knew the woman by name and knew many details of her life, but the patient was completely amnesic for ever having met this person before.

Similarly, it is far outside the range of normal experience for a person to suddenly come out of a blank spell dressed in unfamiliar clothing, driving in a part of town she would never go to alone. If one adds that the clothing appears to be hooker's garb, and there are drugs on the front seat, when the patient is monogamous and has never used drugs or alcohol, then it is clear that this experience is a psychiatric symptom. Such experiences are reported only by DID patients.

Speaking of Oneself as "We" or "Us"

A diagnostic cue for DID that is mentioned throughout the literature is speaking of oneself as "we" or "us." Speaking about oneself in this way can't happen if the presenting personality is unaware of the existence of the other personalities, which may be the case at diagnosis. As in any therapy, patients pick up the jargon of the school of therapy. Patients in a behavioral group for agoraphobia talk about "exposure" and "avoidance." Similarly, DID patients well into treatment talk about "switching" and "integration," and refer to themselves as "we" or "us." I was surprised that this secondary feature was endorsed by 73.5% of our 102 cases because I had assumed that it was more an artifact of therapy than a preexisting symptom, and I am still somewhat suspicious that this is so.

Trance, Sleepwalking, and Imaginary Companions

Although I am skeptical about sleepwalking as an explanation for the murder in Ontario, DID patients report histories of sleepwalking more frequently than patients with schizophrenia, panic disorder, or eating disorders (Ross et al., 1989). This argues for the classification of sleepwalking as a dissociative disorder that may occur as a physiologically based developmental lag in otherwise healthy individuals, or as a feature of a complex dissociative disorder in traumatized children. The author of *Macbeth* considered sleepwalking to be a symptom of profound psychological disturbance. In our series of 102 cases, 55.9% reported sleepwalking, 92.0% going into trances, and 48.0% imaginary companions in childhood.

DID patients enter trance states spontaneously more often than patients from other diagnostic groups. Going into trances may be a good predictor of DID in children (Goodwin, 1985; Kluft, 1985b). The person may look "spaced-out," or as if she is daydreaming. While in this state, the person may be nonspecifically blanked out, or an intense, detailed inner interaction between the alters may be going on.

A third related characteristic of DID patients is imaginary companions in childhood (Schultz, Braun, & Kluft, 1985). DID patients have had imaginary playmates in childhood more often than schizophrenics, or patients with panic, depression, or eating disorders. Childhood companions are developmentally normal, but in the DID patient often persist into late adolescence or even adulthood. Some companions may evolve into alter personalities, some disappear with time, and some persist.

Imaginary companions may be human or nonhuman, and exist on a spectrum from conscious fantasy to dissociative hallucination. I assessed an 8-year-old boy who had a "creature" inside him, and who had been mildly sexually abused. At times, he was aware that "the creature" was "just a story, Dr. Ross," but at times it almost seemed real to him. The creature never took executive control but could be engaged in conversation indirectly by my asking it questions, with the boy telling me what the creature had answered. When I asked for the creature to talk directly the boy talked in a squeaky voice and was obviously "putting it on."

When I asked some particularly disturbing questions of the creature, the boy reported that the creature had immediately taken off in a spaceship, and was out of contact. I understood this creature to be a precursor of an alter personality, but at present an internal imaginary companion. Some imaginary companions seem to be able to shift back and forth from inside to outside, while some are always only one or the other. Monsters under the bed or in the closet are related normal childhood phenomena, but may be linked to severe disturbance in the traumatized child.

Changes in Handwriting

Changes in handwriting frequently occur in DID, especially in diaries and journals. The changes may be subtle or obvious. Some child personalities write in large printed letters with childish spelling errors, letter omissions, and letter inversions; sometimes these seem "a bit much" or "put on." Angry alters may leave furious scratchings, or angry statements in a script that embodies their rage. Slant may switch from left to right, and occasionally personalities write in reverse script that has to be read in a mirror. To a naive person, the different scripts look like the handwriting of distinctly different people.

A related diagnostic clue occurs when the alters sign different names, or different forms of the presenting personality's name. Some clinicians deliberately ask their patients to keep a diary and scan it for changes in handwriting. Often the changes in script will be accompanied by references to the author of previous paragraphs as "she." This is even more suggestive of DID. If the patient is amnesic for part of what is in her diary, and there are passages in the first and third persons, the likelihood of DID must be close to 100%.

Sometimes the changes in handwriting, recognition by strangers, objects missing and present, and other secondary features can result in a degree of paranoid thinking. Not aware that she has DID, the patient may think that an elaborate trick is being played on her. Less extreme explanations include the patient's hypothesis that she must have a "familiar face" or that there must be a lot of people who look like her.

Jane Yank (1991) has published the only study known to me in which objective forensic graphology techniques are used to analyze DID handwriting. Graphological studies should be conducted using simulating controls and factitious and iatrogenic pathway cases. This line of research could be paired with other studies of a cognitive-psychological nature, art therapy investigations, or brain imaging studies of alter personalities. The systematic scientific study of DID handwriting is a grossly neglected area of research.

Extrasensory/Paranormal Experiences

Another aspect of DID that differentiates the disorder from other diagnostic groups is extrasensory experiences. DID patients reported an average of 5.6 (SD = 3.3) different ESP experiences in our series of 102 subjects. These phenomena include mental telepathy, telekinesis, clairvoyance, seeing ghosts, poltergeist contacts, and other classical paranormal experiences. I will discuss this in more detail in Chapter Nine. In a study of college students, we found that ESP experiences clustered with diagnostic criteria for DID, secondary features of DID, Schneiderian symptoms, trances, borderline personality, and sexual abuse as a dissociative factor.

ESP is not "respectable" in mainstream psychiatry, but the experiences will be reported by DID patients if inquired about, have differential diagnostic utility, and are interesting in their own right. Whether they are hallucinations of a dissociative nature, or experiences of reality, is not relevant phenomenologically. The first step is to describe and classify the reported experiences, the second to link them to related phenomena, the third to study their etiology, and the fourth to consider the need for treatment. They should not be enshrined as first-rank symptoms of DID but are worthy of serious study by mainstream psychiatry.

These are the main nonspecific clinical features of DID that are relevant for diagnosis. In the rest of the chapter, I am going to describe the features of the personality system in DID, which is highly variable. This is the phenomenology that is most important to understand in planning treatment and which is diagnostically specific. The DDIS symptom clusters characteristic of DID are shown in Table 6.10. I will discuss the Schneiderian and borderline symptoms in detail in Chapter Eight.

Table 6.10. Symptom Clusters Characteristic of Dissociative Identity Disorder on the Dissociative Disorders Interview Schedule (N = 102)

Item	Mean	SD
Somatic symptoms	15.2	7.3
Secondary features of DID	10.2	3.5
Schneiderian symptoms	6.4	2.8
Extrasensory experiences	5.6	3.3
Borderline personality disorder criteria	5.2	2.3

The more of these diagnostically nonspecific symptoms are present, the more likely it is that the person has DID.

FEATURES OF THE PERSONALITY SYSTEM IN DISSOCIATIVE IDENTITY DISORDER

The specific features of DID are the *DSM-IV* diagnostic criteria and the details of the personality system. Once the diagnosis is made and treatment started, both the general psychopathology of the patient, and the features specific for DID, must be taken into account. Both facets of treatment are indispensable for recovery.

The first problem in treating DID is how to think about the personality system. Some of the resistance to the diagnosis is due to nomenclature. What are we saying when we say that a patient has a number of different personalities inside her?

The most important thing to understand is that alter personalities are not people. They are not even personalities. That might seem obvious, but it is a truth one can lose sight of during therapy. It is probably impossible to construct a satisfactory definition of an alter personality, as Stephen Braude (1995) has pointed out in compelling detail. Alter personalities are highly stylized enactments of inner conflicts, drives, memories, and feelings. At the same time, they are dissociated packets of behavior developed for transaction with the outside world. They are fragmented parts of one person: There is only one person. The patient's conviction that there is more than one person in her is a dissociative delusion, and should not be compounded by a *folie à deux* on the part of the therapist.

There is often a lot of drama in DID. This does not invalidate the diagnosis. It is a fact about a serious and treatable form of human suffering. The second thing to remember about the personality system is that it is driven by pain. Despite the color, complexity, and fascinating theater of the personalities, their wars, love affairs, and internal friendships, they are not people, and they exist to help the patient cope with pain. There is no need to be wistful or regretful about the disappearance of an alter on integration, because that is a step toward healing the pain. The patient may mourn the loss of the alter, but the therapist shouldn't.

DID is an elaborate pretending. The patient *pretends* that she is more than one person, in a very convincing manner. She actually believes it herself. Some DID patients enter therapy aware that the different parts are all parts of one person, but most don't. Someone asked me at a workshop once if integration results in a loss of richness and creativity for the patient. Isn't the patient more interesting as a multiple than as a unified person with problems? My answer was to say that the personality system is driven by pain. DID isn't pleasant entertainment. Part of the problem with the iatrogenesis and social-role explanations (which are really dismissals) of DID is that they imply that patient and therapist are having an interesting tea party together, making up mutually satisfying illusions. Therapy is hard work for both parties.

The alters, put another way, are *devices*. Like any theater, the personality system is based on certain conventions and structural rules. Part of the therapy involves mapping and dismantling these, replacing them with normal, happier, and more functional rules and structure. The patient is acting *as if* she is more than one person, but she isn't. This is different from Hollywood acting because the patient is so absorbed in the different roles that she believes in their reality. When I discussed this point with a drama professor, he said that acting students who are too absorbed in their roles become poorer actors. DID is not acting in the sense that Hollywood actors perform a role.

It only takes a moment's reflection on the film industry to realize this. An actor has to do many takes, jump from scene to scene numerous times in a day, start and stop acting instantaneously, make minute adjustments in posture, tone, and facial expression, and carry out numerous other highly controlled actions. If the actor really felt like a cowboy or science fiction hero, he wouldn't be motivated to act and would probably be perplexed as to where he was and what was going on. The actor who became too absorbed in his role would be disoriented and dysfunctional, like the DID personality who comes out of a blank spell in a bar, surrounded by strangers.

The personality system can be organized in any one of an infinite number of ways, or it can lack structure and definition. Some DID patients have highly structured systems with rigid amnesia barriers, defined switching sequences, sharply demarcated switches, and clear-cut identities for the main alters. Others present more of a shifting sea of partial presences and uncertain identities. It is important for the beginning diagnostician or therapist to realize this; otherwise, he may attribute the lack of clarity in the system to his own inexperience.

What are the most common types of personality in DID? In our series of 236 DID cases, we inquired about nine types of alter personality, which were reported to be present in the frequencies shown in Table 6.11.

Table 6.11 indicates that four personality types occur in about 85% of cases. The child personality usually holds the abuse memories, and carries out the most intense abreactions. The personality of different age may be an adolescent, adult, or older than the chronological age of the patient. The protector usually forms a treatment alliance quite readily, while the persecutor personality is hostile and uncooperative. Most persecutor personalities are in fact helpers who are using self-destructive strategies. Details of alliance formation, contracting with the different personality types, and understanding their function will be discussed in Chapters Twelve through Fourteen.

In the series of 236 cases, the average number of personalities identified at the time of reporting was 15.7, compared with 13.3 in Putnam's series of

Table 6.11. Types and Numbers of Alter Personalities Reported in Two Large Series of Dissociative Identity Disorder Cases

Number of Personalities	Ross (N = 236) (%)	Putnam (N = 100) (%)
Mean	15.7	13.3
Median	8.0	9.0
Type of Personality	Ross	Putnam
Child	86.0	85.0
Different age	84.5	—
Protector	84.0	—
Persecutor	84.0	—
Opposite sex	62.6	53.0
Demon	28.6	—
Another living person	28.1	—
Different race	21.1	—
Dead relative	20.6	—

100 cases. This means that the basic personality types often have more than one representative; there may be a large group of children, several helpers and persecutors, and personalities with ages spanning three or more decades. The more exotic personality types occur less often but are not rare.

Child Personalities

Child personalities are often frightened and untrusting. This characteristic is compounded when the child fears abuse by the therapist. Spontaneous abreactions by "hysterical," terrified child alters are a diagnostic clue for DID, and can be difficult to manage. The child may cower in the corner, curl up in a fetal position, suck her thumb, call for mommy, or simply ask, "Who are you?" Some child alters, on the other hand, are poised, confident, and friendly young adults, despite a claimed age of 7 or 8 years. Others are spontaneous, childish, and delightful. Like alter personalities in general, the children can display the full range of human traits and characteristics. Some children may be relatively full-bodied, and capable of a number of different emotions, attitudes, and behaviors. Others may represent a single memory and mood, and may never express anything else.

Another characteristic of child alters that applies to DID personalities in general, is that they may evolve during therapy. Initially hostile and abusive, a child alter may later become a good friend of the therapist, and an ally in treatment.

Each child personality may be an independent entity, or there may be a suborganization of the children. There may be two or three leaders among the children who control the release of memories, abreactions, and amnesia barriers between different children, and the children and the presenting personality. These leaders may be cooperative, or hostile to each other. Since there are innumerable permutations on all these themes, there is no need to attempt an exhaustive list of examples.

The children, again like alter personalities in general, may exhibit differential aging. One child personality may have been 10 years old when created at chronological age 6, and still be 10 years old at chronological age 33. Another may have been a child alter when created at chronological age 6, but have grown up at the same rate as the presenting personality (who, as far as I am aware, always ages at the normal, real-world rate). Most of the time, personalities do not age, or age at the chronological rate. In my experience, it is unusual for an alter to age faster or slower than chronological time, except during hypnotic rituals.

Other possibilities are an alter who ages at the chronological rate for a while, goes into inner hibernation without aging, then remerges to begin aging again. Sometimes personalities may stop aging at a certain point, while others do not have a specified age, or are unsure of their age. Some personalities, usually not children, claim to be ageless, from another dimension, or thousands of years old. Usually, personalities created in childhood that were older than the chronological age of the patient, are protectors, or carry out a specific function, such as prostitution, physical fighting, schoolwork, or housecleaning. By the time the patient is 35, these alters may still be 10 or 12, but usually seem mature for their age.

Many child alters do not actually function at their alleged age level cognitively. They often understand long words, abstract concepts, and moral dilemmas in a way that would be rare for a normal child of that age. Others do seem to have a childish way of thinking. The cognitive function of alter personalities of different ages cries out for systematic study by developmental psychologists. I predict that there will be mixed findings along the lines I have just described.

A scientific demonstration that child alters do not function cognitively at their alleged age would not invalidate DID. It would only prove that they are not real children. Such evidence, however, would challenge the overliteral view, according to which alters represent a concrete fixation in cognitive development. In my view, child alters are not packets of *childness* retained in a surrounding sea of adult psyche. They are stylized packets of adult psyche. That may seem like a hairsplitting differentiation, but it has implications for therapy and for legal accountability and responsibility. I hold the child alters responsible for their behavior in the same way as the adult host personality.

Freud described alters as being in delirium. This was an error. Child alters may appear delirious or psychotic because of their frightened behavior and belief that the present and the past are the same thing. The vast majority of child alters have a clear sensorium, are alert, and are cognitively intact. Treating the undiagnosed DID patient with antipsychotic medication to control the spontaneous emergence of child alters is a serious clinical mistake.

The emergence of a child alter is usually easy to recognize. There is often a change in posture. The toes may be pointed in, head may be bowed, sideways glances may occur, and the hand movements may become tense, fidgety, or childish in some other way. The facial expression can vary widely, depending on the mood state of the personality, but usually has a childish quality. The speech may be lisping, quiet, monosyllabic, whining, lilting, or display any of countless qualities. Childish vocabulary will be used, and, like the handwriting, grammatical errors, or primitive grammar may be used. The topic of conversation will often be immature, as will the content.

One of the most intense aspects of DID treatment is helping the children through their abreactions. During an abreaction, the child alter may beg the parent to stop, scream, cry, express intense sadness, or clutch her lower abdomen. There may be hand movements to push the father out of her vagina, or motor movements accompanying the abreaction of an oral rape. The genuineness and intensity of the abreactions is one of the most compelling features of DID, but it is not evidence that the abreacted events ever actually took place. I have witnessed intense abreactions of events later proven not to have occurred or retracted as false memories. Retraction does not prove that the events never took place, just as recall does not prove that they did.

Occasionally, the practitioner will meet alters alleged to be less than one year old. These alters are usually said to hold specific abuse memories. For me, this is stretching things too far and emphasizes that alters are enactments rather than literal realities. I have been told about intrauterine alters created because of the trauma of a parental argument: these alters are alleged to have understood who the parents were, that fighting is a bad thing, and even to have worried about what life was going to be like after delivery. Patients can find therapists willing to treat such intrauterine dissociation, but not in my program. One patient who appeared to have a false memory of trauma in a crib at age six months later realized that she had slept in this crib until age three: with this information it appeared that the "false" memory could be accurate. The error was to have misattributed the event to the first year of life based on its occurring in a crib.

The therapist shouldn't believe that child alters are really children, anymore than he believes that demon alters are really demons, or that the patient is really possessed by her dead mother when an alter claims to be the mother. On the other hand, clinicians work within the patient's beliefs and worldview to a varying extent. The child alter personalities are always key components of the personality system in terms of the planning of therapy.

Protector Personalities

Protectors come in many forms and protect in many ways. They are usually older than 10, and often are the same age or a bit older than the chronological age. Protectors tend to overlap with another major class of personalities, the observers. This makes sense because in order to protect one must be aware. Some observers, however, make very few if any interventions or communicate their fuller awareness to protectors who carry out the action.

The protectors that form prior to age 10 are often adolescents; these alters may age at the chronological rate, or not age at all. Many adolescent protectors fall into one of two types: relatively calm and mature, or else volatile and aggressive. The calmer ones tend to help by providing a broader range of more mature coping strategies, by controlling switching, by avoiding situations, and by taking steps to stay out of trouble.

The aggressive adolescent protectors can cause serious trouble during the early phases of therapy. They may be responsible for behavior that meets the A criterion for antisocial personality disorder in *DSM-IV* (to have this diagnosis, one must have exhibited at least three behaviors from a 7-item checklist subsequent to age 15), plus the C criterion, which is the presence of conduct disorder prior to age 15. These alters may destroy property in the office, or assault the therapist. Often their aggression is turned inward as well as outward, so that they are simultaneously protectors and persecutors. They may attempt to kill the host personality in a form of misguided euthanasia, reasoning that she has suffered too much in life. They often abuse substances.

Another group of protectors comprises the avoiders, who have a narrow range of skills. Sometimes these alters are children. For example, I have met a child personality that was skilled at hiding from her sexually abusive father. This was all she did. When she hid on the ward once, it took quite a while to find her. Other personalities may be skilled at out-of-body experience, trance states, inner reverie, or other techniques for surviving trauma. Some protectors have no feelings, are physically numb or anesthetic, or come out to block physical abuse by agitated, rocking behavior. These alters embody one or a few skills from the repertoire that any abused child has potentially available.

Adult protectors tend to be more cognitive and rational in their strategies. They may be excellent consultants to the therapist. Sometimes they control switching, and are in charge of who is out at any given time. They in effect match the alter to the task or situation. Adult protectors tend to be less amnesic than child personalities, but this only a general rule. I have had a patient whose protector had the ability to pull all the personalities in, leaving the patient in a catatonic stupor. Such stupor is not uncommon in DID, must represent a primitive survival mechanism, and is not usually as exquisitely well controlled as in this particular patient.

The observer function of the protector can be split off into a pure observer personality, sometimes called the "Observer." Observers tend to be rarefied, abstract, bloodless entities with little or no feeling. This may be a cultural artifact of popular concepts of artificial intelligence: Perhaps in other cultures the observers act more like mystical entities charged with spirit power. In North American clinical DID, the observers often have no direct stake in the outcome of treatment. They simply record and retain memories.

Some North American observers do have mystical pretensions and may be called the "Inner Self-Helper" or "Center" (Comstock, 1987). Some therapists feel that centers have transcendental abilities including healing and psychic powers. Inner self-helpers are both observers and protectors, although some only help by knowing, not by doing. The observers seem to represent a dissociation of memory, but they usually have only a part of the full phenomenon of memory available to them: they have only the information component, not the feeling, the physiological arousal, or the sensory intensity of the memory. These aspects are parceled out to the children and others.

There is probably a connection between inner self-helpers and hidden observers (Hilgard, 1984). The hidden observer is an experimental artifact of hypnosis experiments rediscovered by Hilgard and rigorously studied by him (see Chapter One). In Hilgard's opinion (1984), which is scientifically cautious, it is a mistake to extrapolate too quickly from his experiments to the phenomonology of DID. However common sense dictates that there must be a connection between DID observers and experimental hidden observers that is more than merely semantic.

Persecutor Personalities

The persecutors are often responsible for suicide attempts, "accidents," self-destructive and self-defeating behavior, and outwardly directed aggression as well. They may be antisocial in other ways, including theft, prostitution, and substance abuse. They are often adolescent, but may claim to be demons, dead relatives, or other figures. They often present as tough, uncaring, and scornful, but this is usually just a front for an unhappy, lonely, rejected self-identity. One typical persecutor I worked with was abusing the other personalities because she felt rejected, because she felt they did not appreciate the hard work she did holding all the anger, and because they were always blaming her for everything that went wrong.

Persecutors carry out their hostile attacks on the other personalities by psychic and physical means. They may burn the host personality with cigarettes, cut her wrists, force her to take pills, or jump in front of a truck, then go back inside just before impact, leaving the host to experience the pain. Their motives can vary widely, as I discuss later in my cognitive analysis of DID. It is quite common for persecutors to have a delusion of separateness, and to believe that they can harm another personality's body without their own body being affected. They usually think it is currently a year from the person's adolescence.

Persecutors also cause internal trouble in a variety of ways. They can make another personality hallucinate, feel frightened or anxious, or be disoriented. They may torture the children by tricking them into believing that the boyfriend is really the abusive father, or by locking them up in a room or closet in the patient's inner world. They can cause muscle twitches, pains, and any other symptom imaginable. They may bully or threaten the alters verbally, and may chase them through internal landscapes. One patient had a persecutor alter that was her dead, sexually abusive father; fortunately, there was a tree the children could go to when he was abusing them. The dead father alter could not come near the tree, so the child personalities were safe there.

Parental introject alters are a particularly interesting form of persecutor. Father and mother introjects are about equally common and are based on the defense mechanism of *identification with the aggressor.* They often believe that they are literally the parent, especially when the parent is dead, and often have no idea that they are in their daughter's body or that the daughter is now an adult. Formation of a treatment alliance with these alters involves direct work on the problem of ambivalent attachment to the perpetrator, which I discuss in Chapter Thirteen. One rarely meets parental introject alters who embody the positive parental transference, which would be a parental introject protector. By convention, *introject alter* is a term reserved for alters who identify themselves as a specific figure from the person's past, though all alters are based on varying mixtures of identification, introjection, and incorporation.

Usually, the persecutor's underlying motivation is actually positive. As mentioned earlier, euthanasia is a common rationale for suicide attempts. Persecutors are probably responsible for more positive borderline criteria and more Schneiderian symptoms than any other personality type. That does not make them easy to work with. Most often, the persecutor is a misguided protector whose behavior makes sense within her own worldview: The first challenge to the therapist is to understand the persecutor's universe, and the laws that govern it.

Personalities of Opposite Sex

These are common. In our series of 236 cases, 62.6% had a personality of opposite sex. Since most patients are female, most opposite-sex alters are male; however, males and females do not differ in the frequencies of any of the nine types of personalities we inquired about (Ross & Norton, 1989a). This means that roughly two thirds of DID patients, regardless of sex, have a personality of the opposite gender. There is often more than one per patient.

In my experience, male alters in female DID patients usually serve one of two main functions: They either act as tough protectors, or embody the homosexual drive of the patient. The latter occurs when a female patient has a heterosexual male alter who is sexually attracted to women. Biologically, this alter's sexual activity is lesbian, but psychologically it is heterosexual. The inverse can occur when a male alter in a female patient is homosexual: This alter is sexually attracted to males, and his behavior is biologically heterosexual. In this case, the alter functions as a denial of the patient's heterosexual drive; the homosexual male alter in a female body may allow good heterosexual function and pleasure to occur in dissociation from the patient's morbid fear of intimacy with men. This is an example of the paradoxical cost-benefit of DID, since the person gets but never gets satisfying sexual relations with men. Sometimes the male alter embodies the self-statement, made during the incest, that "There's no way I'm going to be a girl!"

Female DID patients often have alters who exhibit a form of secondary lesbianism; they can't have normal sexual relations with men because of the past sexual abuse by father, uncle, brother, husband, and father's friends. This is perfectly understandable. The alters are therefore sexually attracted to women, but primarily as a way of getting physical intimacy, affection, and warmth. For these alters, sex is a secondary issue in their sexual activity. This is analogous to male heterosexual rape, in which the real issue is power, anger, and revenge, not sex. If the patient has a problem with a self-identity of being homosexual, she may create a male alter to carry out the sexual relations with women, while remaining heterosexual herself. A same-sex homosexual alter is an "alternate" solution to the same problem.

These solutions to problems of sexuality raise a central puzzle about DID. The creation of a heterosexual opposite-gender alter, or a homosexual same-gender alter, solves the problem of how to have sex with persons of the same gender, while maintaining a heterosexual self-identity. Why is an amnesia barrier required, then? The amnesia seems to be a second level of security in the system. But once the amnesia is in place, why have an alter personality? Why not have pure amnesia for heterosexual activity, without DID? The alter could be a second backup system in case the amnesia barrier fails, I suppose. The unsolved problem is: Why it is necessary to create separate identities, rather than having a single self with complex amnesia?

The same combination of possibilities exists in males, but I have spoken with a comparatively small number of female alters in males. One of them described in *The Osiris Complex* (Ross, 1994b) wanted a sex change operation, which was the reason I was consulted on the case (I recommended strongly against surgical reassignment). In female patients, the tough protector is based on a cultural stereotype of the macho male. These alters present as a two-dimensional caricature of the tough male. The model for the caricature is itself a caricature: the television male cop, trucker, or cowboy. Opposite sex alters in women tend to come from Marlboro country. I wouldn't be surprised if opposite-sex alters in females smoke more than opposite-sex alters in males. When the tough protector gets a bit too tough, the patient can end up getting convicted for assault, or worse.

The repertoire of alter personalities is highly culture-bound, as is the repertoire of therapeutic techniques. In our culture, therapists are at particular risk for one form of bad therapy: relating to alters as if they are real people. This may be more likely to occur in North America than in some other cultures because North Americans are accustomed to two-dimensional caricatures on television, in movies, and in popular books. North Americans, such as movie critics and DID therapists, often do not seem to be able to tell the difference between an implausible caricature of a human being, and a fully created dramatic character.

Therapists will have trouble telling the difference between alter personalities and people, if they respond to a television caricature with intense personal feeling, which actually isn't intense or personal. If you can't differentiate television characters from real people, you are more likely to grant DID personalities independent legal and therapeutic status. This doesn't mean that therapists need to be highbrows; they just need to be able to tell the difference between narrow caricature and full humanity. The characters on leading television programs are actually fragment personalities, not real people, and they have the restricted range, simplicity, and shallowness of DID fragments.

All of this is a matter of degree, not of dichotomous absolutes, of the "real" versus the "fake." These days, there can be as much Hollywood in reality as in Hollywood. It is an everyday occurrence in urban North America to observe gestures and facial expressions, and hear phrases learned from television. The influence of advertising, television, and movies on the phenomenology of DID is a subject unto itself, worthy of serious study.

The tough male alter in a female patient will often exhibit posture, facial expressions, and tone of voice, that are less than convincing portrayals of maleness. This is partly because the women have had such disturbed models of maleness in their lives. Some will accept the existence of male alters without a fuss, others will think it deviant, perverted, or "weird" to have men inside them. On the other hand, it can be comforting to have a personal internal bodyguard around in case of emergency.

Other male alters can be playful children. One female patient also described in *The Osiris Complex* (Ross, 1994b) had a boy personality who had not taken executive control since childhood, until I called him out. He was created in childhood when the patient lived on a farm. Each summer, itinerant farm laborers were hired on her parents' and neighboring farms. Each spring, the patient and her sister had their hair cut short, were dressed in overalls, and were called by boys' names for the summer. This was a deliberate strategy on the part of the nonabusive parents to prevent the girls from being sexually assaulted by farmhands. It worked quite well, in the sense that the patient was only assaulted once. She was a highly dissociative child, however, and created an alter with the name the parents used in the summers. The patient did not require further active DID treatment at the time of consultation, and the boy was content to rest quietly inside indefinitely. There was a girl alter who was the victim of the assault.

Opposite-sex alters are easily sensationalized, but the patient has one gender, and no more has a person of opposite gender inside than she has children, demons, or her dead father. Conflict about sexuality and sexual orientation is universal in complex DID: Consistent with classical analytical theory, the opposite-gender alter is both an expression of the conflict and a defense against it. Opposite-sex alters can be integrated with no disturbing effect on primary gender identity.

Less Common Types of Alter Personality

It is my sense, though there are no systematic data, that the more exotic types of alter personality are more culture-bound. I would expect child, protector, persecutor, and opposite-sex alters to occur in most cultures. If opposite-sex alters are linked to childhood sexual abuse, their prevalence in other cultures would depend on whether sexual abuse is an etiological factor for DID in a given society. There is no shortage of demon alters in our culture, since these occur in 28.6% of cases: One might have thought that the demon alter would be a transcultural phenomenon from our point of view.

The demon alter, I believe, occurs in our culture because of a fundamental dissociation at the root of contemporary Christian religion (Ross, 1995a). It is culturally normal for DID patients to create demon alters to embody irreverent, hostile, and "bad" aspects of themselves, and for the "badness" to be linked to sexuality.

This hypothesis is supported by the evolution of demon alters into unhappy secular persecutors, then therapeutic allies, prior to integration. It is scientifically impossible, however, to prove whether demon alters are or are not demons. There is no diagnostic test to determine whether a patient is possessed by a demon, or has an alter personality identified as a demon. Identification of a demon is a matter of faith and experience, and cannot be confirmed or disconfirmed scientifically. Belief in demons is not unscientific—it is *ascientific*.

If a demon writhes and contorts in response to holy water or oil, this does not prove it is a demon, since a psychological entity will play its role correctly, and exhibit the same writhings. ESP powers do not prove possession because there is no proof that ESP is demonic. Likewise, if an entity disappears permanently following exorcism, this does not prove that it was a discarnate entity: The exorcism may simply have functioned as a culturally sanctioned integration ritual for a purely psychological entity. The inverse is true: Successful secular integration does not prove that a true demon was not present, since an integration ritual may work as an exorcism. This is the same logic as that which limits diagnostic inferences in psychiatry based on response to medication (Ross, 1986a; Ross & Pam, 1985).

There is an important corollary of the preceding logic: Treating entities as demons and exorcising them is not less scientific or respectable than secular DID psychotherapy, or than prescribing medication for schizophrenia. Scientifically, the main concern is empirical: Which approach works better for which patients in which cultures? Until there is a scientific way of identifying demons, a pragmatic treatment-outcome approach is the only correct one. If demons don't exist, no other approach will ever be possible since one can't prove that something doesn't exist by failing to detect it.

The Bible describes a test for demons, which is to expel them into a non-human experimental animal assumed not to be prone to suggestion. So far no one has received a grant for such studies.

The evolution of demonic alters over time, as described in Chapter One, implies that they are culturally determined psychological entities. Demons I have met are secular, except that they claim to be demons. They are angry and irreverent, but in a chip-on-the-shoulder kind of way. Sometimes the therapist will be infected with a demonic chill transmitted by the patient, but I have integrated such chilling entities, and found them to be frightened children who are putting on a tough act. So far I have not observed any phenomena that require a theological explanation, although I am ideologically prepared to make such an explanation if it appears to be the best one in a given case.

I predict that the frequency of demon alters varies with geographic area in North America, with more demons in the "Bible belts." DID patients as individuals are probably more likely to have demon alters if they belong to a fundamentalist church, irrespective of geographic location.

Related to demons are numerous types of discarnate entities. These may be beings from other universes, spirit guides, dead people from long ago, astral entities, psychic intrusions, or relatively undifferentiated beings of uncertain origin. It is important not to react to these with naive enthusiasm. Also, it is not necessary to devise a complex classificatory scheme for alters, since this won't guide treatment decisions in any meaningful way and would simply be a catalog of the types of mythical being known in folklore and mythology.

In all cases, clinicians must try to understand the function of the alter, and its overall role in the personality system, then negotiate toward integration. Personalities of different race are similarly culture-bound: I bet there are far fewer black alters in yellow bodies in China than there are black alters in white bodies in the United States.

Personalities identified as another living person or as a dead relative are slightly different from the other less common personality types. They usually represent a clear-cut identification with a person close to the patient. If the identification is with an abuser, the alter will be a persecutor. If it is with a nurturing grandmother, it will be a protector, as mentioned earlier. One patient had an alter that was a seagull named Jonathan. Not surprisingly, this alter soared in freedom above the patient's troubles, much like Jonathan Livingstone Seagull.

We have exorcised one dead grandmother from a patient, as described in *The Osiris Complex* (Ross, 1994b). She had been an abuser. Prior to exorcism, we did extensive "couple therapy" with the patient and her dead grandmother, resolving long-standing issues between them. The grandmother was formally helped to leave the body and ascend to heaven, and reported while departing that she was going into a bright light, and could see people waiting for her there. She also reported a great sense of peace while departing. The exorcism was conducted jointly by a member of our clinic and a chaplain. In this case, the dead grandmother knew only things about her life which the patient knew, and couldn't remember anything about her life the patient didn't know, despite intact cognitive function.

In another case, I judged the commotion caused by a dead mother at home, which consisted of throwing her daughter off the couch and making hostile statements through her mouth, to be yet another histrionic attempt to stay in therapy indefinitely. I declined to do anything about the problem, which resolved spontaneously: This patient has been integrated for about eight years. I mention these cases here, rather than in the chapters on treatment, because of their bearing on conceptualization of paranormal alters in DID. Papers by Allison (1985), Bowman, Coons, Jones, and Oldstrom, (1987), Kenny (1981), and Krippner (1986) provide further commentary on this aspect of DID. Adam Crabtree's (1985) book is the major source.

Structure of the Personality System

The personality system is often highly complex and detailed in structure. At other times, as mentioned previously, it may be fluid and amorphous. To proceed in therapy, it is necessary to know the structure of the system. Some therapists like to diagram the system on paper, others make a few notes, while others rely more on memory. In one way or another, all therapists make a map of the system. It is important to understand that mapping is simply a term for keeping track of what is going on, and is not a special technique in and of itself.

The simplest system is dual personality, represented by two circles with a name, age, and sex for each circle. Dual personality is uncommon in modern clinical series. Simple DID systems with less than 10 alters are usually relatively easy to map. I am only going to describe a few of the principles of organization of DID systems, because general principles are not clarified by exhaustive examples.

One type of system is a simple linear one. In such a patient, the alters, usually not too many in number, can be represented as integers on a line. In one patient with this kind of system, the primary personality was on the left, while the other alters were arranged in chronological order by date of creation, from left to right. To switch from one personality to another, the patient had to internally switch from alter to alter, then stop at the one she wanted to be in executive control. It was not possible to skip alters, and there was a built-in stop instruction at each end of the register, that the patient didn't have to think about. This kind of system is analogous to the way enzymes read up and down DNA.

In another patient, the system was represented by a large number of circles of varying size. This patient drew diagrams on a regular basis to chart her progress in therapy. The sizes of the circles represented the power of the alters. The relative positions represented coalitions and hostilities in the system, with friendly alters close to each other. Both size and position were constantly shifting. Sometimes circles would go inside other circles, representing temporary protection. Circles disappeared on integration of alters. Sometimes the patient put alters in internal hibernation, which she called "putting them in darkness" or "covering them with darkness": Alters in this condition were darkened circles, rather than empty white ones. One personality was represented as a triangle because its name was the Black Triangle. In this personality system there were no defined switching sequences.

Another polyfragmented woman's system consisted of over 300 entities with names and ages, the vast majority of whom we never met. Her personality system was organized into "teams," with a team leader for each team. The leaders were adolescent or adult alters, while team members tended to be children and fragments. Each team loosely represented a certain theme or conflict. As well, this patient had two Centers who did not belong to any team: the Centers dictated the membership of each team to the patient, who recorded them on a large chart. This may be similar to the experience of William Blake, who said that he was only the secretary, while the real authors of his works were independent beings in eternity.

Another case exhibited two interesting phenomena: layering, and rigid switching sequences. In the initial layer of alters encountered, there was the host, a child, and two adolescents. Actually this set of alters existed in two sublayers. The presenting personality (who was also the host) was amnesic for periods when the other personalities were in executive control, while the other three alters were continuously conscious no matter who was out, and could talk with each other. Technically, there was one-way amnesia between the presenting and alter personalities.

If we wanted to talk to the second adolescent alter, Donna, we had to first talk to Janice, the child alter. One could only gain direct access to Donna by switching from Janice to Donna. If Susan, the other adolescent, was out, and one tried to call out Donna, nothing would happen. Likewise, if we were finished talking to Donna, the only personality we could call out next was Janice. If we tried to call out Susan or the host personality, nothing would happen. Switches between the other three personalities could be done in any sequence. We had trouble remembering this patient's switching rules, but the patient always corrected us when we tried to do a switch that was not permitted by the rules of the system. Later in therapy, we discovered that Donna had not disclosed her complete function and knowledge in the complex personality system that unfolded. She was the only alter on her level who was coconscious with alters on higher levels. She communicated with these other alters in secret, without Susan and Janice suspecting anything. The complete personality system in this patient was organized in successive levels, with a one-way amnesia barrier between each level and the one immediately below it. This meant that, with the exception of Donna, who functioned as a kind of back door in the system, in computer terminology, all personalities were coconscious with alters on their own and lower levels, and amnesic for alters on higher levels. We worked through a number of such levels before the patient was integrated.

Layering is a complex strategy for hiding memories and behavior, and its function is usually not difficult to understand. Kluft (1986b, 1988e) has written most of the published work about layering. The switching rules that some patients exhibit are puzzling. In the patient just described, there was no obvious reason why Donna had to be isolated as she was, in terms of switching, although this seemed to be related to her being coconscious with higher levels. Alters one level above Donna were not coconscious of her awareness of alters two levels up and higher, but could listen in on her conversations with Susan and Janice. The switching rules, in my experience, have the impersonal, psychological quality of laws of physics. They are just structural rules of that universe. In this sense, the switching rules are very different from the psychological content held by the alters, or their observable behaviors, which have obvious intrapsychic and interpersonal functions.

Switching rules and system structures greatly interested the late nineteenth- and early twentieth-century students of DID, as exemplified by Morton Prince (1905/1978). These aspects of DID have shifted to the periphery for me over the past eight years: I now see them as incidental, and make less effort to catalog or inquire about them. Most personality systems do not exhibit rigid switching sequences or rules, but most have complex amnesia barriers that must be taken into consideration in therapy.

When there is a change in the structure of the system, either through integration of alters, or removal of amnesia barriers, the system exhibits a discontinuous change. Old rules are gone and new ones appear. As long as the system is stable in any given configuration, though, the rules are immutable. These phenomena occur only in highly structured systems. The apsychodynamic quality of the switching rules, to my mind, is strong evidence in favor of the reality of DID. The rules cannot be explained by suggestion or role theory, because there is no plausible external place for the rules to originate. Someone building a model of DID de novo, with no prior knowledge of the disorder, would be highly unlikely to construct such switching rules. Where do they come from, then? Where do alter personalities come from, and who or what creates them?

This is the fundamental aspect of DID that prompts transcendental hypotheses. Many observers, from Freud to Myers to Estabrooks have had the impression that there seems to be a higher organizing principle or intelligence responsible for the rules and structure of the psyche, that these rules are not created by the ego or executive self. In philosophy, this line of reasoning is known as *the argument from design*. Ancient philosophers argued for the existence of God by saying that a complex creation like the universe must have a Creator, because so much structure, detail, and aesthetic unity could not arise blindly. The argument from design is regarded as a weak one. Despite that, these patients evoke a sense of higher intelligence in the therapist, as they did in Freud (see Chapter One). This is no less so when the patient has an average IQ. The sense of a higher intelligence at work is evoked by the complexity of the system, and the vast quantity of information it organizes, stores, and accesses.

Such thoughts do not occur in the mind of every DID therapist. They occur in mine, but are not stimulated in me by patients with panic disorder and would be incongruous in a book on panic disorder (Walker, Norton, & Ross, 1991). Whether or not one agrees with the thoughts, something about the reality of DID stimulates them. This quality of DID, I think, is directly connected to the paranormal experiences multiples report more frequently than patients with other disorders (see Chapter Eight).

A patient with prominent factitious pathway elements had a personality system that was organized into two "communities," with an amnesia barrier between communities. Each community had four families, and each family had six personalities. In each family, the six personalities were organized in pairs called "sisters." As well, there was an overseer, Observer personality for each system. The chart of the system prepared by the patient had a horizontal line in the middle of the page: There were four vertical columns above and below the line, with the paired sisters in them. The Observers were positioned above the families in each community. Each family also had a "head," who was an adult responsible for management of that family.

In this system, all the antisocial, acting-out personalities were in one community, while the other community prided itself on "never causing any trouble." Although there were no switching rules in this system, the sequence of integrations was highly structured. Sisters were integrated first; the products of the integration of sisters were then fused so that an entire family was integrated; families were then integrated until there was only one personality plus the Observer in each community; the Observers were then integrated with their respective personalities; finally the two personalities representing each community were integrated. The patient would not allow fusions to be attempted out of sequence and said they would not work.

This system exhibited a common feature, which is protector alters assigned to care for specific children. In this patient, this took the form of adults paired with sister children, or adults caring for a pair of child sisters. The major personalities in the system had clearly defined functions, and although there were no defined switching sequences, there was a specific set of "escalations" the alters could go through. One personality was very critical, verbally hostile, and litigious. When she became too angry or threatened, she would switch to a personality called the Destroyer (a common name for persecutor alters). The Destroyer was self-abusive and assaultive. If the situation was particularly serious, the patient would then switch to Flash, who was extremely assaultive, as described in more detail in *The Osiris Complex* (Ross, 1994b).

There was an interesting derivation for Flash's name. Names often make sense: alters can be named by function (the Observer, the Friend, the Evil One); named after a specific person such as the patient's mother; be given a descriptive name that matches one of their qualities (Universe, Spirit, Dream); have the same name as the host; have variants of the host's name (Beth, Bessie, Liz); have no name; be given temporary names in therapy to keep track of everyone (I called one hostile alter Number Six, because she had no name and was the sixth alter identified); be called by the host's name with a prefix (Little Susan, Angry Susan); have the legal middle name as their only Christian name; or other variants. Names may have been deliberately chosen by the alter herself or other alters, or may just be "there," with no personality seeming to be responsible for choosing the name. Alters can also have more than one name.

According to the patient, Flash was so-called because in early childhood the patient was forced to act in child pornography films by her father. A child alter did the acting. A woman watching the filming used to say, "Is a baby, is a baby," repeatedly, in reference to the patient. This became slurred into Isabella, which became the child alter's name. Flash would come out when Isabella was too disturbed by the events being filmed to tolerate any further executive control. This usually occurred when flashbulbs were going off, or when the bright overhead lights were on, hence the name Flash. During the early and mid phases of preintegration treatment, the other personalities would see a blinding flash of internal white light and feel a surge of rage before Flash came out, and were amnesic for Flash's activities. The patient also had a pleasant adult alter with the same name as the woman who said "is a baby."

This patient had many fantastic and obviously false memories, and her DID may have been purely factitious, or a mixture of childhood-onset and factitious. Since her personality system had many of the qualities that evoke theories of a "higher intelligence," one must bear in mind that the higher intelligence could in some cases be nothing more than the patient's psychopathy.

Mapping the system is a way of keeping track of the conflicts and issues that must be dealt with in therapy. It is not an end in itself. Other attributes of the personalities can be recorded on the map as well, such as height, hair color, and hobbies. Personalities can identify themselves as being prettier than other alters, as older, younger, of different race, or varying in any imaginable way. Another form of mapping is to record the cognitive errors made by each of the personalities, and in the system generally. This is what I will focus on in the next section.

THE COGNITIVE MAP OF DISSOCIATIVE IDENTITY DISORDER

The cognitive aspects of DID have not been written about as much as the psychodynamic, although Kluft (1988e) acknowledges their importance and says that he focuses on them during treatment. Only one paper to date

(Caddy, 1985) has presented a case example of a treatment claimed to be specifically cognitive-behavioral in conceptualization. I believe that most or all therapists deal with DID cognitive errors, however. Consequently, Pam Gahan and I decided to define what we thought was the generic cognitive map of DID (Ross & Gahan, 1988a). Like the map of the system's structure, the cognitive map provides information for treatment planning.

In research on cognitive therapy (Beck & Emery, 1985; Beck, Rush, Shaw, & Emery, 1979; Emery, Hollon, & Bedrosian, 1981; Freeman, 1983), several problems have been tackled with preliminary success. One is to show that certain cognitive errors are specific for certain diagnoses. This is important because a lack of specificity would undermine the rationale for cognitive therapy. The efficacy of cognitive therapy for nonpsychotic unipolar depression has been conclusively demonstrated. The efficacy of cognitive interventions in DID has never been studied beyond the anecdotal clinical level, however. This needs to be done.

Another problem in cognitive therapy research is to demonstrate that specific cognitive errors are present when the disorder is active, and absent when it is in remission. If this cannot be shown, the rationale for the therapy is called into question, even if its efficacy has been demonstrated. Cognitive therapists also hope that correcting the cognitive errors specific for the active phase of an illness improves prognosis by reducing relapse.

DID offers an excellent opportunity to demonstrate all these properties of pathological cognitive errors. In DID, as in depression, a set of assumptions or guiding beliefs appear to underlie and drive the disorder, cognitively speaking. These core beliefs arise from the patient's abusive childhood: Usually the person has been brainwashed into believing them by the abusive parents. The core beliefs, like much about DID, are often paradoxical and related to childhood double binds (DID patients frequently put their therapists in double binds, a phenomenon one could call double-binding transference).

The following are two examples of these paradoxes:

1. I am responsible for the abuse.
   I am not responsible for my own behavior.
2. I deserve punishment.
   Why is this happening to me?

DID patients make these statements directly to their therapists. The cognition's are not something one infers about the patient, they are observed verbal behaviors, to use jargon. Often there is a child alter created to be the victim of the abuse who feels responsible for it. The two examples are generic cognitive errors made by DID and non-DID abuse victims.

The core beliefs of the DID patient may be stated as erroneous syllogisms or logical propositions. The propositions, as in depression, and like double binds, often begin with a moral injunction that illustrates one of the classical cognitive errors such as all-or-nothing thinking, personalization, or overgeneralization. An example is:

1. Good children should love their parents.
2. I don't love my parents.
3. I am bad.
4. I deserve to be punished.

This syllogism is not specific for DID and would be encountered in nondissociative traumatized children, adult children of alcoholics, and other groups.

We have identified eight core assumptions in DID, from which a number of cognitive errors are derived. Some of these are specific for DID. The core beliefs are:

1. Different parts of the self are separate selves.
2. The victim is responsible for the abuse.
3. It is wrong to show anger (or frustration, defiance, a critical attitude . . .).
4. The past is present.
5. The primary personality can't handle the memories.
6. I love my parents, but she hates them.
7. The primary personality must be punished.
8. I can't trust myself or others.

Particular cognitive errors are derived from these core assumptions. This is the general structure of cognitive maps: There is a set of hierarchically superior assumptions, and below them in a diagram, a set of derivative cognitions. This is a bit like the axioms and corollaries in Euclidean geometry.

I will now review each of the core assumptions, and the cognition's derived from them in detail:

1. *Different parts of the self are separate selves.*
   a. We have different bodies.
   b. I could kill (or slash, burn, force to overdose) her and be unaffected myself.
   c. Her behavior is not my responsibility.
   d. The abuse never happened to me.
   e. They're not my parents.

These cognition's are statements made by patients and are evident concretely in their behavior. It is common for persecutor alters to have an entrenched delusion of separateness, without which their self-destructive behavior does not make sense. That feature of DID differentiates it from psychosis, despite the presence of delusions; in DID the delusions are rationally derived from erroneous assumptions and are treatable with psychotherapy. The patient can be argued out of her delusions, although this takes substantial effort. The incorrect assumptions made by the patient are comprehensible in the context of her abuse history, and strike the therapist as mistaken rather than crazy.

I will flesh in the map in more detail in Chapters Twelve through Fourteen. Here I am presenting the abstract bones of the map, so to speak.

2. *The victim is responsible for the abuse.*
   a. I must be bad otherwise it wouldn't have happened.
   b. If I had been perfect, it wouldn't have happened.
   c. She deserves to be punished for it.
   d. I've been abused so much I might as well be promiscuous.
   e. She deserves to die and I might as well die too.
   f. If my parents loved me, it wouldn't have happened.
   g. I deserved to be punished for it.

This set of cognitions is linked to both self-destructive and obsessive-compulsive behavior. One alter tries to be perfect, while a persecutor attempts suicide. The phenomenology of DID can be understood as a dissociative strategy for simultaneously maintaining incompatible cognitions. The crazy-making double binds of childhood are manifested isomorphically in the adult DID patient's cognitions, and in the structure and function of her personality system (Spiegel, 1986b). Creating other people inside is an excellent short-term solution to the abused child's problems.

3. *It is wrong to show anger (or frustration, defiance, a critical attitude . . .).*
   a. When I showed anger, I was abused.
   b. If I never show anger, I will not be abused.
   c. I deserve to be punished for being angry.
   d. If I were perfect, I would not get angry.
   e. I never feel anger—she is the angry one.
   f. She deserves to be punished for allowing the abuse to happen.
   g. She deserves to be punished for showing anger.

Many of the cognitive errors in DID, such as (3a) are accurate observations about the realities of an abusive childhood. They become pathological cognitive errors when they are overgeneralized and extended into adulthood, in linkage with the other cognitive errors I am describing. The third core assumption, from a cognitive perspective, results in the presenting personality entering treatment as a nervous, depleted, depressive person, with a restricted range of affect. This is frequently the case. The intense and conflicting welter of conscious feelings in the patient are stored in the children and the persecutors, and can be readily accessed.

4. *The past is present.*
    a. I am 8 years old.
    b. The abuse is still happening.
    c. I am scared.
    d. The doctor is going to abuse me now.
    e. No one will protect me.

These thoughts are linked directly with abreaction, in which one observes the behavioral and affective consequences of the core assumption. Rather than viewing spontaneous abreaction by child alters as ridiculous, hysterical, or attention-seeking behavior, one should attempt to map the associated cognitive errors. Suppression of the abreactions by behavioral and pharmacological means is not good medicine, if that is all that is done.

5. *The primary personality can't handle the memories.*
    a. We have to keep the memories.
    b. You can't tell her about us.
    c. If she has to remember, we will make her crazy.
    d. If she remembers, she won't like us.
    e. The abuse never happened.
    f. They must be sick to think those things happened.
    g. My parents are not like that.
    h. She is weak—I am strong.

This set of cognitions drives the amnesia barriers. Often, the patient will enter therapy with an idealized picture of the parents and amnesia for the abuse. The amnesia is maladaptive in adulthood because, like other aspects of the disorder, it makes balanced, intimate adult relationships difficult: Only a part of the person is available to become engaged in any relationship. Besides that, negotiating one's way through the day with missing chunks of time is logistically complicated, and difficult to orchestrate smoothly. The alters in the background will often go to great lengths to maintain the amnesia, and to resist the removal of amnesia during treatment. This is why a treatment alliance must be formed with as many alters as possible.

6. *I love my parents, but she hates them.*
    a. She is the bad one.
    b. You have to get rid of her.

   c. Nobody could ever be friends with her (or like her).

   d. She wants to hurt me.

The core assumptions and their cognitions are interlinked and overlap in a complex network. Sometimes the core assumptions appear to be derived from each other, or from their cognitions. For example, the sixth core assumption cannot be made prior to the first, which is the assumption that leads directly to the diagnostic criteria for DID. It is not necessary to make endless decisions about which assumptions and cognitions are primary, and which secondary, because one is dealing with a field, a complex region of positive and negative feedback loops and other regulatory mechanisms.

The different cognitions will be stated sequentially by different alters, with accompanying affect, facial expression, and gesture. The linkages between the different thoughts, their ownership by different alters, and their function in the system, can only be mapped over a series of sessions. Like everything else about the treatment of DID, cognitive mapping takes time.

   7. *The primary personality must be punished.*

     a. It's her fault the abuse happened.

     b. She deserves all the bad things that happen to her.

     c. Everything bad that happens to her happens because she is bad.

     d. She has suffered enough—she would be better off if I killed her.

     e. I can punish her and be unaffected myself.

     f. I (the punishing alter) was never abused.

     g. Nobody would ever want to be close to me (persecutor alter).

     h. I am unlovable.

These cognitions are usually and mostly held by persecutor personalities. They provide good examples of attributional error. An attributional error occurs when one attributes the cause of an event to the wrong thing. Misattributions are influenced by culture, social situation, the individual's cognitive set, and life experience (a short list). The most pervasive misattribution in DID, which is not diagnostically specific, is blaming oneself, or another part of oneself, for the abuse; I call this *the locus of control shift*. The complete analysis of the locus of control shift is reserved for Chapter Thirteen. The locus of control shift-driven attributional errors are associated with ongoing entrenchment in the abuse victim role. They probably occur more frequently among residents of shelters for battered wives, for example, than in the general population.

   8. *I can't trust myself or others.*

     a. People have always abused me.

     b. I always end up choosing abusive relationships.

     c. I want to be abused.

   d. My parents were never consistent with me.
   e. Previous doctors wouldn't believe me (concerning abuse history and diagnosis).
   f. Whenever anybody gets close to me, they leave.
   g. She trusted before and she got hurt.
   h. We won't let anyone get close to her.
   i. I can't trust her—she gets herself in situations she can't handle.

The eighth set of cognitions is more likely to be stated by protectors than persecutors. It also tends to be more pervasively endorsed, in its various permutations, by the entire personality system, which is highly defended against adult intimacy. The issue of trust is a major one throughout therapy; the trustworthiness of the therapist may be tested beyond its breaking point.

This description of DID cognition is an outline of the rich, human detail of therapy. The basic outline of the phenomenology of DID, which has a cognitive aspect, is a necessary, but not sufficient, tool for successful DID therapy. Generous amounts of other principles are also required.

CONCLUSION

DID patients display great variability in their lives, symptoms, cognitions, and personality systems. There are always exceptions, and there is no way that "it has to be." The phenomenology of DID attests to the ingenuity, range, and creativity of the human imagination. Another truth is also important: There are patterns and consistency in the phenomenology that make valid and reliable diagnosis possible. DID has a stable set of core symptoms throughout North America. The instruments for making the diagnosis detect this consistent pattern, and are the subject of the next chapter.

DID can be suspected based on nonspecific symptoms and cognitive errors, diagnosed with virtual certainty based on the specific symptoms and cognitive errors, and then confirmed through direct observation of alter personalities.

CHAPTER SEVEN

Structured Interview and Self-Report Measures of Dissociation

A number of publications describe instruments developed for the self-report measurement of dissociation (Bernstein & Putnam, 1986; Riley, 1988; Ross, Norton, & Anderson, 1988; Sanders, 1986), and one instrument has been presented at a conference only (Dyck & Gillette, 1987). Two structured interviews for diagnosing dissociative disorders have been tested and published, one of which is the Dissociative Disorders Interview Schedule (DDIS) developed by my team in Winnipeg (Ross, Heber, Norton, et al., 1989). Marlene Steinberg, a psychiatrist at Yale, developed the Structured Clinical Interview for *DSM-IV* Dissociative Disorders (SCID-D) (Steinberg, 1987, 1993, 1994, 1995; Steinberg, Howland, & Cicchetti, 1986).

I am going to focus on four of these instruments, the Dissociative Experiences Scale (DES: Bernstein & Putnam, 1986; Ross, Norton, & Anderson, 1988), the Structured Clinical Interview for *DSM-IV* Dissociative Disorders (SCID-D: Steinberg, 1995), the Dissociative Disorders Interview Schedule (DDIS) and the Dissociation Questionnaire (DIS-Q: Vanderlinden, 1993; Vanderlinden, Van Dyck, Vandereycken, & Vertommen, 1991). Although more replication studies using these instruments are required, together they provide an effective, easy-to-use, practical standardized assessment battery for the clinician.

Self-report and structured interview questionnaires are required in psychiatry for a number of reasons. First, such measures are essential to establish the reliability of a given psychiatric diagnosis: One must show that different people in different places are talking about the same disorder when they present findings on DID. More important, the diagnosis must have validity. There are different subtypes of validity, but making the diagnosis must mean something in terms of differentiating the condition from other disorders. There should be a difference in prognosis, treatment, function, or some other meaningful aspect of the patient's life; otherwise the reliable diagnosis is clinically useless.

The DDIS, SCID-D, DES, and DIS-Q can be used in a number of ways. In a forensic case, they would strengthen the assessment of a DID patient. They can be used in screening clinical and nonclinical populations for DID. They can be an aid to diagnosis, and they provide detailed systematic information for clinical use. In my practice, I have used the DES and the DDIS in consultations and assessments in Step 1 of the assessment, then made a general clinical assessment in Step 2.

DISSOCIATIVE MEASURES BESIDES THE DDIS, DES, DIS-Q, AND SCID-D

The Perceptual Alteration Scale (PAS)

The PAS developed by Sanders (1986) is not yet ready for widespread clinical use. It has a number of weaknesses that make it less useful than the DES. The PAS is a self-report scale derived from the MMPI. It has good initial reliability, but it has not been tested in a clinical population. Thus its utility in screening for DID or documenting the symptoms of patients with dissociative disorders has not been demonstrated.

Many of the MMPI questions in the PAS do not seem to have much to do with dissociation and the questions in the different factors do not always seem to be related to the name of the factor. For example, "I feel that my mind is divided," is an item in the factor called Modification of Affect, but doesn't refer to affect as such. "Even when I have missed several meals, I find that I am not hungry," is an item in a factor called Modification of Cognition, but doesn't seem to have anything in particular to do with dissociation, unless it represents a dissociation of hunger, which would be an example of dissociation of sensation, not cognition.

With more work, the PAS may demonstrate that it has some clinical utility. Because many of the questions are not examples of clinical dissociation, as usually described, the PAS may yield surprising or unexpected insights into dissociative psychopathology, by showing a relationship between classical dissociative symptoms and other phenomena.

The Questionnaire of Experiences of Dissociation (QED)

Riley (1988) developed the QED as a self-report measure of dissociation. It consists of 26 items in a true-false format. The QED appears to have good psychometric properties, but it has not been used in published research to anywhere near the extent of the DES (Dunn, Ryan, Paolo, & Miller, 1991; Gilbertson, Torem, Cohen, Newman, & Radojicic, 1992; Gleaves, Eberenz, Warner, & Fine, 1995). QED scores correlate well with DES scores, but it is not clear what the QED adds to using the DES alone. Since I have not used the QED myself, I will not comment on it further, except to say that its utility and future place in the field are uncertain.

The Phillips Dissociation Scale (PDS) of the Minnesota Multiphasic Personality Inventory (MMPI)

David Phillips (1994) developed a 20-item dissociation scale based on the MMPI that appears to be very promising. The MMPI-2 items that form the scale include items such as "I have had blank spells in which my activities were interrupted and I did not know what was going on around me"; "My memory seems to be alright"; "I often feel as if things are not real"; "Evil spirits possess me at times"; and "I *often* (commonly) hear voices without knowing where they come from."

It is not surprising that criteria for diagnosing DID are already embedded in the MMPI without their pattern being recognized by the MMPI scoring rules. The MMPI is based on the dominant conceptual system of late twentieth-century psychiatry, for which the DID symptom pattern is unrecognizable. The symptoms themselves have been observed and studied for decades, but not understood.

In his study, Phillips compared a sample of 20 patients having diagnoses of DID or DDNOS with 20 general psychiatry patients: The dissociative group had an average score of 11.1 (SD 4.6) on the PDS, compared with 2.2 (SD 2.0) for the general group ($t = 7.99$, $df = 38$, $p < .001$). There are enormous MMPI archives around the world that could be reanalyzed in conjunction with thorough clinical reassessment of patients for dissociative disorders, including many MMPIs from long before the upsurge of interest in dissociation in the 1980s. Review of MMPIs from the 1950s or 1960s in conjunction with diagnostic reassessment in the 1990s would yield a vast quantity of valuable information, and would almost certainly demonstrate that diagnosable DID was common in clinical settings three to four decades ago.

USE OF THE MMPI, SCL-90, MCMI, AND THE RORSCHACH FOR ASSESSING DISSOCIATION

The Minnesota Multiphasic Personality Inventory (MMPI) is the most widely used psychological test in the world; the Hopkins Symptom Checklist-

Revised (SCL-90) is one of the most widely used self-report measures of general psychopathology; the Millon Clinical Multiaxial Inventory (MCMI) is also widely used; and the Rorschach is well known even to laypeople. I discuss these tests together because none was developed to measure dissociation or contains dissociative norms or scoring rules in its manual.

Some work has been done with the Rorschach (Lovitt & Lefkof, 1985), but it does not yet have the status of a specific diagnostic tool for dissociation. Coons and Fine (1988) and Coons (1992) demonstrated that the MMPI can be used effectively for screening for DID, prior to development of the Phillips Dissociation Scale. Their study involved diagnostically blind raters of the MMPI and showed that the MMPI hit rate for DID is as good or better than for many other disorders. Further work may yield a more specific DID profile, but differentiation of DID from borderline personality disorder using the MMPI is problematic. The MMPI scoring manuals do not include rules for diagnosing DID.

We administered the SCL-90 to 144 subjects with DID in order to establish norms for DID. Like all other research measures, the SCL-90 shows that DID patients report high levels of symptoms across a wide range of psychopathology. No specific pattern or profile emerged other than a pan-elevation across all SCL-90 subscales, with prominent elevation of the anxiety, depression, interpersonal sensitivity, and psychoticism subscales. In a regression analysis on 119 subjects who also completed the DDIS, the SCL-90 global score, called the global severity index, predicted the number of perpetrators of physical abuse with a beta weight of 0.28 ($r = 0.11$, $p < .003$). Many different forms of psychopathology correlate with many different elements of childhood trauma in a variety of different statistical analyses, using a variety of different measures; reducing this to stable underlying relationships will require a lot more research.

In a study of 96 DID patients who completed the MCMI (Ellason, Ross, & Fuchs, 1995), we found a pattern similar to that on the SCL-90: The most elevated Axis I scales were dysthymia, depression, thought disorder, and anxiety disorder, and the overall pattern was one of wide-ranging severe psychopathology. A reasonable conclusion to reach concerning the MMPI, MCMI, SCL-90, and Rorschach, based on the existing data, is that a pattern of global severe psychopathology should raise the index of suspicion for DID. None of these tests, based on their standard scoring rules, can differentiate dissociation from psychosis.

DISSOCIATIVE MEASURES FOR CHILDREN AND ADOLESCENTS

I am an adult psychiatrist and this is a book about adult DID, therefore I will not review child and adolescent measures. The development of reliable measures of dissociation in children and adolescents has lagged behind that for adults by at least half a decade. Preliminary data on a number of different measures have been published, but none have been subjected to replication studies involving large numbers of subjects. Over the next decade, I expect that the key contributors will develop reliable and valid self-report and interviewer-administered measures of comparable utility to the DES, DIS-Q, DDIS, and SCID-D.

I refer the reader to papers by Reagor, Kasten, and Morelli (1992), Tyson (1992), Branscomb and Fagan (1992), Evers-Szostak and Sanders (1992), Hornstein (1993), and Peterson and Putnam (1994) for discussion of child diagnostic criteria and measures. For descriptions of child and adolescent cases, the reader should consult Bowman, Blix, and Coons (1985), Kluft (1985b), Dell and Eisenhower (1990), Hornstein and Putnam (1992), and Vincent and Pickering (1988): These papers and the references they contain will lead the reader into the literature.

THE DISSOCIATIVE EXPERIENCES SCALE

The Dissociative Experiences Scale (DES) is a 28-item self-report instrument that can be completed in 10 minutes, and scored in less than 5 minutes. It is easy to understand, and the questions are framed in a normative way that does not stigmatize the respondent for positive responses. A typical DES question is, "Some people have the experience of finding new things among their belongings that they do not remember buying. Mark the line to show what percentage of the time this happens to you." The respondent then slashes the line, which is anchored at 0% on the left and 100% on the right, to show how often he or she has this experience. The DES contains a variety of dissociative experiences, many of which are normal experiences.

A newer form of the DES has a format in which the responses are made by circling a percentage ranging from 0% to 100% at 10% intervals. The advantage of the new form of the DES is that it is easier to score. It appears to have excellent convergent validity with the original form of the DES, and to be interchangeable with it (Ellason, Ross, Mayran, & Sainton, 1994).

The DES has very good validity and reliability, and good overall psychometric properties, as reviewed by its original developers (Carlson, 1994; Carlson & Armstrong, 1994; Carlson & Putnam, 1993; Carlson et al., 1993). It has excellent construct validity, which means it is internally consistent and hangs together well, as reflected in highly significant Spearman correlations of all items with the overall DES score. The scale is derived from extensive clinical experience with and understanding of DID. In the initial studies during its development and in all subsequent studies, the DES has discriminated DID from other diagnostic groups and controls at high levels of significance, based on either group mean or group median scores. In most samples, the mean and median DES scores for DID subjects are within 5 points of each other.

As reviewed in Chapter Six, the higher the DES score, the more likely it is that the person has DID. In a sample of 1,051 clinical subjects, however, only 17% of those scoring above 30 on the DES actually had DID (Carlson et al., 1993). The DES is not a diagnostic instrument. It is a screening instrument. High scores on the DES do not prove that a person has a dissociative disorder, they only suggest that clinical assessment for dissociation is warranted. This is how we report DES scores in our consults, as within or not within the range for DID, and as consistent or not consistent with the clinical and DDIS diagnosis of DID. DID subjects sometimes have low scores, so a low score does not rule out DID. In fact, given that in most studies the average DES score for a DID patient is in the 40s, and the standard deviation about 20, roughly about 15% of clinically diagnosed DID patients score below 20 on the DES.

The DES is the only dissociative instrument that has been subjected to a number of replication studies by independent investigators. We found in our original replication (Ross, Norton, & Anderson, 1988) that it discriminated DID from other groups very well, with scores similar to those found by Bernstein and Putnam (1986), and this pattern has persisted in all subsequent research.

In another study (Ryan, 1988; Ryan & Ross, 1988), we administered the adult form of the DES to 345 college students with a median age of 24 years, and 168 adolescents ages 12–14. We found that DES scores decline with age on a curve similar to the decline in hypnotizability scores with age (Berg & Melin, 1975; Gordon, 1972; Morgan & Hilgard, 1973; Spiegel & Spiegel, 1978). The 12-year-olds had a median scores of 20.2, the 14-year-olds a median score of 14.8, and the college students a median of 7.9. The difference between 12- and 14-year-olds was significant at $p < .00001$.

Hypnotizability and dissociation are linked to each other, so it is not surprising that the DES yields scores that vary with age the way hypnotizability does. In both the adolescents and the college students, every item on the DES correlated with the overall scores for that group at $p < .001$ by Spearman correlation. This suggests that the adult form of the DES is a good screening instrument in subjects as young as 12; an adolescent form of the DES is in development.

In the same study, we wanted to find out if the DES is a useful screening instrument in a nonclinical population. We therefore administered the DDIS, the SCL-90 (Derogatis, Lipman, Rickels, Uhenhuth, & Covi, 1973), and the Millon Clinical Multiaxial Inventory (MCMI; Millon, 1977) to 20 high scorers and 22 low scorers on the DES, among the college students.

The high- and low-DES scorers differed on each subitem and the overall score of the SCL-90. They differed on 15 of 20 scales on the MCMI, and they differed drastically on the DDIS. There were 25 different dissociative disorder diagnoses made in the high group, for example, and none in the low. This means that the DES can predict who will not, and who may have a dissociative disorder with high accuracy. As well, the DES taps into the dissociative component of general psychopathology, as evidenced by the SCL-90

and MCMI findings. This is consistent with everything in the clinical literature about dissociative disorders (see Chapter Six). The DES is not just picking out a dissociative anomaly that is unconnected to anything else.

This study helps to validate the DDIS. An interesting finding was noted
when we did an analysis to see which sections of the DDIS best predicted
DES score. The section of the DDIS that best differentiated the high- and
low-DES scorers was the section called Secondary Features of Dissociative Identity Disorder. The items in this section are very similar to many
questions in the DES, but were independently derived. We had not seen the
DES before constructing the DDIS. This means that the two instruments
are measuring the same phenomena, one by self-report and one by structured interview.

In another study (Ross, Miller, Reagor, et al., 1990), we found that in 82
DID subjects who completed both the DES and the DDIS, the Secondary
Features of DID section predicted DES scores with a beta weight of 0.61 in
a stepwise regression analysis, and was the only DDIS section to enter the
regression equation at $p < .05$. This was consistent with the findings in the
college student study.

A study by Draijer and Boon (1993) validated the DES against the SCID-
D using a receiver operating characteristics analysis and found that the self-
report and structured interview measures worked well together, and
validated each other. These three independently developed measures, the
DES, DDIS, and SCID-D, each based on distinct logic and scoring rules, all
seem to be measuring the same domain in a reliable and valid fashion.

Because of these properties of the DES, and its extensive research base,
it is the best self-report instrument for measuring dissociation available.
The complete scale is available in the original paper (Bernstein & Putnam,
1986), except that question 25 is inadvertently missing. Question 25 reads,
"Some people find evidence that they have done things that they do not remember doing. Mark the line to show what percentage of the time this happens to you." The new form of the DES, with no questions missing, is
available in Carlson and Putnam (1993). The DES has been translated into
many different languages and used in published research by many different
researchers, many of whom are not primarily identified with the dissociative disorders field.

Van Ijzendoorn and Schuengel (in press) recently completed a meta-
analysis of over 100 published DES studies involving 11,914 subjects.
Their analysis involved 827 DID subjects from 30 different studies who
had a mean DES score of 45.1 compared, for example, with 811 subjects
with personality disorders from 12 different studies who had a mean
DES score of 18.0. The meta-analytic data confirmed the robust psychometric properties of the DES, especially its ability to discriminate DID
from other diagnostic groups.

An important result of the meta-analysis was that in 10 studies involving
2,513 subjects the combined effect size for the relationship between dissociation and hypnosis was only $d = 0.27$, which is very modest, and classified

as a weak degree of convergent validity between the measures: Moderate effect sizes are above 0.50, and strong ones above 0.80. By comparison, the combined effect size for pooled studies comparing DES scores of DID subjects to those with epilepsy was 1.16.

THE DISSOCIATION QUESTIONNAIRE (DIS-Q)

The DIS-Q was developed by Johan Vanderlinden in Belgium (Vanderlinden, 1993; Vanderlinden, Van Dyck, Vandereycken, & Vertommen, 1991). Vanderlinden and his colleagues have published widely in Europe in a variety of different languages, as well as in North America, and this work is referenced in Vanderlinden (1993). In his 1993 monograph, Vanderlinden describes the development and psychometric properties of the DIS-Q in detail.

The DIS-Q was developed as an expanded version of the DES with a different response format. It also drew on the PAS, the QED, and clinical experience in Europe. The DIS-Q contains 63 items with a response format in a Likert-type scale ranging from 1 to 5: 1 = not at all, 2 = a little bit, 3 = moderately, 4 = quite a bit, and 5 = extremely. Typical DIS-Q questions include: "At times it appears that I have lost contact with my body"; "Sometimes I discover that I have done something without remembering anything about it"; and, "I have the feeling that I am made up of two (or more) persons."

The average DIS-Q score for DID is 3.5 (*SD* 0.5), for DDNOS is 2.9 (*SD* 0.6), for schizophrenia is 2.0 (*SD* 0.6), and for nonclinical normal controls is 1.5 (*SD* 0.4). Vanderlinden has done DIS-Q studies involving large samples in a variety of clinical populations, in different countries and languages, and in the general population. His psychometric studies of the DIS-Q are thorough and rigorous, and indicate it is a reliable and valid measure. I revised the English of the DIS-Q for usage in North America and used it in one unpublished study in which I found that it correlated with the DES at a high level, and performed in North America much like it does in Europe in terms of discriminating DID from other diagnostic categories.

The DIS-Q will continue to make a significant contribution to our understanding of dissociation, especially in Europe. The major research in the field outside North America comprises the work of Boon and Draijer (1993) in the Netherlands; of Vanderlinden in several European countries including Belgium, the Netherlands, and Hungary; and of Tutkun, Yargic, and Sar (1995) in Turkey.

THE DISSOCIATIVE DISORDERS INTERVIEW SCHEDULE

The Dissociative Disorders Interview Schedule, *DSM-IV* Version (DDIS) (Ross, Heber, Norton, et al., 1989) is reproduced in Appendix A along with its consent form, and scoring key. The DDIS was developed because every area of psychiatry requires a valid and reliable structured interview, both for research and clinical purposes. Also, findings from structured interview are essential for publication and establishing the dissociative disorders as a legitimate area of study. Although more replication work is required, I feel that the DDIS has shown that DID is a valid and reliable diagnosis, that it has a consistent set of features, and that it is worthy of serious attention.

The DDIS can be administered to a normal subject without an abuse history in less than half an hour. Interviews with complex multiples can usually be completed in 45 minutes. The overall interrater reliability of the DDIS in its original development was 0.68, which is as good as the standard psychiatric structured interviews. The DDIS has been used in 23 published studies by my research group listed in the references and reviewed throughout this book, and these papers have appeared in 12 peer-reviewed journals.

The DDIS has been translated into French, Dutch, Italian, Hebrew, Spanish, Japanese, Turkish, and Polish, and has been used in its English version in North America, Australia, and Great Britain.

The DDIS has good clinical validity. In its initial development, 10 subjects with both clinical and DDIS diagnoses of DID were interviewed by a psychiatrist blind to their diagnoses. She was aware only that anywhere from 0 to 10 of the women could have DID. She diagnosed DID in 8, and "atypical dissociative disorder—rule out DID" in two women. These two women had had full DID in the past but were in remission at the time of interview. The validity of the DDIS is further demonstrated by the cumulative weight of all the published studies employing it.

As of 1995, the DDIS had been administered to over 500 subjects with nondissociative clinical diagnoses, with a false-positive DDIS diagnosis of DID occurring in less than 1% of cases. The sensitivity of the DDIS for the diagnosis of DID (the true positive rate) in a series of 196 cases of clinically diagnosed DID was 95.4% (Ross, 1995b). Pooling the 500 nondissociative patients with the 196 DID patients, the overall kappa value for the rate of agreement between clinician and DDIS for the presence or absence of DID is 0.96. This is superior to the performance of any other structured interview for any other psychiatric disorder, except for the SCID-D, as will be discussed.

In the first paper showing that the DDIS could differentiate DID from other diagnostic categories (Ross, Heber, Norton, & Anderson, 1989a), kappa for the rate of agreement between clinician and DDIS on the presence or absence of DID was 0.95. This value was not reported in the paper but can be calculated from the published data. In terms of the most difficult diagnostic differentiation, that between DID and DDNOS, the DDIS performs well: A discriminant function analysis correctly assigned 94.1% of the DID subjects to the DID category in a study involving 166 subjects with DID and 57 with DDNOS (Ross, Anderson, Fraser, et al., 1992).

When we did Spearman correlation coefficients of symptom clusters in the DDIS with overall DES scores in our college student study, we found very high correlations for four items: secondary features of DID (0.78), Schneiderian symptoms (0.67), borderline personality disorder criteria (0.67), and extrasensory experiences (0.67). These Spearman correlations demonstrate with a different statistic the strong relationship between the major DDIS symptom clusters and DES scores.

A self-report version of the DDIS is currently under study, and appears to correlate well with the interviewer-administered version in the preliminary data. I would also like to develop a computerized version. Future studies will involve administering the DES, DDIS, SCID-D, and other measures to large numbers of clinical subjects with and without dissociative disorders: The subjects will also receive clinical diagnostic interviews from clinicians skilled in diagnosing dissociative disorders. The DDIS, SCID-D, and clinical interviewers will be independent and blind to each other's findings. The data published to date strongly support the conclusion that the DDIS is a valid and reliable structured interview that can discriminate DID from other diagnostic categories with a high level of accuracy.

THE STRUCTURED CLINICAL INTERVIEW FOR *DSM-IV* DISSOCIATIVE DISORDERS (SCID-D)

The SCID-D makes all of the five dissociative disorder diagnoses. It is specifically designed to fill a gap in the SCID, the Structured Clinical Interview for *DSM-III-R*, which makes many *DSM-III-R* Axis I diagnoses, but does not inquire about dissociative disorders. None of the standard psychiatric structured interviews make dissociative diagnoses. The SCID-D has been published by the American Psychiatric Press (Steinberg, 1995) and is readily available. It makes a detailed and comprehensive assessment of dissociation, and has excellent initial reliability and validity. SCID-D trainings are provided by Marlene Steinberg on a regular basis.

The main drawback of the SCID-D is that its administration is time-consuming and not straightforward to learn. It cannot be administered by an untrained person, requires skilled clinical judgments for its scoring, and can take longer than 90 minutes to administer. These are also the strengths of the SCID-D: It provides a detailed, rich, and probing documentation of dissociative symptomotology. The development of the SCID-D has been supported by grants from the National Institute of Mental Health, and the interview has been analyzed with advanced statistics. It is the only measure of dissociation that has been the subject of an entire book (Steinberg, 1995) and it is also the foundation of a second book (Boon & Draijer, 1993).

The SCID-D has an interrater agreement of 0.95 for the diagnosis of DID, and can discriminate DID from other psychiatric disorders very effectively. Steinberg recommends that the SCID-D be used as part of a multistage assessment process, in the same way as I use the DES, with a DES screening, then a structured interview, then clinical interviewing.

Marlene Steinberg's decade of work on the SCID-D is a major body of programmatic research. The next decade will see published SCID-D research from many different cultures and languages. The work of Boon and Draijer (1993) in the Netherlands using the Dutch version of the SCID-D is the major piece of research on dissociation done outside North America. My review of the SCID-D is relatively brief because Steinberg (1994, 1995) has reviewed it at length elsewhere.

CONSISTENCY IN THE FEATURES OF DISSOCIATIVE IDENTITY DISORDER USING THE DES, DIS-Q, SCID-D, AND DDIS

A large body of cross-linked research studies using the DES, DIS-Q, SCID-D, and DDIS, indicate the validity, reliability, and consistency of DID and its associated features. This consistency in the phenomenology of DID was first evident in our study of 236 cases reported to us by 203 different clinicians throughout North America (Ross, Norton, & Wozney, 1989). The findings in this study are remarkably consistent with those of Putnam et al. (1986). Putnam's study was done four years earlier using a different instrument, which we had not seen. The findings in these two studies are consistent with all subsequent published studies and the clinical literature. For example, Gray and Braun (1986) reported that 126 DID patients averaged 6.9 years in the mental health system prior to diagnosis, while ours averaged 6.7 years and Putnam's 6.8 years.

The DID cases assessed in North America by self-report and structured interview are very much like DID cases similarly assessed in Turkey, Japan, the Netherlands, Puerto Rico, and Norway.

CONCLUSION

We now have instruments available that are practical, easy-to-use, clinical tools for the diagnosis of DID. They are useful in research, for screening purposes, in confirming clinical diagnoses, in forensic work, and as data for third-party insurers. To demonstrate the efficacy of a treatment, it is necessary to show that a reliable and valid disorder is being treated; that a specific treatment is being delivered; that the treatment is cost-effective and can be taught to others; and that both a general and a specific beneficial response occurs. These are challenges that will face the field over the next decade.

CHAPTER EIGHT

Dissociative Identity Disorder and Other Psychiatric Disorders

The main purpose of this book is to describe the clinical features and treatment of dissociative identity disorder (DID) in detail. The second is to place DID in the context of general psychiatry. DID would be interesting if it were a rare curiosity, but it is much more than that. Freud's early patients were dissociative and included cases of classical DID (see Chapter One). It is mainly dissociative patients who exhibit symbolic conversions, sexually driven somatization, and other defenses Freud first analyzed and classified. Freud discovered the mechanisms, repudiated their traumatic etiology—which, simplified, is trauma plus autohypnosis, as stated by Breuer (Breuer & Freud, 1895/1986, p. 329)—and then devised a set of secondary metapsychological theories to explain his patients' problems.

Freud's repudiation of the seduction theory concealed the traumatic foundation of the disorders from which his theory originally developed. The dissociative disorders became an obscure corner of psychiatry, rare and irrelevant to the mainstream, in part because of Freud's influence. There is a mutually exclusive relationship between the repudiation of the seduction theory and the understanding of trauma-driven dissociation. That is one reason there is so much resistance to the diagnosis of DID: Dissociative identity disorder necessitates a revision of Freudian theory, such that the foundation of the classical defense mechanisms in trauma is recovered and brought back into focus. Put another way, modified, corrected psycho-analysis is what I and others in the field practice.

For most of the 20th century, Freudian and biological psychiatry have maintained a mutually advantageous homeostasis, despite their mutual disdain. In twentieth-century psychiatry, the biologists, who were virtually all biomedical reductionists, claimed certain phenomena as their own. One example of this is Schneiderian first-rank symptoms of schizophrenia (Kluft, 1987b), which are widely held to be symptoms of biologically driven major mental illness, though not unique to schizophrenia. DID patients have numerous Schneiderian symptoms that can be cured with psychotherapy. DID patients demonstrate that much supposedly hard-core biological symptomatology is trauma-driven and treatable with psychotherapy. At the same time, DID necessitates revisions in Freudian theory and therapy.

This is why DID is an important diagnosis. Study of dissociative disorders will lead to changes in the official diagnostic scheme, in our understanding of phenomenology, and in therapeutics. Many of these changes will probably not occur until *DSM-VI.* The challenge to specialists in dissociation is to generate data, tools, and therapies that have a solid scientific basis. If this doesn't happen, dissociation may again fall into obscurity: This time, it would probably be discredited by biological psychiatry, which dominates the field today.

In this chapter, I will discuss at length borderline personality disorder and schizophrenia, which are the leading items in the *DSM-IV* differential diagnosis of DID. I will also review a number of other psychiatric diagnoses: It is important to understand the relationship between DID and other psychiatric disorders in order to make a differential diagnosis and plan treatment. Also, study of DID can teach us a great deal about how to classify, and treat other disorders in *DSM-IV.*

A SECTION OF TRAUMA DISORDERS IN *DSM-VI?*

As described in Chapter Six, DID patients also meet diagnostic criteria for other psychiatric disorders, including depression, borderline personality disorder, somatization disorder, substance abuse, bulimia, panic disorder, and others (Atlas, 1988; Markowitz & Viederman, 1986). It is common for a DID patient, in the course of her lifetime, to meet *DSM-IV* criteria for 15 different disorders, and for more than five of these to be active at the same time. This doesn't make any sense. It violates a principle of science called *Occam's razor,* according to which, "Entities are not to be multiplied without necessity" (Russell, 1945). Occam's razor means that the simplest explanation consistent with the facts is the best explanation and that entities are not to be postulated if they are not required to explain a phenomenon.

In nineteenth-century physics, there was a great deal of theorizing about a substance called ether, which was thought to fill the universe. Experimental attempts were made to measure the ether wind, which was thought to result from the drift of ether through the universe. If there was an ether wind, it would be blowing in opposite directions relative to an observer on the surface of the earth, at intervals six months apart, because the earth would be on opposite sides of the sun. No such effect was detectable. The main reason ether was dropped from physics, though, was that it became an unnecessary postulate and fell before Occam's razor.

In Ptolemaic astronomy, a vast machinery of cycles and epicycles was invented to explain the motion of the stars and planets. The cycles and epicycles were circular mechanical pathways that exerted force on the heavenly bodies and interacted like gearwheels to coordinate their motions. After Kepler, the entire machinery was simply dropped. There are no epicycles in nature. Although Ptolemy was a genius, his astronomical theory is best described as antiquated.

The history of gross anatomy is also instructive. The anatomy of Galen dominated medicine for over 1,500 years, until new discoveries pushed it into decline. For hundreds of years, however, professors of anatomy taught that dissection was unnecessary because one could refer to Galen. To dissect was in fact heretical, because it implied that there was a need to check on Galen. This was the ultimate appeal to authority. Those who wanted to make dissection of cadavers part of medical training often suffered political consequences.

When dissection was introduced in a few medical schools, some professors contended that when the anatomy of a cadaver differed from that of Galen, it was the cadaver that was wrong. One example of such a difference involved details of the blood supply to the uterus, which Galen described based on incorrect theory about the cause of menstruation. The idea, popular in nineteenth-century medicine, that hysteria is caused by a wandering uterus, is derived from the same theory. The terms hysterectomy and hysteria come from the Greek word for "uterus." Indeed, hysterectomy was recommended as a treatment for certain female psychological disorders as late as the nineteenth century (Veith, 1965), as were marriage and sexual intercourse (marriage was the necessary social structure for intercourse to occur, intercourse being the curative agent). Theoretical errors in medicine may have far-reaching practical consequences.

Freudian repudiation of the seduction theory is supported by a similar appeal to authority—to question it may be heretical. In contemporary medical schools, derisive dismissals of DID are common. These may originate from either of the two main camps in twentieth-century psychiatry, Freudian or biomedical reductionist. Returning to Occam's razor, DID doesn't fit into *DSM-IV* properly, in part because DID patients have numerous concurrent diagnoses and thus need a parsimonious single diagnosis that encompasses all of the symptomatology. DID accounts for only a small part of the specific dissociative symptoms of these patients. Part of the problem is the conceptual base of *DSM-IV.*

DSM-IV can be described as a Newtonian document. It is based on classical Cartesian psychiatry. In *DSM-IV,* psychiatric disorders, or at least groups of disorders, are related like the billiard balls in nineteenth-century physics metaphors. According to *DSM-IV* rules, one can have a mood disorder, anxiety disorder, dissociative disorder, eating disorder, and personality disorder (probably borderline) all at the same time. There is no necessary or conceptually compelling relationship between all these independent entities.

This Newtonian logic leads to futile but common debates about whether bulimia is an epiphenomenon of mood disorder, or whether DID is an epiphenomenon of borderline personality disorder, among a long list of such debates. Bulimia and depression are viewed as independent billiard balls in such thinking, with a causal, linear relationship between the two. The depression billiard ball has specified position and momentum and causes secondary movement in a billiard ball we call bulimia. Treat the depression billiard ball, to correct its disordered momentum, and the disordered movement in the bulimia billiard ball will not occur. Many studies are designed to elucidate the relative positions and momenta of psychiatric disorders on this single plane.

Single plane? *DSM-IV* has five Axes, someone will reply. That doesn't matter. Axis II is a vestigial remnant of the biological-Freudian homeostasis. The personality disorders are separated out on Axis II because Freudian and biological theory have not been integrated. Axes III through V are not diagnostic axes. DID patients demonstrate that the diagnostic system doesn't make sense. DID patients are an anomaly that cannot be incorporated into the dominant twentieth-century psychiatric paradigms. Hence the resistance to DID, which is a resistance to paradigm shift.

The first step in rewriting *DSM-IV* is the coining of a new diagnostic term that will take all the features of DID into account. The diagnostic term should be politically acceptable, conceptually sound, and result in DID being integrated into the mainstream. What is DID? It is a polydiagnostic disorder of childhood onset, arising from childhood trauma, at least on its primary pathways.

What is the relationship between different diagnoses such as depression, panic disorder, bulimia, and borderline personality disorder within the polydiagnostic chronic trauma syndrome? If chronic childhood trauma disorder is present, none of these other diagnoses should be made as a freestanding entity. They must be listed as subdiagnoses of the inclusive disorder. This doesn't mean that the bulimic behavior doesn't exist, but the patient has only one disorder. That is the formal relationship between the DID patient's many different concurrent diagnoses. What about the dynamic relationship?

DID stands in a hierarchically inclusive relationship to depression, substance abuse, and the other diagnoses within the overall trauma syndrome. The other disorders occur lower in a hierarchy depicted in Figure 8.1. One

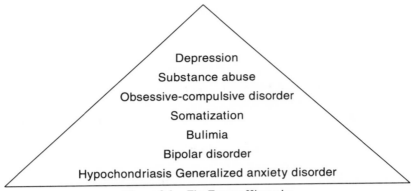

Figure 8.1.   The Trauma Hierarchy

passes vertically up the hierarchy as a function of two variables: increasing severity and chronicity of trauma (one variable with two subcomponents), and dissociative ability. The most severely abused and dissociative patients develop DID. Others who are less severely traumatized, or who are less gifted at dissociation, develop drug habits, personality disorders, and depression. There is no necessary or invariable relationship between the disorders lower in the hierarchy, which can occur in different combinations in different patients.

The relationship between the subdiagnoses of this chronic trauma disorder is best understood using a metaphor from quantum mechanics. Chronic trauma disorder is a single field, with distinct regions. These different regions are called mood disorder, eating disorder, and so on. DID teaches us that numerous regions of the field can be activated simultaneously in a given patient. Phenomenologically, movement from one region of the field to another takes the form of transitions through a continuum of changing density, rather than discrete jumps from one billiard ball to the next. The subregions of the field (DID, bulimia, drug abuse) do not interact according to Newtonian principles; rather they are interrelated by complex postclassical mechanisms.

What difference does this make clinically? I predict that if one attempts to treat, say, the depression in a chronic trauma patient, without diagnosing the DID, the patient's response is often unsatisfactory. If one makes the diagnosis of DID, however, and treats the DID, the hierarchically lower diagnosis of depression goes into remission, or responds much more cleanly to antidepressants if it recurs postintegration. This is why the trauma diagnosis makes a difference. Chronic trauma disorder brings conceptual order to the data available in the literature. I have listed many specific predictions of this trauma model in *Pseudoscience in Biological Psychiatry* (Ross & Pam, 1995).

The hypothesis that treating hierarchically lower disorders is ineffective and has no effect on the hierarchically superior DID is based on treatment failures subsequently diagnosed as DID and successfully treated with special DID techniques. What about the treatment successes? I mean the patients with DID whose DID was never diagnosed, but who went into remission when they were given antidepressants, group therapy for substance abuse, cognitive-behavioral therapy for bulimia, or some other hierarchically lower treatment. If such patients exist, DID specialists never see them. The therapeutic utility of chronic trauma disorder as a diagnosis depends on such patients not existing or being a small minority in the overall universe of DID.

All possible combinations of treatment response and failure could be tested in properly designed trials, although this would be logistically difficult. For example, chronic trauma patients could be entered into a randomized, double blind, placebo-controlled trial of an antidepressant, and response of all the subdiagnoses and symptoms could be monitored. The hypotheses generated by the diagnosis of chronic trauma disorder are all testable, scientific hypotheses.

Geri Anderson and Sharon Heber (Ross, Anderson, Heber, & Norton, 1990) administered the DES and DDIS to 20 subjects with DID, 20 prostitutes, and 20 strippers. We did this because we knew that 19.1% of DID patients in our series of 236 had worked as prostitutes. We also knew that at least 50 % of prostitutes had been sexually abused as children (Silbert & Pines, 1981, 1982, 1983, 1984). We therefore expected to find abuse histories and dissociative disorders in prostitutes. Strippers were included for several reasons. Women shift back and forth between stripping and hooking or do both at once, so strippers should also be dissociative.

In our study, the degree of dissociation was clearly linked to the severity and chronicity of abuse. The DID patients had an average duration of physical abuse of 15.0 years, compared with 4.2 years for the prostitutes and 4.3 years for the strippers. The DID subjects had an average of 2.5 different physical abusers, compared with 0.7 for the prostitutes and 0.6 for the strippers.

In terms of sexual abuse, the DID patients had an average duration of sexual abuse of 12.7 years, compared with 2.7 years for the prostitutes and 2.1 years for the strippers. They had an average of 1.7 different sexual abusers compared to 0.8 for the prostitutes and 0.7 for the strippers. Finally, the DID patients had experienced an average of 3.6 different forms of sexual abuse compared with 1.4 for the prostitutes and 1.5 for the strippers. The DID subjects differed from the prostitutes and strippers on all these measures of trauma at $p = .02$, or greater.

The DID patients were also more dissociative. They had more dissociative diagnoses and scored much higher on the DES. They had many more secondary features of DID and Schneiderian symptoms. However, there were no differences between groups in the frequencies of depression, substance abuse, or borderline personality disorder. The hypotheses underlying chronic trauma disorder were supported. All three groups had trauma histories, but the group with the most severe trauma had the most dissociation. Hierarchically lower phenomena did not differ between groups.

I expect these preliminary findings to stand up across studies and centers with a variety of subject groups. Dissociative features and diagnoses are hierarchically superior elements of the chronic trauma disorder. Dissociative symptoms include secondary features of DID, Schneiderian symptoms, ESP experiences, and borderline diagnostic criteria. In the study of prostitutes and strippers, ESP experiences and borderline personality did not differentiate groups. This suggests that there may be hierarchical structure even within the dissociative cluster, but further studies are required to examine this possibility.

The name of the polydiagnostic trauma disorder in *DSM-VI,* if it enters the manual, is not yet known. Whatever the eventual name, it should appear in a trauma section that includes the dissociative disorders, posttraumatic stress disorder (PTSD), acute stress disorder, and borderline personality disorder.

THE RELATIONSHIP BETWEEN DISSOCIATIVE
IDENTITY DISORDER AND OTHER TRAUMA DISORDERS

It wouldn't make sense to create a new trauma section of *DSM-VI* and not define the relationships of the disorders within the category. PTSD is currently defined in *DSM-IV* as an anxiety disorder, although it has more dissociative features than anxiety symptoms (Brende & Benedict, 1980; Spiegel, 1984, 1986a, 1986b; Spiegel, Hunt, & Dondershine, 1988; Young, 1987). *DSM-IV* PTSD is much more dissociative, both in its criteria and in the discussion section, than *DSM-III* PTSD. Spiegel, Hunt, and Dondershine have done work on the dissociative aspects of PTSD, as has Spiegel alone (1986a, 1986b). These and other studies will probably result in PTSD being shifted out of anxiety disorders. It would be an error to shift it into dissociative disorders, however.

Concerning the anxiety disorders, both PTSD and obsessive-compulsive disorder are classified as anxiety disorders but neither has anxiety as a cardinal feature, any more than do DID or schizophrenia. For both, anxiety is an epiphenomenon. Both should be taken out of the anxiety disorders, leaving generalized anxiety, panic, and the phobias as a truly related group of disorders. Some cases of obsessive-compulsive disorder are dissociative in nature (Ross & Anderson, 1988) and are presenting features of the chronic trauma disorder. Others could be assigned to mood, delusional, or other diagnostic groups. At any rate, obsessive-compulsive disorder is not primarily an anxiety disorder, and neither is PTSD.

The trauma disorders could be subdivided into acute and chronic trauma, childhood and adult onset, and dissociative or nondissociative, bearing in mind that dissociation occurs on a continuum. It is likely that mild trauma, such as that which usually precedes adjustment disorders, can be handled without the mobilization of dissociative defenses except in individuals who have chronic trauma disorder. They use dissociation all the time.

It is possible that dissociation is the strategy par excellence for coping with severe trauma and that even otherwise nondissociative individuals will mobilize their evolutionary ability to dissociate if the trauma is extreme enough. This would result in more dissociative symptoms occurring in a population exposed to extreme trauma than in one exposed to intermediate trauma, assuming that pretraumatic DES scores were the same in both groups. These hypotheses could be tested by measuring dissociation in all military inductees and following those persons who did and did not enter combat. Such a study might eventually lead to selection of combat soldiers at lower risk for adult onset PTSD and better preventive interventions for those high dissociators who do have to enter combat. Maybe nobody with a DES score over 30 should become a marine. On the other hand, healthy high dissociators might make the best marines, because they could dissociate terror, cold, and fatigue, and maintain their function. The issue might be separating healthy from pathological dissociators.

I mention these possibilities to indicate the potential utility of the reorganization of *DSM-IV*. Such a reorganization was inherent in the thinking of therapists treating DID in the 1980s. It will not directly affect the *DSM* system until the twenty-first century, with a lag time of at least 20 years, which is roughly the period of time required for the resistant generation of psychiatrists to retire and die.

Within the trauma category, the different diagnoses could be related to each other in a variety of different ways: Since no such category exists in *DSM-IV* and probably will not in *DSM-V,* there is no need to suggest an organizational principle now. Further relevant research will have been published before any *DSM* committee has to draft the category rules.

BORDERLINE PERSONALITY DISORDER

Borderline personality disorder is one of the most controversial diagnoses in psychiatry, although it is much more accepted, studied, funded, and diagnosed than DID (Kernberg, 1975; Masterson, 1976). In a symposium of nine papers on borderline personality in the *Canadian Journal of Psychiatry* (Links, 1988), DID is not mentioned once. DID, dissociation, and childhood trauma had virtually no effect on the clinical thinking of mainstream psychiatrists about borderline personality disorder in the 1980s. However, this situation began to change in the 1990s. To understand borderline personality disorder, one must review the history of the diagnosis and the origins of the term itself.

As described in Chapter Two, DID fell into disrepute following Freud's rejection of dissociation, the seduction theory, and hypnosis;

other contributing factors were the ascendancy of Bleuler's schizophrenia and the transfer of academic energy into behavioral studies. Schizophrenia means "split mind disorder," which is actually the correct term for DID, not for schizophrenia. Many DID patients were misdiagnosed as schizophrenic and mistreated within biological psychiatry because of the mistaken term.

Alternatively, DID patients were treated psychoanalytically for their disordered oedipal fantasies and hysterical symptoms. Shortly after World War II, however, Hoch and Polatin (1949) noticed that many patients were atypical and did not fit in with dementia praecox or psychoneurosis. Hoch and Polatin described these patients as suffering from "pseudoneurotic schizophrenia" (p. 276), a term similar to "hysterical psychosis, "hysterical schizophrenia," and other related terms. The choice of pseudoneurotic schizophrenia was odd because it could as easily have been neurotic pseudoschizophrenia. In any case, the coined phrase did not stick. Hoch and Polatin conclude their paper by saying, "A few of these 'borderline' cases are described and their symptomatology analyzed. It is suggested that these patients be classified 'pseudoneurotic form of schizophrenia'" (p. 276). Although the term pseudoneurotic schizophrenia did not stick, "borderline" did.

Hoch and Polatin present five cases of pseudoneurotic schizophrenia. Their patients had undiagnosed DID and suffered from posttraumatic dissociative disorders, as did the patients in *Studies on Hysteria* described 54 years earlier by Breuer and Freud (1895/1986). Hoch and Polatin note that their patients suffered from all the symptoms of neurosis, had no thought disorders, had "incestuous ideas" (p. 253), exhibited complex sexual conflicts, and often had extensive amnesia for childhood. In addition they had "brief psychoses" (p. 253), which is why they were called schizophrenic.

Hoch and Polatin's Case 2 is quoted as saying of herself, "I'm divided. Part of me is here and part of me is floating away" (p. 264). Case 3 was quoted as saying:

> My subconscious mind plays tricks on me. I was in a trance. I seemed to be separated from my body. My conscious mind has to pass on everything my subconscious mind does. My subconscious mind tries to do and say things that other people have in their minds. I feel what they think. The words I cannot understand are "positive" and "negative." It means that I'm trying to be certain about things. I feel like I'm hypnotized. Did you hypnotize me? At times I have the feeling as if a voice was telling me to go to sleep and act like a child and be babied. (p. 267)

In another passage about Case 3, Hoch and Polatin write, "I have a male mind and a female body and I don't like women" (p. 268). Asked how long she had been hearing the voice, she said, "On and off for about 2 years" (p. 268). Sometimes it was a real voice, sometimes she thought it was her own ideas "which became loud" (p. 269). Of Case 3, Hoch and Polatin note that "early memories were blocked" (p. 268). Case 4 was a male with DID. Case 5 presented with:

> . . . marked self-recriminatory ideas, a feeling that she is two persons, a desire to kill members of her family and a fear that her husband might kill her . . . . She also complained about hearing motors roaring in her ears; began to think of herself at times very objectively; and she would smile at her own activities and reactions. She also could hear herself talk to herself as if there were two persons. At times she would laugh at her own feelings. She had a sensation of voices inside her head repeating things she had previously thought of, or reminding her of what she had done. She realized that these voices were products of her own thinking, nevertheless she could not control them; she felt obsessed by them. (pp. 272, 274)

In Chapter One, we saw that demon possession, obsession, dissociation, and DID are the same phenomena, in different cultural-historical contexts.

Hoch and Polatin's patients often gave them the diagnosis of DID directly and explained the dissociative nature of their symptoms. Hoch and Polatin couldn't hear because they were trying to fit the patients into a preconceived conceptual system that couldn't accommodate them. The history of psychoanalysis and the history of borderline personality disorder both start with small series of DID and DDNOS patients.

Within the Freudian-biological homeostasis, the undiagnosed DID patients, partially recognized by Hoch and Polatin, presented a problem. They appeared to have more than a personality disorder but less than a major chronic psychosis. They did not fit into either subparadigm very well. They were on the borderline between personality disorder (the Freudian camp) and psychosis (the biological camp). The attempts to account for these patients involved extensive metapsychological theorizing, on the one hand, and efforts to classify them as *formes frustes* of biological psychosis on the other. In the end they were called borderlines.

Today, many clinicians regard borderline personality disorder as a legitimate diagnosis. Looking at DID patients from the borderline vantage point, they hold that DID is an epiphenomenon of borderline personality. Basically, the argument is that DID specialists create a DID artifact in borderlines. Such clinicians rarely diagnose DID because they deal with the "real" disorder, borderline personality, without introducing an additional hysterical illusion. In this context, "hysterical" has theoretical pretensions but really means hysterical in the sense of a hysterical woman screaming about a mouse in the closet. The woman needs a slap on the face and settling down, while a man takes care of the mouse.

One doesn't have to look far in the borderline literature to find cases of undiagnosed DID. In a paper called "Prolonged Psychotic States in Borderline Personality Disorder," Lotterman (1985) describes eight borderline patients with "hysterical psychoses" (p. 36). He addresses the problem of how to account for borderline patients having personality disorders and psychotic features at the same time. This is an unreal problem because borderlines don't have either personality disorders or psychoses: They have a chronic trauma disorder.

In the longest case history, Lotterman describes a 27-year-old female inpatient with auditory hallucinations, depression, depersonalization, derealization, fugue states, sleepwalking, pseudoseizures, self-abusive behavior, suicide attempts (including ingestion of 4 grams of amitriptyline in one overdose), "autohypnotic trance-like states" (p. 38) alternating with lucid states, absence of a thought disorder, alternating homosexual and heterosexual states, and a fantasy of chopping up her parents. Lotterman does not comment on whether she did or did not have an abuse history. The patient failed to respond to large doses of chlorpromazine and haloperidol, or to a course of 20 ECT treatments. Lotterman comments: "A factor which appeared to exacerbate her symptoms was the fact that in her first two months of treatment, she had four separate psychotherapists, due to the rotation of psychiatric residents on her unit. For this adopted woman, this was probably a particularly potent stressor" (p. 38). The patient's diagnoses were changed prior to successive trials of different treatments and included depression, hysterical personality (on psychological testing), borderline personality, hysterical schizophrenia, and schizophrenia. Lotterman is to be thanked for his detailed account of the failure to diagnose DID in this patient and the numerous errors of omission and commission in her treatment.

The other seven patients in Lotterman's report also had auditory hallucinations, courses of 20 or more ECT treatments with transient response, sexual delusions and hallucinations, and other features common in the histories of undiagnosed DID patients. Not all of the patients described in the series sound strongly dissociative, but one had been cutting and scratching herself since the age of 8: "One important feature of this patient's history, was incestuous relations with her father. This fact emerged only after several years of treatment" (p. 41). It is important to emphasize that I am not singling Lotterman out for fault. In fact the reverse is true: He is to be commended for his scholarship, his efforts to diagnose and treat his difficult patients, and his frank discussion of what, for classical psychiatry, is their "inexplicable" symptomatology. Lotterman writes of his patient: "Throughout this time, something still seemed inexplicable" (p. 37).

The classification of borderline personality disorder in *DSM-IV* is an artifact of the Freudian-biological homeostasis. In *DSM-IV,* most adult psychiatric disorders, including DID, are diagnosed on Axis I. The personality disorders are separated out on Axis II and are widely regarded as being psychodynamic in nature. Axis I is the territory of the biologists, Axis II that of the psychoanalysts, although each camp tries to claim the other's territory, in an insoluble struggle over disputed desert. So-called neurotic disorders also occur on Axis I, but the bioreductionist view is that they are either mild biological illnesses or not psychiatric disorders and better left to social workers. In their efforts to explain the inexplicable, analysts try to move DID onto Axis II, and biologists try to reduce it to chemicals on Axis I.

Perhaps Axis I should be renamed Chemical Axis, and Axis II, Freudian Axis. The neurotic Axis I disorders could be reclassified as social work disorders rather than psychiatric disorders.

There is a precedent for moving a disorder from Axis II to Axis I. In *DSM-II*, dysthymic disorder was classified as "dysthymic personality disorder," along with the other personality disorders. In *DSM-III*, it is a poorly operationalized affective disorder on Axis I. In *DSM-IV*, it is a well-operationalized mood disorder on Axis I. The percentage of dysthymic patients treated with antidepressants has gone up, and the percentage treated with psychoanalysis gone down, in conjunction with this nosologic shift. There is a precedent, then, for moving a psychoanalytic disorder off of Axis II onto Axis I, despite a metapsychological investment in "characterological depressions." Borderline personality should be moved off of Axis II onto Axis I.

In the sparse metapsychological literature on borderline personality and DID (Benner & Joscelyne, 1984; Buck, 1983; Clary et al., 1984; Fast, 1974; Gruenewald, 1977, 1984; Horevitz & Braun, 1984; Ross, 1985; Young, 1988), a distinction is made between splitting and dissociation. Splitting is held to be the foundation of borderline personality, and dissociation the basis of DID. This means that the distinction between the two disorders is real only if the distinction between splitting and dissociation is real, which it isn't. Young (1988) unintentionally points this out in reviewing the relevant literature. He refers to Kernberg's (1975) definition of splitting as "alternative activation of contradictory ego states" (p. 33) and defines dissociation as a defense that "maintains conflict-laden material and painful affects in dissociated states" (p. 33).

In Young's reading of the literature, the distinction between splitting and dissociation hinges on two points: Splitting is based on contradictory ego states, whereas dissociated states are incompatible but not necessarily contradictory; splitting is based on splitting of introjects, whereas dissociated states need not be linked to introjects. Young therefore concludes that DID and borderline personality are distinct entities. The first problem is that these distinctions are very difficult if not impossible to demonstrate empirically with any interrater reliability.

Young makes three arguments in favor of the distinction between DID and borderline personality: Not all DID patients are borderline; not all alters are based on introjects; and in many patients there are too many alters for them all to be based on contradictory states.

There is an error of reasoning here. Contradictory states are a subset of incompatible states. That is why some alters are based on contradiction, but not all. In addition, incompatible states are not necessarily linked to introjects. That is why some alters identify themselves as specific other living or dead people, but many don't. Splitting is a subset of dissociation.

This being the case, it is not surprising that DID and borderline criteria exist in the same dissociative cluster.

The same holds true phenomenologically. The borderline patient switches states. In fact this is the metapsychological hallmark of her disorder. In one state, she disavows her affect and behavior while in other states. It is as if she has an amnesia at the level of affect and behavior, but not at a cognitive or informational level. The borderline patient has a severely impaired continuity of identity across states. If the amnesia barrier was made complete, and the sense of separate identity of the split states elaborated a little, one would be dealing with an alter personality. Phenomenologically, alter personalities are elaborations of borderline splitting.

This dissociative model of borderline personality is consistent with Braun's (1988a, 1988b) BASK model of dissociation. In the BASK model, dissociation can occur in four continua: behavior, affect, sensation, and knowledge. The borderline patient dissociates in all but knowledge, although there is impairment even in that continuum. The DID patient has completed the dissociation of knowledge, or informational awareness. The BASK model of borderline personality is in turn consistent with Gunderson's (Gunderson, Carpenter, & Strauss, 1975; Gunderson & Kolb, 1978; Gunderson, Kolb, & Austin, 1981; Gunderson & Singer, 1975) phenomenological observations about the frequency of dissociative features in borderlines. The problem with Gunderson's analysis is that he makes dissociation a subfeature rather than the core of borderline personality.

Gunderson also writes about the brief psychotic episodes experienced by borderlines. These are probably dissociative. This is partly a matter of definition: In my vocabulary, psychotic symptoms are features of a chronic major mental illness of presumed biological etiology, or of delirium; dissociative symptoms belong to a cluster including hypnosis, absorption, imaginative involvement, and fantasy, and are usually posttraumatic in origin. Dissociative and psychotic symptoms may be indistinguishable phenomenologically. This is accepted to be the case for symptoms of mania and schizophrenia—a given symptom may occur in identical fashion in either disorder. Diagnostically, this means that clinicians cannot reliably distinguish mania and schizophrenia on cross-sectional mental status examination alone. They must consider course, family history, treatment response, associated features, premorbid personality, and other factors in making a diagnosis.

The same is true for distinguishing dissociation and psychosis. In this regard, I will discuss the interview techniques relevant to the differential diagnosis of auditory hallucinations later in this chapter under schizophrenia.

The point I am making about DID and borderlines is that DID is not a rare, obscure diagnosis of little relevance to mainstream psychiatry. It is common, especially in patients diagnosed as borderline, and has numerous implications for psychiatric nosology, theory, and therapeutics. Are there any data supporting the idea that borderline criteria are part of a dissociative cluster?

In the first empirical study of the relationship between DID and borderline personality, Horevitz and Braun (1984) found that 70% of 33 cases of DID also met criteria for the Axis II disorder. Their feeling was that borderline personality is a measure of the overall function of the patient, but not necessarily related to the DID. I have published many studies that provide data on the relationship between the two disorders and consistent evidence in favor of a dissociative model of borderline personality. In this body of research, borderline diagnostic criteria function as an Axis I trauma symptom checklist that correlates with the severity and chronicity of abuse, and the other DDIS symptom clusters.

In an initial study (Ross, Heber, Norton, & Anderson, 1989a), we interviewed 20 DID, 20 schizophrenic, 20 eating disorder, and 20 panic disorder patients with the DDIS. The only difference between groups in frequency of borderline personality was that the DID group met the criteria more often than the panic patients, $p = .01$. This showed that borderline personality was no more characteristic of DID than of schizophrenia or eating disorders, in our sample. Based on our data, it is inconsistent to dismiss DID as an artifact of borderline personality, unless one makes a similar dismissal of schizophrenia, which no one would do. Gunderson, Carpenter, and Strauss (1975) and others (Sheehy, Goldsmith, & Charles, 1980) have shown that borderline personality and schizophrenia can be reliably differentiated, just as we have shown is the case for DID and schizophrenia. Although it is always good to have more data, there is really no doubt that DID is not an artifact of borderline personality disorder.

In our study, of the eight *DSM-III* borderline criteria, only one, instability of affect, differentiated DID from all three other groups. Two items, identity disturbance and unstable relationships, did not differentiate DID from any other group. To have borderline personality disorder, according to *DSM-III* rules, one must be positive for five or more of the eight criteria.

A very different picture emerged when we compared the groups on number of positive borderline criteria. The DID subjects had a mean of 5.3 positive borderline symptoms, eating disorder 3.4, panic disorder 2.4, and schizophrenia 3.0. In this comparison, DID differed from each of the three other groups at $p = .003$ or greater, while none of the other groups differed from each other. These data show that "borderline personality" as a discrete entity does not differentiate DID from other disorders very well. However, "borderlineness," as one form of dissociation, does. Psychiatric patients who are more dissociative are more borderline. This supports the idea of borderline criteria being items on a spectrum of increasingly severe dissociation, rather than criteria for a freestanding entity. The DID subjects had much more severe trauma histories than the other three groups.

In a second study (Ross, Anderson, Fraser, et al., 1992), we increased the number of DID patients interviewed with the DDIS to 166: Of these, 61.4% met criteria for borderline personality. This is close to the 70% of Horevitz and Braun. The percentage of DID patients who meet criteria for borderline personality disorder is probably lowest in a private practice in which clients pay fees themselves and highest in tertiary care hospital-based practices like mine and Braun's. In our experience, borderlineness is a measure of the behavioral difficulty, intensity, and complexity of double binds, acting out, and involvement with social agencies we can expect during treatment.

In a subsequent study (Ellason, Ross, & Anderson, 1996), we compared 206 DID patients with concurrent borderline personality to 90 DID patients without borderline personality disorder on the DES and DDIS. The borderline multiples were much more dissociative and reported more severe trauma histories. They had more Schneiderian symptoms, more secondary features of DID, and higher DES scores. I mention these studies to illustrate the relationships between borderline personality disorder criteria, dissociation, and childhood trauma that show up in a large number of different studies in different clinical settings, using a variety of different statistical methods.

If subjects in a borderline clinic were interviewed with the DDIS and DES, a highly dissociative subgroup could be readily identified. This subgroup would have more DID, secondary features of DID, Schneiderian symptoms, positive borderline criteria, and ESP experiences. They would probably have more somatic symptoms as well. They would have more severe abuse histories. For future research, three groups need to be identified and compared:

1. DID with borderline personality disorder.
2. DID without borderline personality disorder.
3. Borderline personality disorder without DID.

These groups would exhibit childhood trauma, DES scores, and levels of DDIS symptomatology in the pattern $1 > 2 > 3$, or the pattern $1 > 2 = 3$.

Another study on the relationship between DID and borderline personality was the study of 345 college students (Ryan, 1988) described in an earlier chapter. Of 345 university students who completed the DES, 20 students scoring above 22.6 and 22 scoring below 5.0 completed the SCL-90, Million Clinical Multiaxial Inventory (MCMI), and the DDIS. In this study, we were comparing nonclinical high dissociators and low dissociators. Items occurring more frequently in the high group might therefore be part of a dissociative cluster.

The same pattern of dissociative cluster items was found in this study. The high group had more somatic symptoms, Schneiderian symptoms, secondary features of DID, ESP experiences, and positive borderline criteria than the low group. They also had higher rates of sexual abuse. It appears that somatic symptoms are clearly dissociative although they are less consistent discriminators of dissociative and nondissociative subjects than the other items in the cluster.

We (Ryan, 1988; Ryan & Ross, 1988) did two other analyses of the college student data that were consistent with all our other findings. We did

Spearman correlations of items on the DDIS with DES scores and found that four items on the DDIS correlated at $p = .0001$. These were secondary features of DID ($r = 0.78$), Schneiderian symptoms ($r = 0.67$), borderline criteria ($r = 0.67$), and ESP experiences ($r = 0.59$).

When we did a regression analysis of the data, we found that the item on the DDIS that best predicted DES score was secondary features of DID (beta weight $= 0.60$). This finding validates the DDIS against the DES, because the secondary features section contains dissociative experiences inquired about by the DES but in different wording. There were seven factors in the regression model. In the order they entered the model, these were secondary features of DID, trance states, psychogenic amnesia, DID, borderline personality disorder, childhood sexual abuse, and Schneiderian symptoms.

There is a strong and clear pattern in these data. The reason the different sections of the DDIS are in the DDIS is that clinicians have been observing the dissociative cluster in their DID patients for the past 15 years.

One final piece of data on the college students: The high and low groups did not differ on the narcissistic, histrionic, and antisocial subscales of the MCMI, but they differed at $p = .0001$ on the borderline subscale. This suggests that DID and dissociation are not linked to histrionic personality style and that borderline criteria belong to a dissociative cluster rather than to the group of personality disorders on Axis II referred to as Cluster B. Cluster B includes borderline, histrionic, narcissistic, and antisocial personality disorders. This conclusion is also supported by other research reviewed in Chapter Six.

In my experience, the diagnosis of borderline personality disorder doesn't usually have much to do with the *DSM-IV* criteria in any case. It is very rare to see documentation on a chart of which criteria the patient meets and which she doesn't. If one asked a random sample of residents and psychiatrists to list the *DSM-IV* criteria for borderline personality, very few could list all eight, and many could list only two or three. In practice, I think that many clinicians diagnose a patient, usually female, as borderline, when they can't even say what the criteria for diagnosis are or which ones the patient meets. This is very different from the clinical diagnosis of depression, which is usually based on detailed inquiry about specific diagnostic criteria, with good interrater reliability. Data to support the contention that most residents cannot list sufficient criteria from memory to diagnose borderline personality disorder are presented in *Satanic Ritual Abuse*.

What is the clinical diagnosis of borderline personality disorder based on, then? Gut feeling, I think. The gut feeling is based on not liking the patient. When a patient is called borderline, in my experience, it usually means that the diagnostician finds her difficult and annoying to deal with. It also means that the clinician is stuck in one or more double binds. A typical double bind is the following: If you send me home, I will kill myself; if you admit me, I will deteriorate. The patient states only the first half of the bind.

The clinician on call in emergency, usually a resident, is then put in a second double bind by the system: If you send her home and she kills herself, that shows poor judgment on your part; if you admit her, it shows you can't handle borderlines in emergency. Next the patient is put in a counter-double-bind: We don't admit borderlines because they deteriorate and disturb the milieu; if you act out enough, we will certify you. The resolution of the double bind usually involves a compromise, which can be an overnight stay in emergency, referral to the outpatient department, a short-term prescription for medication, or contact with the therapist by the resident, all of which demonstrate the benevolence of the resident.

The patient diagnosed as borderline is usually the victim of negative characterological attributions by mental health professionals. For example, instead of attributing the borderline's refusal to attend group therapy to untreated panic disorder with agoraphobia, the patient is described as manipulative and acting out. The agoraphobia does not get treated, and the staff decides to "set limits" on the patient. The patient responds by threatening suicide. It is impossible to work with intensely borderline patients without getting endlessly caught up in such power struggles.

Often, if the dissociative, anxiety, and depressive symptoms of the borderline patient are successfully treated, the borderline personality will melt away. I have had the experience of watching apparent borderline personality disorder with concurrent major depressive episode vanish after several weeks of therapeutic doses of antidepressant, concurrently with remission of the depression. And I have seen a nonborderline bipolar man become severely narcissistic-borderline while hypomanic, then transform back into a well-adjusted person on lithium, with concurrent remission of his hypomania. This could be called the epiphenomenology of borderline personality disorder.

Borderline, in actual clinical reality, doesn't refer directly to *DSM-IV* criteria. Borderline is a term describing a general way in which the patient-mental health professional system is organized. The core of this organization is the double bind. In fact, "borderline" has nothing in particular to do with "personality," a widely used but nebulously defined term in psychiatry. Borderlines do not have something wrong with their personalities. Neither do DID patients. Both have dissociative disorders involving numerous psychic functions, including affect, behavior, memory, cognition, and perception.

"Borderline" organization is characteristic of many different systems. Consider the legal system. The legal system has borderline personality disorder: It is perverse, destructive, and prone to aggressive acting out. It thinks in dichotomized categories. Supposedly, the legal system is a system of justice designed to protect honest citizens and punish criminals. In practice, one is actively rewarded for fraudulent affidavits, unethical behavior, self-interested abuse of other citizens, and psychopathic opportunism. This is called a "defense" in legal terminology. One is punished for honest and decent behavior, which is not "smart" according to the rules of the system. To be "smart" and to "win" in the justice system, one must be a legal criminal.

Clinicians who dismiss DID patients as "just borderlines" are in error. Neither diagnosis has anything in particular to do with "personality," neither is a psychosis or a personality disorder, and both are aspects of chronic trauma disorder in the majority of patients treated by mental health professionals. Borderline personality and DID are overlapping facets of one polydiagnostic syndrome. All the available data support that contention: There are no disconfirming data.

SCHIZOPHRENIA

DID is often mistaken for schizophrenia (Putnam et al., 1986; Ross, Miller, Reagor, et al., 1990; Ross & Norton, 1988; Ross, Norton, & Wozney, 1989). In this section, though, I am going to discuss the relationship between correctly diagnosed schizophrenia and correctly diagnosed DID. Schizophrenia, which is probably a group of illnesses rather than one disorder, may be an organic disease of the brain and a medical illness in the strictest biomedical sense of the term, although that has not been proven. The comprehensive treatment of schizophrenia involves intensive psychosocial interventions, however (the same is true for rheumatoid arthritis). The ultimate goal of current schizophrenia research is to find biological methods for treating and preventing it. DID, on the other hand, could be prevented by stopping childhood trauma. This means that primary prevention of schizophrenia is more likely than the eradication of DID.

DID may be roughly as common as schizophrenia. It probably causes about as much morbidity for the individual, economic cost for society, and emotional cost for friends and relatives of the patient, although the quality of all these is different from that in schizophrenia. At the present time, DID is more treatable than schizophrenia.

I think that when DID and severe schizophrenia coexist in the same patient, the DID often gets lost in the fragmentation and disorganization of the patient's psyche. Psychotherapy for the DID is probably of limited or no use in such cases, of which I have encountered a number. The patient should probably be treated as a schizophrenic, even in an ideal world of unlimited resources. In a finite world of severely limited resources, such patients should not get psychotherapy when there are better prognosis candidates on the waiting list.

There may be a dissociative subtype of schizophrenia, however. This subtype may have a different prognosis or treatment response. One of my research goals is to attempt to identify such a subtype. If it exists, it should be incorporated into future *DSM*s, along with catatonic, paranoid, and other subtypes.

Dissociative schizophrenia is probably characterized by Schneiderian symptoms, ESP experiences, bizarre somatic delusions, borderline criteria, and childhood trauma. The patients may have a borderline premorbid character, rather than schizoid-schizotypal. Or the "mystical" adolescent interested in demonology, who retires into his bedroom for months before his first psychotic break, may be highly dissociative. I don't know.

My main prediction is that the positive symptoms occurring in schizophrenics are dissociative in nature. The main features that differentiate DID and schizophrenia are the negative symptoms of schizophrenia and the posttraumatic dissociative features of DID. The negative symptoms of schizophrenia are occupational and social deterioration, emptiness, loss of drive, and the other "burnout"-type features. The negative symptoms appear to be irreversible deficits in brain function caused by a progressive biological illness. Antipsychotic medications have no effect on the negative symptoms of schizophrenia.

In a very simple model, which is no simpler than the dopamine theory of schizophrenia, the deterioration of the schizophrenic brain causes positive symptoms during acute flare-ups and in the initial years of the illness. These are due to the irritation of the brain by the etiological agents of the illness, which might be a virus and dysregulated immune cells in one patient, endogenous toxins in another. The brain of the schizophrenic gets "feverish" during acute phases. In this model, the neuroleptics are nonspecific firehoses that cool the brain off temporarily, until the "fever" subsides. Their clinical site of action could be in the walls of cerebral capillaries as easily as in the synapses.

Patients who develop the biological illness of schizophrenia should be more likely to display dissociative features if they have abuse histories. One would want to compare three diagnostic groups and nonpsychiatric controls on the DES and DDIS: dissociative schizophrenia, paranoid schizophrenia, and DID. This study would yield four clusters: abuse-dissociation-schizophrenia (dissociative subtype of schizophrenia), no abuse-no dissociation-schizophrenia (paranoid schizophrenia); no abuse-dissociation-no schizophrenia (normal dissociation); and abuse-dissociation-no schizophrenia (DID). I when I say no abuse, I mean no more abuse than in controls without psychiatric disorders.

A question would arise concerning the group with dissociative schizophrenia. Do they have two diagnoses or one? Do they have dissociative schizophrenia only, or do they have schizophrenia and DID concurrently? Unlike the question about whether borderlines have a psychosis or a personality disorder, that would be a real question.

Although one cannot infer etiology from treatment response in psychiatry (Ross, 1986a; Ross & Pam, 1995), pragmatically, the question is whether patients with dissociative schizophrenia benefit from psychotherapeutic interventions derived from the DID literature. Historically, the psychotherapy of schizophrenia has been more or less abandoned, although Meichenbaum (1977) has shown that cognitive-behavioral interventions can reduce delusional statements made by schizophrenics. It may be that the positive features of dissociative schizophrenia can be treated at least partially with psychotherapy, though. Because schizophrenia carries such severe morbidity, this is a possibility worth investigating. The first step is to determine whether a dissociative subtype of schizophrenia exists and to show that it can be reliably differentiated from other subtypes.

Research I have published to date (Ellason & Ross, 1995a; Ross, Anderson, & Clark, 1994; Ross & Joshi, 1992b; Ross, Miller, Reagor, et al., 1990; Ross & Norton, 1988) supports the conclusions that positive symptoms of schizophrenia are more common in DID than in schizophrenia; can be arrived at through a trauma pathway; are more common in schizophrenics reporting childhood abuse than in those not doing so; and cluster with other DDIS symptom clusters in the dissociative subtype of schizophrenia. Additionally, negative symptoms of schizophrenia are more common in schizophrenia than in DID.

For example, in one study (Ross, Anderson, & Clark, 1994) 83 subjects with long-standing clinical diagnoses of schizophrenia were interviewed with the DES and DDIS and then divided into those reporting childhood physical and/or sexual abuse ($N = 37$) and those ($N = 46$) not reporting childhood abuse. The abused schizophrenics reported many more symptoms in all the DDIS symptom clusters including Schneiderian first-rank symptoms of schizophrenia. The abused schizophrenics endorsed an average of 6.3 Schneiderian symptoms compared with 3.3 for the nonabused schizophrenics ($t = 3.9$, $df = 81$, $p < .001$). The abused schizophrenics had an average DES score of 21.6 compared with 8.5 for the nonabused subjects ($t = 4.8$, $df = 79$, $p < .001$)—DES data were missing for two subjects.

Although these are data from a single study with methodological limitations, they point to the possibility of a dissociative subtype of schizophrenia, and justify further investigation. The relationship between childhood sexual abuse and positive symptoms is also very strong in the general population (Ross & Joshi, 1992b). In a stratified cluster sample of 502 respondents in the general population, there were 397 subjects reporting no Schneiderian symptoms and 35 reporting 3 or more: of the non-Schneiderian subjects, 8.1% reported childhood abuse compared with 45.7% of the Schneiderian subjects. The relationship between childhood trauma, other dissociative symptom clusters and positive symptoms of schizophrenia was borne out by a number of other statistical analyses including a stepwise regression analysis.

Globally in psychiatry, I think, we have become sloppy clinicians in our study of schizophrenia because of the bioreductionist model of the illness. The tendency now is away from spending any amount of time talking with the schizophrenic patient in an attempt to understand his or her mind. Once we check off a few symptoms, make the diagnosis, and start medication, detailed study of the psychosis becomes clinically irrelevant, in much of daily practice. One monitors the patient only carefully enough to track treatment response, which is usually not very carefully. There is no reason to try to understand the patient's mind in detail, as there is in a long-term psychotherapy case, because the symptoms are just biologically driven craziness that needs to be suppressed with medication.

These remarks are directed at the general tendency of most clinical practice in North America. The medical treatment of schizophrenia isn't really psychiatric these days, although the physicians who provide it are called psychiatrists. It is really neurological, and the physicians are psychiatric internists. Within the biomedical camp, this is viewed as highly desirable. But I think we have become third-rate phenomenologists of schizophrenia. We should consider putting the psychiatry back into schizophrenia treatment, not just with educational groups, social support, and similar interventions, but with mind interventions that are specific for the illness and effective. This would have to involve something very different from conventional psychoanalytic psychotherapy.

DID taught me something about the clinical examination of auditory hallucinations. Contemporary psychiatry is like a cardiology in which one examines the radial pulse but never listens to the heart with a stethoscope. In the clinical examination of auditory hallucinations, a major feature is simply left out of all the standard textbooks. In the routine clinical assessment of auditory hallucinations, the diagnostician should determine whether it is possible to talk to the voices. This exercise is an important method for subtyping dissociative schizophrenia, or at least I think it will become that. As things stand now, the only people who talk to patients' voices are DID therapists. In mainstream psychiatry, this doesn't even occur to the examiner as a possible intervention.

Although one must avoid tautological definitions, it is possible that one cannot talk to psychotic voices, but only to dissociative voices. If one can hold conversations with the voices of a patient who has correctly diagnosed schizophrenia, this would be evidence in favor of a dissociative subtype. There are two main ways to talk to voices.

The first steps in the clinical examination of auditory hallucinations are those of conventional psychiatry. One must find out if there are voices, the number of different voices, what they say, the tone or mood of their speech, their association with other symptoms, and the patient's understanding of them and response to them. The voices may talk directly to the patient; if they order her to do things, that is called a command hallucination. Or the voices may talk to each other, in a cooperative, argumentative, or other fashion. The voices may comment on the patient and her thoughts, feelings, and actions in the third person.

Voices can do other things. They can repeat the patient's thoughts out loud or say them just before the patient was going to think them. They can perform thought insertion and thought withdrawal. It is important for the examiner to think about the voices as if they are actual people and try to find out what they are like, what they are doing, and what their motivation seems to be. In other words, one should examine all auditory hallucinations as if they come from alter personalities, in order to positively rule dissociation in or out. This applies no matter what the clinical diagnosis.

In severe acute schizophrenia, the voices are often bizarre and irrational. The patient may describe CIA agents talking in his testicles, or Martians talking through a microphone implanted in his brain. The content of the voices' speech may be incoherent, irrational, or bizarre. Such voices tend to be psychotic, rather than dissociative. One cannot engage them in conversation, nor can the patient. Often they do not come from inside the patient's head, whereas dissociative voices tend to. All these distinctions are based on clinical experience, not on designed studies.

Psychotic voices tend to be associated with thought disorder and acute phases of a psychotic illness, whereas dissociative voices tend to be chronically present even when the patient is functioning well. All these distinctions are only general rules of thumb. The distinction between psychotic and dissociative voices may be semantic. Psychotic, in this regard, may be a subset of dissociative, because dissociation must occur in some form for a mind to hear part of itself talking and to experience that as nonself talking. If that is the case, psychotic voices are a form of dissociation with certain characteristics, one of which is that they occur in a chronic major mental illness of presumed biological etiology. But there are other differences.

I examined a young native man with schizophrenia. He had numerous severe negative symptoms, inappropriate affect, poverty of speech and movement, a psychotic sister, and a supportive, warm, nonabusive family. But I could talk to his voices. He had two main voices with whom he held conversations. Both spoke in English and were white, although other minor voices spoke in Cree. He described one as good and one as bad. The bad one wanted him to assault people and generally act in an unpleasant manner. The good one tried to soothe him and advised more socially acceptable behavior. The bad one sometimes claimed to be the Devil.

Previous to my examination, a social worker had talked directly with the Devil briefly, when he had taken executive control spontaneously. I was unable to induce a switch, but I had a long rational conversation with the two voices. They both gave their points of view on the patient and each other, spoke politely, and would be described as "cooperative to examination" in a conventional mental status examination report. The voices in this patient were more than chaotic symptoms of insanity. They were in fact sane. Schizophrenic voices tend to be crazy.

In this patient, his dissociative features did not lead to any novel interventions or any change in the standard biomedical therapy, or in the broader biopsychosocial management of the case, which included periodic family meetings with the parents, the patient, and the psychotic sister. The parents reported transient positive improvement after a series of traditional native medicine interventions.

To engage the patient in such a conversation with the voices, one explains in a straightforward fashion that sometimes it is possible for the doctor to ask the voices questions. One then explains simultaneously to the patient and the voices how the procedure works:

> I am going to ask the voices some questions now. What I want the voices to do is listen, then answer to John. John will tell me what the voice said, then I will ask another question. If any of the voices want to ask me a question, they should feel free to: John will tell me what was asked, and I'll try my best to answer. First I want to talk to the voice John calls the white voice. The first question I have is, white voice, can you hear me and understand what I'm saying?

If the patient reports that the voice answered, "Yes," one proceeds with whatever line of questioning seems required. If the voice said, "No," I might reply:

> Because the voice said, "No," I know that means he can hear me and understand me. I can't force you to talk, white voice; in fact, I don't even want to try to force you to do anything. I would like to talk to you a bit, though, because what you have to say might help me understand John better and figure out how to help him. What do you think of that, white voice?

I use various strategies to try to engage the voice. If none work, I leave open the possibility of talking to me or another doctor later. All this is done with no formal induction of hypnosis, in a straightforward fashion and in a normal tone of voice. If there is no response from the voices of any kind, one can fish a bit in various ways, just as one might with a hostile adolescent who won't talk.

When trying to talk to the voices, with or without success, it is always important to monitor the patient's affective and physiological state. There may be no answer, but the patient may feel a wave of anger coming from somewhere, or may get tense or frightened. These are signals that dissociated affect is linked to the psychic region from which the voices emanate. This is suggestive evidence that a substantial amount of psyche has been dissociated and that it has internal structure. Simple psychotic voices often don't appear to have any psychic structure linked to them.

Psychotic voices probably come from very small fragments of psyche, too small even to be "fragments" in the sense of fragment personalities. I lean toward a continuum of increasingly small amounts of psyche dissociated (Ross, 1985) as one passes downward from personalities, to fragments, to psychotic voices.

Hierarchically, the next step after engagement of the voices in conversation, with the patient as intermediary, is inducing a switch of executive control and talking directly with the voices while they have executive control. Techniques for doing this are described in Chapter Fourteen. Here is another example of a patient whose voices I talked with indirectly. This man was amnesic for a rape-murder and two rapes with attempted murder committed 8 years prior to examination, for which he was eventually found guilty 16 years after the crimes. He had been in a mental hospital since the crimes and had been unfit to stand trial. In the past, he had had numerous conversion and dissociative symptoms. He had two female voices, one friendly and one extremely hostile. They were difficult to engage in conversation because of the hostility of the bad voice.

Whenever the patient got too close to a woman, including female staff, the bad voice started instructing him to perpetrate a violent sex crime on her. The voices were not affected by his antidepressant and antipsychotic medication. I could not talk with the voices very long because of the hostility of the bad voice and therefore could not rule DID in or out. For a man like this, and for society, there are two options, if one excludes capital punishment: (1) He can stay in hospital or prison until he dies; (2) regular intensive psychotherapy can be conducted for years. From Option 2, there are two possibilities: He can be cured and set free eventually, or he is untreatable and can never be safely released. In practice, he could eventually be released neither treated nor safe.

The bad voice is the portal of entry into that region of the man's psyche that holds the memory and motivation for the crimes. Even if classical DID isn't present, the only possibility for cure lies on the other side of the amnesia barrier, with the voice. The cost of the psychotherapy would be a minute fraction of the total cost of housing this man in hospital or prison. In addition, knowledge of other unsolved crimes and the fate of unlocated missing persons may be locked away behind the amnesia barrier. To me these are possibilities that warrant aggressive investigation.

DID potentially can teach us much about schizophrenia and psychotic features that occur in schizophrenia, mania, delirium, and other organic brain syndromes. The examination of auditory hallucinations is incomplete if the assessor does not try to talk with the voices. For these reasons, DID should not be ignored by conventional psychiatry. A patient who reports chronic auditory hallucinations may have either DID or schizophrenia: The differential diagnosis is based on features other than the positive symptoms of schizophrenia, because these symptoms alone do not differentiate the two disorders.

MALINGERING

According to *DSM-IV*, DID "must be distinguished from Malingering in situations in which there may be financial or forensic gain and from Factitious Disorder in which there may be a pattern of help-seeking" (p. 487). The Kenneth Bianchi (Allison, 1984; Orne et al., 1984; Watkins, 1984) and Ross Carlson (Weissberg, 1992) cases provide evidence in support of that caution. In the forensic context, malingering is always in the *DSM-IV* differential diagnosis, no matter what the symptoms are, but there is no evidence indicating that DID is faked more often than other disorders in forensic settings.

Despite its rough utility in forensic situations, the conceptual system of the late twentieth century concerning malingering and factitious disorders rests on unscientific and untestable foundations. This failure in *DSM-IV* causes problems in understanding the relationship between DID and malingering.

In *DSM-IV*, malingering is categorized under "Other Conditions That May Be A Focus of Clinical Attention" and cannot be diagnosed on Axis I or II because it is not a legitimate psychiatric disorder. It is therefore given a V code and listed on page 683 as V65.2:

> Malingering differs from Factitious Disorder in that the motivation for the symptom production in Malingering is an external incentive, whereas in Factitious Disorder external incentives are absent. Evidence of an intrapsychic need to maintain the sick role suggests Factitious Disorder.

This differentiation is repeated on page 471 of *DSM-IV* where the Axis I category of factitious disorder is explained:

> Factitious disorders are characterized by physical or psychological symptoms that are intentionally produced or feigned in order to assume the sick role. The judgment that a particular symptom is intentionally produced is made both by direct evidence and by excluding other causes of the symptom . . . . In Malingering, the individual also produces symptoms intentionally, but has a goal that is obviously recognizable when the environmental circumstances are known . . . in contrast, in Factitious Disorder, the motivation is a psychological need to assume the sick role, as evidenced by an absence of external incentives for the behavior.

On page 449 of *DSM-IV*, in the text for somatization disorder, the reader is instructed as follows:

> In Factitious Disorder with Predominantly Physical Signs and Symptoms and Malingering, somatic symptoms may be intentionally produced to assume the sick role or for gain, respectively. Symptoms that are intentionally produced should not count toward a diagnosis of Somatization Disorder.

These distinctions between factitious disorder, somatization disorder, and malingering are unscientific for several reasons. They violate *DSM-IV* system rules, which state that diagnostic criteria must be based on phenomenology, not theory. The distinction between conscious and unconscious motivation, between "intrapsychic need" and "external incentives," lies outside the bounds of observable behavior. Conscious-versus-unconscious is an inference made from patient reports and observed behavior, and is neither a symptom nor a sign, which means it cannot be a criterion for a medical diagnosis. There is no evidence that psychiatrists can make the conscious-unconscious distinction with any degree of interrater reliability and there is no literature documenting any experimental effort by psychiatrists to differentiate conscious and unconscious symptoms. The key *DSM-IV* difference between a somatic symptom and a factitious symptom is unscientific.

The *DSM-IV* distinction between malingering and factitious symptoms is an artifact of the accident that the distinction is being made by a doctor. Faking symptoms for gain in the medical setting is diagnosed as a legitimate Axis I disorder, but faking them in all other contexts is called malingering. The idea that the sick role does not involve "obvious, external incentives," while faking in the rest of the world does, is far from self-evident. Many social psychologists and behaviorists hold that the sick role, like all human behavior, is "motivated by external incentives."

There is no scientific evidence that psychiatrists can make the differentiation between fakery with external incentives and fakery based on intrapsychic needs. The distinction implies that human behavior can be separated into these mutually exclusive categories based on metapsychology, which is implausible. The *DSM-IV* rules for malingering, somatization, and factitious disorder are derived from Freudian theory but are simplistic from a psychoanalytical perspective. The problem with them is not that they are Freudian, but that they are unscientific.

Many symptoms common in DID patients are listed in the *DSM-IV* criteria for somatization disorder, including amnesia, which occurs in all cases of DID. According to *DSM-IV* rules, a psychiatrist must assess the amnesia in a DID case and determine whether it is conscious, in which case it is factitious or malingered, or unconscious, in which case it is a symptom of either a somatoform disorder or a dissociative disorder. There are no rules for deciding between dissociative and somatoform. If the amnesia is judged to be conscious, the criterion for differentiating malingered from factitious is entirely artifactual, as I have pointed out.

There's something curious about malingering getting boldface emphasis in the differential diagnosis of DID, when it isn't even mentioned in many other sections of *DSM-IV*. Why is that? It occurred to me that there must be some dynamic reason why malingering is emphasized in the *DSM-IV* differential diagnosis of DID. What does lying have to do with DID? Wondering about this, it occurred to me that lying is a form of dissociation. To lie, one must dissociate.

What is a lie? A lie is a deliberate untrue statement. One consciously intends to lie and when caught is morally responsible. Liars get punished or at least admonished. Lying is not "okay," in conventional morality. Lying about one's innocence is not a defense in a court of law: There is no defense called "not guilty by reason of lying." Lying is not insanity or a sign of illness. It is more like a sin. Most people would agree with this view of lying.

Is Santa Claus a lie? When a parent tells his young child that Santa is coming, that is a deliberate untrue statement. But it is not a lie. No one calls the parent a liar.

What about Munchausen's syndrome, which can be a presenting feature of DID (Goodwin, 1988)? The Baron von Munchausen was a delightful liar (lying can be lots of fun for both liar and audience), but patients with his syndrome are not delightful. Munchausen's patients fake illnesses, change their names, and trick doctors into unnecessary surgery, investigations, prescriptions, and hospitalizations. But are they lying? Munchausen's patients seem to be at least partially victims of that well-known malady, "believing your own bullshit." Where is the dividing line between lying and delusion? What about lying to yourself? Where is the transition point between lying and self-deception?

Deciding what is a lie, what is a delusion, and what is misinformation can be a very difficult clinical problem. There is no set of well-defined clinical categories that provide a differential diagnosis of lying. If a patient makes a statement that might be a lie, what else could it be, clinically? A delusion, an overvalued idea, an obsession, a misattribution, what else? This isn't something one gets taught about in psychiatric training.

To lie, one must dissociate. To dissociate is to split apart and separate psychic states and contents. To lie, one must do this. In a lie, one disavows reality and knowingly substitutes a falsehood. The liar places reality, and his knowledge of it, to one side. This is a mild, minor, consciously controlled form of dissociation. Like other dissociative phenomena, it occurs on a spectrum from normal lying through to pathological dissociation.

An alter may state that her biological father is not her father, while acknowledging that he is the biological father of the body and of the presenting personality. Is this a lie? Should one tell the alter to "Smarten up, and stop lying"? No. This is a dissociative symptom of a treatable mental illness. It is not surprising, then, that malingering, which is the clinical term for lying, occurs in the differential diagnosis of DID. The creation of alter personalities is an extreme extension of the normal psychic mechanism of everyday malingering: From this perspective, dissociative disorders are malingering that deceives the malingerer.

Item 10 on the Dissociative Experiences Scale reads, "Some people have the experience of being accused of lying when they do not think they have lied. Mark the line to show what percentage of the time this happens to you" (Bernstein & Putnam, 1986, p. 733). This item is in the DES because DID patients disavow behavior for which they are amnesic. People accuse them of lying because they don't realize that there is amnesia involved. Like all other items in the DES, this item has a Spearman correlation of $p = .0001$ with overall DES scores in both adolescents and college students, which suggests strongly that it is a dissociative symptom.

Item 10 is one of the most elevated items on the DES among normal adolescents (Ross, Ryan, Ross, & Hardy, 1989). Why? I'm not exactly sure. But there seems to be a developmentally normal form of dissociation that occurs in young adolescents and makes them appear to others to be lying. This is different from getting caught lying. There is a potential field of study that involves the normal developmental relationship between dissociation and lying, and the pathology of lying at various ages. Confabulation in Korsakoff's patients, for instance, is an organically driven symptom that might be related to the high scores of normal adolescents on DES Item 10. Both involve the substitution of falsehood for reality, but neither are lying.

These are speculations, but I think there is some inner necessity or logic to the fact that malingering is in boldface in the differential diagnosis of DID in *DSM-IV*. There is more to it than historical artifact, forensic caution, and confused thinking. This is what I mean by a dynamic relationship between lying and dissociation. My experience of iatrogenic and factitious pathway cases of DID is that neither can be understood in terms of conscious-unconscious or environmentally strategic-nonstrategic dichotomies.

Skeptics about DID sometimes complain that the dissociative disorders are based on unproven theory. This charge actually applies to malingering and factitious disorders, which skeptics use to dismiss DID, while the diagnostic criteria in the dissociative disorders section require no metapsychological assumptions. The *DSM-IV* system rules prevent a meaningful differentiation of malingered and "real" DID. One could say that real cases of DID are malingered, that DID is never real, that malingering is a real form of factitious disorder, and that factitious disorders are malingered, and therefore not real. The four pathways to DID described in Chapter Three provide an organized, testable way of making the necessary distinctions.

OBSESSIVE-COMPULSIVE DISORDER

As suggested earlier, obsessive-compulsive disorder is not an anxiety disorder, contrary to its classification in *DSM-IV*. Anxiety is a minor secondary feature of the disorder. In some cases, it is probably a variant or feature of depression, Tourette's syndrome, schizophrenia, or another primary diagnosis. Other obsessive-compulsive patients appear to have a free-standing disorder limited to the specific obsessions and compulsions. Historically, obsession was related to demon possession, which is a dissociative phenomenon.

I have done one small study that demonstrates the existence of a dissociative subtype of obsessive-compulsive disorder (Ross & Anderson, 1988). During the course of our clinical work in Canada, we did sodium amytal interviews on two obsessive-compulsive patients refractory to treatment. Under sodium amytal, both manifested entities like alter personalities, who claimed responsibility for the patients' obsessions and compulsions. Neither of these entities ever took executive control outside the sodium amytal interview, but both used copresence to inflict symptoms on the patients. Neither was a full alter personality.

We were able to differentiate these two patients from a third obsessive-compulsive patient on a variety of measures. The third patient did not manifest an alter-personality-like entity on sodium amytal interview. We also compared the three obsessive patients with three DID patients on the measures used. The two dissociative obsessive patients resembled the DID patients more than the nondissociative patient.

The measures used in this study were the DDIS, DES, the Anxiety Disorders Interview Schedule, the SCL-90, and the Lynfield Inventory for obsessive-compulsive disorder. The nondissociative patient had lower scores on all measures and met criteria for far fewer diagnoses. Although this was only a small pilot study, it provides the measures and ideas for definitive identification of a dissociative subtype of obsessive-compulsive disorder. One of the dissociative-obsessive cases is described in detail in *The Osiris Complex* (Ross, 1994b).

One would give these measures to, say, 100 consecutively seen obsessive-compulsive patients, with enrollment at several Anxiety Disorders Clinics. Next, a DID specialist blind to the results of the interviews and self-report questionnaires, would attempt to contact an alter personality-like entity using sodium amytal. The measures would predict which patients would clinically dissociate under sodium amytal. The patients could then be triaged into controlled behavioral and pharmacological treatment outcome studies, in a blind, randomized fashion. Clinicians assessing the treatment response of the obsessive-compulsive disorder would be blind to the measures of dissociation and the results of sodium amytal interview.

I expect that such a study would identify a dissociative subtype of obsessive-compulsive disorder that is harder to treat with serotonergic antidepressants or behavioral techniques. Conversely, screening out patients with the dissociative subtype would yield a better differentiation of placebo and active treatment response rates in nondissociative obsessive-compulsive disorder.

The presence of highly dissociative individuals in a wide variety of diagnostic groups is probably confounding studies of many kinds in psychiatry, including nosologic, treatment outcome, and biological marker studies. They are increasing the variability, narrowing the gap between placebo and active treatment, and increasing the percentage of nonresponders. Screening out these people should be of great interest to the pharmaceutical industry, if no one else.

Clinically, obsessions and compulsions are much like the Schneiderian symptoms in DID. They arise from a large, structured, dissociated portion of psyche. Until I worked intensively with DID patients, it never occurred to me to ask where obsessions and compulsions come from. I was taught that they are "ego alien" and heard some implausible psychoanalytic discussion of their site of origin. But by and large, where the symptoms come from was never asked. It didn't seem to be an important question: The obsessions just came from "out there," somewhere. Out there was perfunctorily assumed to be "the unconscious," and there wasn't much else to say about it.

To me, having worked with DID patients, where the obsessions come from is a crucial clinical question. The dissociative view of general psychopathology flows inevitably from intensive work with DID, if one listens to the patients. If you work with multiples a lot, all patients start to sound dissociative. This is similar to the specialist in depression, for whom everyone seems to be depressed. I expect the reader and the field to take my bias into account and to weigh my data and argument accordingly.

Like much else in general psychopathology, obsessions and compulsions seem to arise from dissociated aspects of the psyche. They must, otherwise they wouldn't be experienced as obsessions and compulsions. The therapeutic question is whether it is necessary, or helpful, to work directly with the dissociated psyche in order to alleviate the symptoms. This is the case in DID. Why not in obsessive-compulsive disorder? In practice, the expedient approach might be to do a sodium amytal interview in all patients who fail to respond to adequate trials of antidepressants and/or behavioral treatment. Depending on the findings on sodium amytal interview, dissociative interventions could be attempted next.

If the patient has DID, however, the hierarchically superior treatment should be instituted first, and the obsessive-compulsive symptoms should remit by the late preintegration phase of therapy.

CONVERSION DISORDER

Once one begins to think dissociatively, conversion disorders appear to be dissociative in nature. In fact, conversion disorders are classified as dissociative disorders in the International Classification of Diseases (World Health Organization, 1992). I'm not sure why North Americans have a problem seeing the correctness of this. In my clinical experience, conversion disorders occur in two forms: as isolated conversions in the absence of overt severe general psychopathology, or as features of a chronic complex dissociative disorder.

According to the model of dissociation outlined in Chapter Six, dissociation can occur in any area of the brain, with the function corresponding to that brain region being dissociated. A pure, simple dissociation of memory is psychogenic amnesia; a dissociation of motor or sensory function, a conversion disorder. To me this is self-evident. I am trying to make it other-evident.

In *DSM-IV*, conversion is classified as a type of somatoform disorder. This is the case for two reasons: first, because the body is involved; second, because of the vestigial influence of Freudian theory. Freud attempted to make distinctions between repression, conversion, and somatization that are untestable and not clearly thought out.

Conversion disorder is called conversion disorder because Freud said it was based on conversion. If it was based on somatization, it would be called somatization disorder; if on repression, repression disorder with physical symptoms, I suppose. Conversion disorder couldn't be called somatization disorder in *DSM-IV* because that name is used for Briquet's hysteria (Mai & Merskey, 1980). The symptoms of Briquet's hysteria are part of the dissociative cluster, however. The somatoform disorders need extensive reorganization. As they stand, they are a group of heterogeneous disorders thrown together as a group of illnesses because they have physical symptoms.

The necessary reorganization would bring greater conceptual consistency to the field and would group things as they are grouped in nature. In nature, similar treatments are effective for similar disorders. The etiology, natural history, and treatment of conversion disorder and dissociative amnesia are very similar. For conversion disorder and hypochondriasis, they are very different. Yet conversion is classified in a group of somatoform disorders that includes hypochondriasis. This makes sense only as the outcome of a set of unresolved historical forces, not as a scientific classification.

Some cases of *DSM-IV* pain disorder may represent positive dissociative symptoms. Dissociation can result in something being present that is usually absent or something being absent that is usually present. Dissociative headache is a good example of dissociative psychogenic pain. Pain disorder is probably a heterogeneous group of disorders, with some cases actually being organic pain of unrecognized etiology. There may be a dissociative subtype.

INTERMITTENT EXPLOSIVE DISORDER

I have never seen a case of intermittent explosive disorder, but I have met quite a few intermittently explosive alter personalities. This diagnosis is a dissociative disorder by definition, regardless of etiology. It is defined as intermittent switching to explosive states. *DSM-III* notes that there can be partial or complete amnesia for the explosive state, a fact highly suggestive of undiagnosed DID, but all discussion of amnesia has been removed in *DSM-IV* and the dissociative disorders are not mentioned in the differential diagnosis. The general drift of the *DSM-IV* text for intermittent explosive disorder is that it is caused by organic brain dysfunction.

If a series of patients with alleged intermittent explosive disorder were reviewed by a DID expert, I believe that many would have partial or full DID. In many, a switch of state could be induced quite easily by hypnosis, sodium amytal, or experimental oral alcohol.

The Cartesian mind-body dichotomy in psychiatry is evident in opinions that intermittent explosive disorder is a form of epilepsy or other organic brain illness (implying that the patient is not legally responsible for the explosive behavior). This results in acting-out adolescents being treated with medication to control their "seizures." That is fine if the medication works, but the dissociative phenomenology of the "illness" has not been explored, consequently neither have curative psychotherapeutic possibilities derived from the DID literature.

TEMPORAL LOBE EPILEPSY

Related to the issue of whether intermittent explosive disorder is a form of epilepsy is the idea that temporal lobe epilepsy should be seriously considered in the differential diagnosis of DID. It shouldn't. I am discussing it in this chapter because there is no chapter on DID and neurological disorders. Temporal lobe epilepsy is classified as complex partial seizures in the official nomenclature. I will refer to it as temporal lobe epilepsy because readers are likely more familiar with that name.

The inclusion of temporal lobe epilepsy in the differential diagnosis of DID, in the DID literature, is based on a few reports of small series of patients with concurrent DID and temporal lobe epilepsy (Benson, Miller, & Signer, 1986; Cocores, Bender, & McBride, 1984; Mesulam, 1981; Schenk & Bear, 1981).

The first trouble with the alleged cases of DID/temporal lobe epilepsy in the literature is that many of them don't have DID. These are in fact the only false-positive cases of DID I know of in the psychiatric literature prior to 1988 (Coons, 1988a). That is curious, because these papers are sometimes thought to discredit DID as a legitimate psychiatric diagnosis. In Benson, Miller, and Signer's (1986) paper, for example, the "DID" consists of intermittent psychotic states with Capgras's syndrome. These probably represent status epilepticus. The states have none of the structure, rationale for existence, or function of alter personalities. There is no evidence of childhood abuse. In other papers, some of the cases don't have full DID.

There isn't a single case in the literature of classical DID responding to antiepileptic medication. Collective clinical experience in North America, if it were assembled in a single report, would document hundreds of DID patients with blood level-controlled trials of epilepsy medication with no effect on the DID. In fact, not a single case of an adequate trial of epilepsy medication in a well-described case of DID, with adequate observation of symptom-response is documented in the literature.

In the only study comparing DID patients with and without temporal lobe epilepsy, Putnam (1986a) found no difference between the two groups in abuse histories or features of their DID. In the only study comparing groups of DID ($N = 20$) and temporal lobe epileptic patients ($N = 20$) with reliable structured interviews, we found that the two disorders differed on all dissociative sections of the DDIS, and on the DES, at high levels of significance (Ross, Heber, Anderson, et al., 1989). The 20 temporal lobe epileptics did not differ from 28 controls with other neurological disorders, except that they more often met criteria for depersonalization disorder. We interpreted the finding on depersonalization as evidence that it is not a freestanding disorder, but a symptom of other disorders, in this case of epilepsy.

The data show that DID and temporal lobe epilepsy can be clearly differentiated on a large number of clinical features at high levels of significance.

A study by Loewenstein and Putnam (1988) using the DES confirms this. As well, temporal lobe epilepsy has no effect on the features of DID in patients who have both disorders. This shows that the relationship between DID and temporal lobe epilepsy is a research dead end. Clinically, there are no positive reasons to consider temporal lobe epilepsy in the differential diagnosis of DID any more than any other neurological disorder. Perhaps this piece of reductionist-driven clinical lore can be laid to rest.

ALCOHOL IDIOSYNCRATIC INTOXICATION

Alcohol idiosyncratic intoxication is also called pathological intoxication. It is defined as abrupt "maladaptive" changes of behavior markedly atypical for the person when not drinking. The changed behavior is usually aggressive or assaultive and occurs "within minutes of ingesting an amount of alcohol insufficient to cause intoxication in most people" (*DSM-III-R*, p. 129). The differential diagnosis includes temporal lobe epilepsy and malingering. The disorder is regarded as an organic mental disorder (Goodwin, Crane, & Guze, 1969) but has been dropped from *DSM-IV.*

Alcohol idiosyncratic intoxication is basically intermittent explosive disorder triggered by pharmacologically insignificant doses of alcohol. Yet the two appear in unrelated sections of *DSM-III-R* and neither is mentioned in the differential diagnosis of the other. This doesn't make sense. It shows that *DSM-III-R,* like *DSM-IV,* has DID: Its sections were produced by dissociated fragment committees, many with two-way amnesia barriers between them.

The authors of the discussion section of alcohol idiosyncratic intoxication in *DSM-III-R* try to account for the observed fact that a pharmacologically meaningless dose of alcohol is involved by postulating a lowered biological threshold of sensitivity to alcohol. They suggest several mechanisms for this including subclinical temporal lobe epilepsy, encephalitis, brain injury, debilitating physical illness, and old age. This is pushing biological explanations a long way. Interestingly, Goodwin, Crane, and Guze (1969) note one individual in their series of 100 cases who "believed he could produce a blackout at will, as a kind of 'self-hypnosis'" (p. 1036). This suggests that careful screening might have yielded more cases of psychogenic dissociation.

What doesn't get consideration is psychological dissociation triggered by the psychosocial context and meaning of alcohol ingestion. Pathological intoxication is basically a state-switching disorder triggered by the social act of drinking alcohol. Placebo alcohol in the same social setting would probably work just as well. Like intermittent explosive disorder, many people with idiosyncratic alcohol intoxication probably have partial or full DID: All have angry states dissociated from their host states. Accessing and interviewing these dissociated states would probably be technically straightforward.

The exclusively biological account of alcohol idiosyncratic intoxication in *DSM-III-R* is an example of bioreductionist ideology creating a dissociated diagnostic system. It is also symbolic of a general bias in the field of substance abuse. People with different forms of substance abuse experience altered states and amnesia on a regular basis. Much of this is no doubt biologically driven. But much is probably psychological and dissociative in nature. Everything tends to get written off as a result of drugs, however. If I am correct, the phenomenology of substance abuse disorders needs major revision.

Some alcohol blackouts start before alcohol ingestion—is this retrograde organic amnesia or a switch to a substance-abusing alter? At least some chemically dependent patients refractory to the usual treatments probably have DID: In such cases the addicted alter never gets treatment and sits scornfully coconscious in the background while the host personality dutifully attends treatment. The patient never gets better because the wrong "person" is in treatment. The therapist might as well be treating the patient's brother, uncle, or neighbor.

Alcohol idiosyncratic intoxication patients are dissociative patients who give themselves in vivo placebo sodium amytal interviews using pharmacologically insignificant amounts of alcohol. Successful treatment might result from the doctor doing the interviewing, rather than the patient.

EATING DISORDERS

In our series of 236 cases of DID (Ross, Norton, & Wozney, 1989), 16.3% had a previous diagnosis of an eating disorder. This is an underestimate of the prevalence of pathological eating behavior in DID, which was present in 38.3% of 107 of cases interviewed with the SCID. Eating disorders are related to sexual abuse (Goodwin & Attias, 1988; Goodwin, Cheeves, & Connell, 1988) and to DID (Torem, 1986, 1987, 1988), but only in a subgroup of patients. The majority of eating disorder patients probably arrive at their clinical conditions through pathways other than trauma and dissociation.

Anorexia and bulimia can both have specific dissociative mechanisms. Goodwin and Attias (1988) have described such specific dissociative mechanisms with great depth and clarity. The distortion of body image in anorexia nervosa can have a dissociative basis and can be caused by the copresence of an alter personality in some cases. Somatic memories and behavioral enactments of specific abuse incidents can underlie binging, vomiting, purging, and other behaviors.

I am not going to say much about eating disorders and dissociation, other than to note that there is undoubtedly a dissociative subgroup of such patients. Some of these have frank DID, some don't. These patients are an excellent population for study because they have discrete behavioral symptoms that can be monitored in treatment. The efficacy of dissociative interventions could be readily demonstrated in a subgroup of patients in treatment for eating disorders.

I have emphasized the concept of a dissociative subgroup of eating disorders because there is likely a mood disorder subgroup, among others. As in all sections of *DSM-IV,* the challenge is to identify specific diagnostic subgroups that respond differentially to different well-defined treatments. One of the subgroups that should be considered throughout psychiatry is the dissociative.

PSYCHOSEXUAL DISORDERS

Many of the psychosexual disorders are dissociative disorders. Take the man who is impotent with his wife, but not with his mistress, during masturbation, or while dreaming. There is nothing wrong with his penis or with the nerves and hormones connecting his penis and his brain. He has dissociated his ability to have an erection in one particular social context.

The same is true for psychogenic frigidity in a woman who reaches orgasm easily with a vibrator. Such a woman has dissociated her ability to be aroused and fulfilled sexually. Impotence and frigidity occur on a spectrum. At one end of the spectrum are pure biological forms, at the other pure psychological forms, and in the middle are mixed forms. This is analogous to the classification of asthma as intrinsic, extrinsic, or mixed.

The psychosexual disorders of arousal and orgasm are like conversion disorder and psychogenic pain: Psychogenic impotence is clearly dissociative, whereas dyspareunia (painful intercourse for the female) may be. The disorder of absent function is clearly dissociative, whereas the disorder of abnormal pain is not so clearly dissociative.

Another group of psychosexual disorders involve sexual orientation and gender identity. In the absence of any research data, I can only speculate that ego-dystonic homosexuality and transsexualism may be dissociative in some cases. Evidence in support of this possibility is the frequent existence of homosexual and opposite-sex alters in DID. This does not mean that a substantial proportion of transsexuals are dissociative, but the possibility is worth investigating. In *The Osiris Complex* (Ross, 1994b), I have described one man with an incorrect diagnosis of schizophrenia who wanted a sex-change operation. His female personality was easily contacted and wanted to get rid of the male host, everything he stood for, and his genitals. The female alter saw this as a power struggle for control of the body.

The most important possibility is that many sex criminals have dissociative disorders. Bliss (1985) has provided preliminary evidence that this is the case, but no definitive study has been conducted. We know that many abusers were themselves abused. It would make sense that many sexual criminals have dissociative disorders. One such man is described in the discussion of schizophrenia. Enough is now known about dissociation that it is imperative, from the point of view of the social responsibility of the psychiatric profession, to investigate whether sexual criminals are often dissociative and whether treatment techniques from the DID literature would reduce recidivism.

BIPOLAR MOOD DISORDER

Manic-depressive illness is called bipolar mood disorder in *DSM-IV*. I believe that, like schizophrenia, it is likely a biological brain illness, that the primary treatment is medical, and that psychosocial interventions are required. This is the majority, mainstream view in contemporary psychiatry. Manic-depressive illness is a disorder of switching. Patients with the disorder switch states in a pathological manner. Their problem is severalfold: They switch into states, switch out of states, and get stuck in states in an abnormal manner.

There is a severe discontinuity of mood, speech, thought, and behavior across states. What about identity? And memory? A distortion in memory is characteristic of depression, and depressed patients ignore their positive achievements and qualities while selectively focusing on the negative (Beck et al., 1979) when in the depressed state. Little attention is paid to the discontinuity of identity that must occur across states, as patients switch from depression to mania. This is an interesting area for research.

I am not suggesting a reclassification of mania or depression as dissociative disorders. They are mood disorders. But the discontinuity of identity across states in DID might shed light on the switch process in manic-depressive illness. The situation might be a little different with nonpsychotic unipolar depression. This disorder might have prominent dissociative mechanisms.

I have done successful classical cognitive therapy with a few unipolar depressive patients. In my experience, which is representative, depressed patients can be transiently converted to a normal affective state with cognitive interventions even in the first few sessions. Often less than 10 sessions are required to switch the patient out of depression for a long period. What does this mean? It tells us that the normal mood, thoughts, and behavior of depressed patients are not lost. They are not simply absent due to a chemical deficiency in the brain. In fact, they can be recovered psychotherapeutically quite quickly.

This is like the recovery of normal mood in DID by switching from a depressed to a nondepressed alter, and it suggests to me that in unipolar depression the patient's normal mood is dissociated. It must be, otherwise how could one get it back so quickly? The machinery that maintains the separateness of alter personalities can be analyzed cognitively, and many of my interventions in DID are cognitive. Perhaps in unipolar depression the depressogenic cognitions are the psychic machinery for maintaining a dissociation of normal mood. Dismantle the machinery, and the normal mood comes back. This is what happens in cognitive therapy, according to Beck (Beck et al., 1979).

A corollary of this view of unipolar depression is that the antidepressants are actually antidissociatives. The standard view of the antidepressants is that they work by correcting a deficit that is thought to be a deficiency in noradrenalin or serotonin function in the brain. Maybe antidepressants actually work by dampening down and suppressing an excess of dissociation. Neurochemically, this would mean that the antidepressants reduce levels of one or more neurotransmitters by an actual reduction in synthesis or release of transmitter, an increase in reuptake or degradation, or a modulation of receptor density or sensitivity. Both mechanisms, dissociative and depletive/depressive, could be at work in subgroups of mood disorders, which would account for the contradictory results in biological marker studies—dissociative depressed patients have an excess of transmitter; nondissociative have a deficiency. Some patients presenting with depression, of course, actually have DID (Frances & Spiegel, 1987).

This reasoning is an example of how the study of DID can lead to novel hypotheses in biological psychiatry. These hypotheses could lead to experimentation and insight at the basic and clinical levels. The view that the antidepressants are actually antidissociatives would make sense of the fact that chlomipramine, a tricyclic antidepressant, is effective for obsessive-compulsive disorder (Ross, Siddiqui, & Matas, 1987), which is dissociative in nature in a subgroup. This line of thought leads to the opposite prediction of that made in the section on obsessive-compulsive disorder: Chlomipramine could be most effective in the dissociative subtype of obsessive-compulsive disorder, rather than least effective. The two possibilities could be studied in the same clinical trial.

A similar trial could be carried out for unipolar depression. Depressed patients could be divided into high and low dissociators on the DES and DDIS. Half of each group could be given imipramine, and half chlomipramine, in a randomized double-blind fashion. Imipramine is less effective for obsessive-compulsive disorder than chlomipramine, but the two are equally effective, overall, for depression. If obsessive-compulsive disorder is dissociative, and if chlomipramine is the most antidissociative tricyclic, then chlomipramine should be more effective than imipramine in the high-dissociative depressed group and equally effective in the low-dissociative depressed group.

Similarly, if cognitive therapy is an antidissociative treatment, it should be more effective in high-DES unipolar depression. I want to emphasize that I am advocating a way of thinking about psychopathology and classifying psychiatric illnesses that leads to testable hypotheses in both biological and psychological psychiatry.

A final additional speculation. Methylphenidate (Ritalin) is effective in slowing down hyperactive children, although it is a stimulant. This is paradoxical. Similarly, some people react to benzodiazepines, which are sedatives, with hyperalertness, arousal, and agitation. Why should a stimulant slow down a hyperactive child? Perhaps the children are hyperactive because they can't dissociate irrelevant stimuli effectively. Perhaps methylphenidate helps them dissociate better.

As for the people who fly into a rage on diazepam, perhaps the drug interferes with their ability to maintain their rage in a dissociated state. This would make sense, because sodium amytal increases the ease with which one can access dissociated states, and it is a sedative. Similarly, one can sometimes transiently reverse catatonia in a schizophrenic with benzodiazepines like diazepam and lorazepam.

Clinically, I've had the experience of curing the catatonic state of a woman with a psychotic unipolar depression in five minutes with sodium amytal. This woman had been unable to eat or drink, was mute and fearful, and was catatonically posturing in the seclusion room. Within five minutes of starting the intravenous sodium amytal, she began tearfully but coherently giving me a full history of the prodrome and onset of her depression. After the interview, she went to the washroom and had lunch. I attempted to but could not engage her voice in conversation. Such dramatically effective interventions arise from looking at the world through dissociative-colored glasses.

CONCLUSION

The purpose of this chapter has been to elucidate the relationship between DID and selected other psychiatric disorders, with a focus on borderline personality disorder and schizophrenia. I have also argued for a reorganization of *DSM-IV*. Many disorders currently scattered around *DSM-IV* should be reclassified within a category of trauma disorders. Others have dissociative aspects that should be studied scientifically, or they include a dissociative subgroup with distinct features. Thinking dissociatively leads to novel testable hypotheses in both biological and psychological psychiatry.

Dissociative Identity Disorder and Nonclinical Dissociation

The mind of an individual psychiatric patient is embedded in the collective mind, language, and history of his or her culture: Clinical dissociation arises out of the everyday, nonpathological dissociation occurring in a given society. This means that dissociative identity disorder (DID) is a microcosm of our culture, and that history must be taken into account in studying DID (Carlson, 1981, 1984; Crabtree, 1985, 1993; Drew, 1988; Hawthorne, 1983; Rosenzweig, 1988). When I say "our culture," I am taking about urban literate English-speaking North America of the late twentieth century.

The philosophical foundation of our culture is Cartesian dualism. The evolution toward this dualism, which is a fundamental dissociation of mind and body, began in ancient Greece. The dualism is fundamental in the sense that it is the *dynamic,* living foundation of our culture. It is concretely present in our art, science, and religion. The philosophical doctrine expounded by Descartes is not the *cause* of this dualism—it is an expression of it, and a reinforcer of it.

In conjunction with this basic dualism, the history of Western civilization is a history of increasing fragmentation and specialization of function. The shaman has dissociated into many fragments, including doctor, priest, poet, entertainer, weatherforecaster, psychotherapist, and politician. The fragmentation is not all bad: It has led to modern medicine and the highest material standard of living in human history. It is also not all good.

In this chapter, I am going to examine everyday nonclinical dissociation, and the relationship between extrasensory perception (ESP) and dissociation. The purpose of this chapter is to embed the study of DID in a broad, general context. I discuss the theme of Cartesian dualism as a fundamental dissociation of mind and body at length in *Satanic Ritual Abuse* (Ross, 1995a). I have mentioned dualism here to establish a link with *Satanic Ritual Abuse,* and to emphasize that the necessary context for the study of dissociation is historical, philosophical, and anthropological—at a minimum.

EVERYDAY NONCLINICAL DISSOCIATION AND THE SPECTRUM OF DISSOCIATION

Anxiety, depression, and dissociation are common features of everyday life. Dissociation isn't recognized as much as the other two, just as dissociative disorders are diagnosed less often than anxiety and mood disorders. Before reviewing some of our research data on ESP, I am going to provide several examples of nonclinical dissociation. These will provide a feel for the importance and prevalence of dissociation as a major aspect of normal mental function. As for any psychiatric disorder, understanding of clinical dissociation must be based on a more general psychology of normal mental function.

At a movie theater, one can get so absorbed in a movie that one enters a dissociative state. While dissociated, the moviegoer does not realize that he is in an altered state of consciousness. It is only when the movie hits a dull patch, someone gets up to go for popcorn, or the person in the next seat makes a romantic hand maneuver, that one comes out of trance (the third example can provoke a rapid switch to another altered state). The experience is a bit like waking up and then realizing that you have been asleep, but are now awake. This experience occurs within the absorption/imaginative involvement factor of the DES.

Another example is the dissociation that occurs while reading a child's book aloud for the hundredth time. The child and the other parent can be attentively listening to the story, and may not notice the slightest change in the reader's voice. The reader suddenly returns to consciousness, aware that he has completely blanked out for the last three pages, without any interruption in his reading. This doesn't happen with new books, and is more likely to happen at the child's bedtime in a dim room, lying on a bed, with a bedtime book. This is an example of normal amnesia, and belongs to the second DES factor.

I remember hearing that a well-known Canadian folksinger is amnesic for all of every performance: This is an extension of the normal process of reading several pages in a trance, with posttrance amnesia. Of course, the singer might have DID, which is a further extension of normal dissociation. Similarly, many people who drive cars have had the experience of coming to, suddenly aware that he or she is amnesic for the last few blocks. This can be dangerous at night on a lonely road if the trance state shifts into sleep.

It is normal for the world and one's self to become unreal as one falls asleep, when very tired, during extreme traumatic events, under the influence of prescription, over-the-counter, or street drugs, during a fever, or in conjunction with jet lag. All these experiences fall within the depersonalization/derealization factor of the DES.

Dissociation can increase an individual's functional level. I remember walking long distances in Rome while visiting a friend there in the 1960s. I didn't have a map and didn't know the city. I found my navigation more effective when I paid less attention to it, letting my unconscious slide along the grooves I had cut during previous walks. Every athlete is aware of this process and of the need to cultivate it. A light trance state with diversion of attention from the task at hand can produce a better performance.

Everyday dissociation occurs at a more mundane level. Divided consciousness is required, for example, to talk on the phone, scan the newspaper, and stir the spaghetti sauce at the same time. Everyone daydreams, which is a dissociative state. There are several multibillion-dollar industries in North America that exist because their products induce altered states related to daydreaming. The products include novels, magazines, movies, television, pornography, alcohol, and cocaine. In fact, much of the crime in North America is driven by the desire to enter altered states of consciousness, primarily through drugs and sex. This could be called the social pathology of artificially induced dissociation.

The desire for intense dissociated states must be built into our DNA: Without the desire for orgasm, the race would not be propagated. Such states are wonderful, desirable, and healthy, in their natural form. But there is nothing wonderful about the chemical ecstasy of the heroin-addicted HIV-positive ghetto prostitute. This is why there is a psychiatry of dissociation, the goal of which is to substitute healthy, normal altered states for self-destructive, painful ones. The goal of the treatment of DID is not to produce someone who never dissociates. That would be like giving someone a lifetime prescription for an antidepressant to prevent the person from feeling sad when loved ones die. Such a prescription would be a clinical error for two reasons: It is a misconceived goal of treatment; and the antidepressants don't have that effect anyway.

Studies have established that hypnotizability, which is linked to but not identical to normal dissociation, is distributed on a bell-shaped curve in the general population (Berg & Melin, 1975; Gordon, 1972; Laurence, Nadon, Nogrady, & Perry, 1986; Morgan & Hilgard, 1973). Only about 10% of people are excellent hypnotic subjects. High hypnotizability has nothing to do with being gullible, easily influenced, hysterical, or dumb. It is a skill that requires conscious focusing and willing participation, except in highly charged situations such as war, sustained brainwashing, natural disaster, or sexual assault, during which an individual becomes vulnerable to involuntary dissociative symptoms.

The major forms of psychopathology all occur on a spectrum from normal to pathological, although psychiatrists and psychologists debate whether disorders like panic disorder are discrete disease entities or extensions of normal with no sharp cutoff between normal and pathological. This debate continues for virtually all psychiatric disorders, including the dissociative disorders.

Take alcoholism, for example. Anyone can differentiate a teetotaler from someone who consumes 26 ounces of vodka a day, and it is no great surprise that psychiatrists can make this distinction with structured interviews. However, this is not how alcohol consumption is distributed in the general population. Some people don't drink at all, some have an occasional cocktail, some a glass of wine with most meals, and some drink six to eight beers on a weekend. At some point along the spectrum there is a gray zone in which it is a matter of judgment whether a given person is an alcoholic or just someone who enjoys drinking a lot.

Many *DSM-IV* diagnostic criteria sets require that the symptoms interfere with function or cause significant personal distress before a diagnosis can be made. This requirement does not solve the gray zone/cutoff problem because impairment and distress also occur on a spectrum and are a matter of degree. The same analysis of normal anxiety and sadness can be made in regard to the anxiety and mood disorders, which also occur on a spectrum of severity.

My view is that dissociation, anxiety, depression, and substance use all occur on spectra from normal to pathological, that there is no sharp cutoff, and that extreme cases are in a discrete and separate category nevertheless. Everyone without an anxiety disorder uses their experience of normal anxiety to understand anxiety disorders, and the same should be true for the dissociative disorders. We all have a bit of the addict and a bit of the multiple inside us.

EXTRASENSORY PERCEPTION AND DISSOCIATION

The exclusion of ESP from serious mainstream psychiatry is antiscientific. This is true whether or not ESP is real. If ESP is real, then its exclusion from mainstream scientific study is based on prejudice, not a scientific attitude. On the other hand, if ESP is illusory, it should be studied just like any other set of symptoms, delusions, or hallucinations. Psychiatrists do not make fun of schizophrenic delusions, and refuse to study them—yet that attitude toward ESP predominates in the field. Regarding ESP as a serious subject of study is discouraged through a million little social mechanisms.

Freud, the father of twentieth-century psychiatry, excluded ESP, and broke with Jung partly because of Jung's interest in the paranormal. Why did ESP get excommunicated?

ESP got discredited along with hypnosis in part because of its accidental historical connections with charlatans and cranks. Respectable scientists didn't want to be seen in the company of quacks, so they rejected both the individual men involved, and the paranormal as a field of study. The exclusion of ESP from mainstream psychiatry was culture-specific, and determined by the social prejudices of a particular phase of our civilization. In addition, ESP was rejected because of scientific conservatism, much like the medical establishment's initial rejection of the stethoscope, antiseptic surgical technique, the dissection of cadavers, smallpox vaccinations, and the circulation of the blood. With ESP, there is another factor at work.

ESP is closely linked to dissociation (Braude, 1995; Crabtree, 1985; Estabrooks, 1943; Jung, 1902/1977; Myers, 1903/1920; Rogo, 1986a). The ESP-dissociation linkage is like the findings of quantum mechanics and relativity theory, which destroyed the certainties of nineteenth-century physics. If ESP actually happens, it means that the relationship between mind and body is different from that postulated by contemporary reductionist science. If ESP actually happens, the physics of the universe, and the interaction of mind and matter, are far from fully accounted for; the same is true of the *dynamics* of the psyche. If telekinesis is real, mind is a physical force in the universe, as real as electricity, magnetism, or gravity. Psychiatry then becomes the physics of the mind. If DID is real, the model of the mind must change, independently of the reality of ESP, therefore the ESP-dissociation linkage is a double threat to reductionist dualism.

If ESP experiences were obviously delusional, they could be incorporated into contemporary psychiatry easily, along with other delusions. The difficulty is that they aren't obviously delusional. Before ESP was banished to the fringes of psychology, subjects with dissociative and paranormal experiences were widely studied in Europe. In the nineteenth century, many leading physicists and psychologists devoted a lot of time and energy to the study of ESP. Among these men was Carl Jung, who wrote a thesis in medical school dealing with the paranormal and dissociation, although he didn't use those terms (Jung, 1902/1977).

In the second half of the twentieth century, in North America and Russia, paranormal phenomena have been taken seriously, in terms of research funding, primarily by intelligence agencies. For instance, William Gates, former Director of the CIA, confirmed on the ABC television program *Nightline* on December 12, 1995, that the CIA and other intelligence agencies had spent 20 million dollars on ESP research from the 1950s through 1984. This financial support included the CIA's MKULTRA Subproject 136, which was funded for $8,579 on August 23, 1961: The title of the project was "Experimental Analysis of Extrasensory Perception." I obtained a copy of MKULTRA Subproject 136 documents through the Freedom of Information Act. The intelligence agencies were using psychics in operations at least up until 1984, according to Gates and an unidentified CIA employee whose job was oversight of ESP research and operations by other intelligence agencies and the military. No information was provided concerning activities after 1984.

The nineteenth-century mediums displayed many features of DID. This doesn't mean that they had DID—we don't know if they had abuse histories and created alter personalities to cope with it, or not. But there is a close relationship between DID and mediumship (Braude, 1995). The young women studied by Jung entered trances, during which "controls," dead people, and other entities took executive control of their bodies. Some of the women had somatic and other "hysterical" symptoms outside their trance states.

Most of the paranormal phenomena of nineteenth-century spiritualism can be readily understood as purely psychological in nature. Late twentieth-century DID patients often have alter personalities who claim to be dead people, spirits, astral beings, or other entities. It is clear that these are dissociated parts of the patient's mind. Often, though, the alters provide an initially compelling picture of paranormal power. The demons can be very chilling, until one discovers that they too are abused children. The question is, whether some mediums, and some DID patients, actually do have ESP. There is lots of psychological trickery, subterfuge, and theater, but in the midst of all that, is there actually some real telekinesis, clairvoyance, and telepathy? I'm willing to believe that there is, but I haven't yet seen the evidence, as illustrated by a case in *The Osiris Complex* (Ross, 1994b). It is peculiar that an expert in the paranormal like Rogo (1986b) can write a book on poltergeists, spend hundreds if not thousands of hours tracking them, yet never once have witnessed a poltergeist firsthand. That's a bit like my writing a book on DID, never having met an alter personality. If poltergeists exist, why are they so hard to document?

In analyzing the relationship between ESP and dissociation, a simple decision tree can be constructed. The first step is to establish that dissociation and paranormal phenomena coexist in a person. This is evident from nineteenth-century spiritualism, as documented in Jung's thesis. My research team in Winnipeg interviewed a series of "alternative" therapists who use a variety of new age techniques but aren't formal mediums, to determine whether they have dissociative features and/or abuse histories on the DES and DDIS (Heber, Fleisher, Ross, & Stanwick, 1989).

The 12 alternative therapists reported more Schneiderian first-rank symptoms, secondary features of DID, and paranormal experiences than a comparison group of 19 psychiatry residents, but not more childhood trauma or overall psychopathology. The alternative therapists reported an average of 7.8 (*SD* 2.5) ESP/paranormal experiences on the DDIS, compared with 0.9 (*SD* 0.7) for the psychiatry residents. The three elevated symptom clusters were all understood by the alternative therapists as being positive and valued spiritual attributes that they used in their practices. Therapists using paranormal abilities are easy to find in North America, resemble the mediums studied by Jung, exhibit the link between dissociation and ESP, and do not appear to be mentally ill.

I will assume that ESP and dissociation are linked phenomenologically. The first branch in the decision tree leads to two possibilities: One is that ESP is not real. If ESP is not real then it is one more set of symptoms in the dissociative cluster (first-rank symptoms of DID). If the second possibility is true and extrasensory phenomena are scientific realities, a more complicated and interesting relationship between psychic ability and dissociation must be present. ESP seems to be specifically linked to dissociative disorders, and to be less common in other psychiatric illnesses, as confirmed in the entire body of research conducted with the DDIS.

The DDIS study focusing specifically on the relationship between childhood trauma, dissociation, and ESP is an analysis of data from the general population survey in Winnipeg, discussed in Chapter Five (Ross & Joshi, 1992a). Like other surveys, we found that paranormal experiences are common in the general population: Of 502 respondents, 17.8% reported experiencing precognitive dreams, 15.6% mental telepathy, 5.2% contact with ghosts, and 0.6% possession by a demon. Only 34.3% of the sample reported no paranormal experiences and 5.1% reported five or more, with 12.6% reporting three or four paranormal experiences.

The ESP experiences fell into three factors accounting for 44.0% of the variance on principal components analysis: The first factor included classical ESP experiences such as mental telepathy and precognition, plus contact with ghosts and spirits, and knowledge of past lives; the second was a possession factor; and the third consisted of demon possession and contact with poltergeists. I consider poltergeist phenomena to be a form of externalized possession, so the composition of the third factor makes sense to me.

When the sample was divided into 63 individuals reporting childhood physical and/or sexual abuse and 439 not reporting abuse, the abused group reported twice as many ESP experiences. In a Pearson correlation matrix, a number of different DDIS abuse variables correlated significantly with the number of ESP experiences at $p = 0.20-0.26$. Finally, in a regression analysis, significant predictors of the number of ESP experiences included childhood physical and/or sexual abuse (beta weight 0.21), the amnesia (activities of dissociated states) factor on the DES (beta weight -0.20), Schneiderian symptoms (beta weight 0.19), and age (beta weight -0.17).

The existing data clearly support a consistent relationship between childhood trauma, dissociation, and the paranormal, which is more evident in younger people. Richards (1991) also found a significant relationship between paranormal and dissociative experiences in a study using the DES. However, Richards and I agree that this is only part of the story: Childhood trauma and dissociative disorders are accompanied by increased rates of ESP experiences, but the relationship is weak in the opposite direction. That is, most people who are psychic do not exhibit dissociative or other psychopathology, although they describe many benign dissociative experiences.

I have constructed a model of the relationship between dissociation and ESP. I have invented a cultural dissociation barrier that separates paranormal experience from normal perception; in most Western people the barrier is impermeable (Ross, 1991b). Logically, six combinations of dissociation and ESP are possible:

1. No dissociation; no ESP.
2. No dissociation; ESP.
3. Normal dissociation; no ESP.
4. Pathological dissociation; no ESP.
5. Normal dissociation; ESP.
6. Pathological dissociation; ESP.

Most people in North America have no dissociation-no ESP (by which I mean zero or one ESP experience on the DDIS, and DES scores in the normal range). What is it that opens a window to the paranormal in the cultural dissociation barrier? I hypothesize that severe, chronic childhood trauma interrupts the closing of the window to ESP: This window is usually closed developmentally in our culture. In our culture, paranormal experience is suppressed and ignored, as it is in mainstream psychiatry (Ross, 1991b, 1994b). That is why childhood trauma, pathological dissociation, and ESP are linked in North America: The window is closed during "normal" development in the absence of trauma.

ESP and normal dissociation are closely linked in nature and therefore tend to be elevated together in the absence of trauma and pathology. One would predict from this model the following frequency relationships between the preceding configurations in the general population in North America: $1 > 2$; $3 > 4$; and $6 > 5$. A larger sample size is required to provide a test of this model. I also predict that in polytheistic cultures which value normal dissociation and ESP but lack endemic childhood trauma, the most common configuration would be 5, and the least common 6, whereas in our culture 1 is the most common. It appears that Bali is a candidate for such a polytheistic culture (Suryani & Jensen, 1993)

According to many Christian fundamentalist exorcists, ESP is demonic. Vulnerability to ESP is vulnerability to the devil. This vulnerability, according to the exorcists, is often caused by childhood trauma, especially sexual abuse. It is perpetuated by sinful living. The exorcists have recognized the three DDIS ESP factors and their relationship to childhood trauma within their fundamentalist worldview. The demons are exorcised at the beginning of the fundamentalist treatment program, which involves recovery of dissociated abuse memories and working through of abuse-linked conflicts. This sounds very similar to our treatment of DID, except that our "demons" are integrated rather than exorcised, and the integration occurs late in treatment.

The differences in technique are interesting. So is the difference in conceptualization. Here I want to focus on the common observation made from distinctly different philosophical perspectives: Dissociation and ESP occur together in people who have been traumatized as children. The trauma seems to keep open a window in the child's mind, through which paranormal information enters. The dissociative mind seems to be very open to unusual experiences. If ESP is real, no complete psychology can ignore the relationship between ESP and dissociation, which reveals fundamental properties of the mind and the physical universe. Here arises another paradox of DID: If ESP is real, the most dissociated members of our society are most open to experiences characteristic of less dissociated cultures.

An observation that needs to be made, is whether integrated DID patients lose their ESP experiences. They lose much of their psychopathology. If the ESP goes with it, does that imply that it was delusional? Perhaps our cultural suppression of ESP has been strengthened and reinforced during the therapy. If the ESP remains, does that mean it is real, or that the patient is incompletely treated? None of these questions can be resolved unless ESP is definitively shown to be real. If that happens, half the decision tree is knocked out. In the absence of such proof, we are left with ifs, ands, buts, and ideology. The outcome data reviewed in Chapter Eleven indicates that treatment of DID to integration results in a significant reduction in ESP experiences, but that does not tell us whether the ESP was illusory, or a window to real ESP gets closed with integration.

If ESP is delusional, it is important that we study it like any other psychopathology. If ESP is real, it is necessary to bring it into mainstream psychiatry initially as symptomotology, in the absence of scientific proof of its reality. Otherwise it won't get in at all. This is a Trojan horse maneuver for getting ESP established as a legitimate field of mainstream study. DID patients are probably the best population for testing for extrasensory perception in our culture.

ESP experiences differentiate DID patients from subjects with schizophrenia, panic disorder, eating disorders, temporal lobe epilepsy, other neurological disorders, multiple sclerosis, and migraine headache in studies we have conducted to date. Schneiderian symptoms also differentiate DID from all these other groups, including schizophrenia. Considered as delusions, ESP experiences are highly specific for the presence of a severe dissociative disorder. In turn, all patients we have assessed with complex DID have had extreme childhood trauma. This means that ESP experiences should generally be considered indicators of dissociation and trauma, rather than psychosis (see the discussion of schizophrenia in Chapter Eight).

Extrasensory perception is a legitimate area of clinical study. In view of the enthusiasm in our culture for trance channelers, *ersatz* enlightenment, and levitation in six easy lessons, scientific caution in the endorsement of ESP as a field of study is necessary. On the other hand, ideological rejection of ESP as a clinical phenomenon is just that, ideology, not science. Let me give a concluding vignette that illustrates the problems of dealing with ESP in inpatient psychiatry.

A single Eskimo man in his late 20s was admitted under my care because of suicidal ideation. He belonged to the highest risk group for suicide in the Canadian Arctic: acculturated, educated single Eskimo males. He had several severe psychosocial stressors, and a diagnosis of adjustment disorder with depressed mood. I discharged him after a few days and he was still alive two years later.

This man's father and paternal grandfather were both shamans. He himself had experienced bending plants with his mind, several other forms of telekinesis, and several episodes of clairvoyance. There were no psychotic features or hallucinogen abuse. He wanted me to take away his suicidal ideation and to prevent him from having any more ESP experiences. On one level, he seemed to perceive me as a powerful shaman who could cure his symptoms of craziness. I did not seem to impress him with my attempts to normalize his experiences as culturally acceptable, to explain that many people from all cultures and races believe in the reality of such experiences, and to point out that they are not necessarily symptoms of mental illness.

I was thus in the position of being requested to denigrate his culture to make him feel better, while being aware that the denigration of his culture and its shamanism was a major factor in his emotional disturbance. This man is intelligent, articulate, and far more successful at securing grants than any psychiatrist at my medical school. I think that clinicians should be perplexed and uncertain about how to handle ESP experiences in their patients, except in the most floridly psychotic patients. We should not devalue these experiences, because if they are real that would be bad medicine, akin to the devaluing of trauma histories as oedipal fantasy.

CONCLUSION

Twentieth-century psychiatry has grossly underestimated the amount of dissociation in the normal population, and in clinically disturbed individuals. Everyday dissociation needs to be studied thoroughly, in its pathology, its mundane aspects, and in the superior performance of gifted individuals. It is as if modern academia has a blind spot for one of the major themes of human psychology, an amnesia, one might say. DID patients are providing the stimulus for the reversal of this amnesia in North America in the late twentieth century. The relationship between childhood trauma, ESP, and dissociation requires much more study.

CHAPTER TEN

Skeptical Criticisms of Dissociative Identity Disorder

Dissociative identity disorder (DID) is the most controversial disorder in psychiatry. However, the quality of argument used by DID skeptics is evidence of the failure of liberal arts education in the English-speaking world. None of the published critiques of DID have any base in research or data, and all are characterized by elementary errors of logic and scholarship. The level of skeptical scholarly discourse about DID is lower than would be tolerated anywhere else in psychiatry. The standard of analysis I expect, but have never seen, from critics of DID can be found in my book *Pseudoscience in Biological Psychiatry* (Ross & Pam, 1995).

In this chapter, I will review a selection of recent critiques of DID published in 1994 and 1995. Choosing references from these years ensures that the critics have had the opportunity to review modern scientific research data and the major clinical writings in the field. I will review two studies on psychiatrists' and psychologists' beliefs about DID, catalog the main errors of logic, scholarship, and argument in the skeptical literature, and then review individual skeptics one by one.

HOW COMMON IS EXTREME SKEPTICISM ABOUT DISSOCIATIVE IDENTITY DISORDER?

Two studies have surveyed psychiatrists and psychologists on their beliefs and experience concerning DID (Dunn, Paolo, Ryan, & Van Fleet, 1994; Mai, 1995). Dunn and colleagues surveyed 1,120 Veterans Administration psychologists and psychiatrists and found that 97% believed in dissociative disorders and 80% in DID; 12.3% did not believe in DID, and 7.7% were undecided. Respondents not believing in DID tended to be older, not to have seen a case personally, and to be psychiatrists rather than psychologists at $p < .05$.

Mai, a DID skeptic, surveyed 180 psychiatrists in Ontario, Canada, and found that 66.1% believed in DID, 27.8% did not, and 3.3% were unsure, with 2.8% of the data missing; 56.7% had seen a case of DID; the average number of cases seen per psychiatrist was 3.78 (*SD* 10.26); and the number of newly diagnosed cases per psychiatrist was 1.21 (*SD* 5.02).

These data lead Mai to conclude, "It appears, therefore, that the diagnosis of MPD is made by a small number of psychiatrists who make a relatively large number of new diagnoses of the condition" (p. 156); and "Responses to this questionnaire study of Canadian psychiatrists confirm that a substantial minority doubts the existence of MPD as a diagnosis" (p. 157). Mai does not change his position even when his own data disagree with him, and he inverts the fact that the majority of psychiatrists surveyed believe in DID to report that a substantial minority disbelieve. If the data were that 66.1% did not believe in DID, would Mai have written that a substantial minority believe in the diagnosis, and viewed this as evidence in favor of its validity?

There are about 2,000 psychiatrists in Canada, a country of 26 million people. For illustration, if we assume Mai's data to be representative of Canadian psychiatrists as a whole, and if 66.1% believe in DID, this is 1,320 psychiatrists; if the average number of newly diagnosed cases per psychiatrist is 1.21, this is 2,420 cases, almost all of which were probably diagnosed since 1985; 1,134 psychiatrists have actually seen a case themselves. If we then extrapolate to the United States, which has about 30,000 psychiatrists, 19,830 American psychiatrists believe in DID; 17,010 have actually seen a case; and American psychiatrists have newly diagnosed 36,300 cases.

On the other hand, if Mai's data are idiosyncratic and not generalizable, they don't mean anything. Mai's data either mean nothing or indicate that almost 40,000 cases of DID were newly diagnosed in North America by over 18,000 different psychiatrists from 1985 to 1995. Mai's data are useful in putting the skeptical position into perspective.

The Canadian Psychiatric Association recently formed the Canadian Psychiatric Association Research Network to promote psychiatric research, and in a 1995 announcement listed the specialty areas of its first 307 members: 32 individuals listed dissociative disorders; 28 eating disorders;

21 AIDS/HIV disease; 19 geriatric psychiatry; and 7 substance abuse. These numbers indicate that there is as much serious research interest in the dissociative disorders in Canadian psychiatry as in eating disorders, AIDS, geriatric psychiatry, and substance abuse, which contradicts Mai's viewpoint.

TWENTY-FIVE ERRORS OF LOGIC, ARGUMENT, AND SCHOLARSHIP IN THE SKEPTICAL LITERATURE

The DID critics never review the literature adequately. They make massive overgeneralizations without discussing relevant papers published in leading journals. No critic has ever made a detailed analysis of methodological problems in dissociative research, and all argue exclusively at an anecdotal, ideological level. I have published more weighty criticisms of my own research than any critic has published concerning any work in the field. Some critics make major errors in their references on a repeated basis. Other critiques of the skeptics include ones by Braude (1995), Barton (1994a, 1994b), Kluft (1995), Martinez-Taboas (1995), Putnam (1995), and Ross (1990a). The 12 cognitive errors I identified in my 1990 paper are included in the 25 errors listed here, with some changes in wording and emphasis.

The skeptical errors are:

1. *Arguments Are Applied Only to DID That Could Just as Well Be Used against All Other Psychiatric Disorders.*

This is a pervasive strategy in the skeptical literature. DID will be dismissed as a hypnotic or cultural artifact with no data or argument as to why this analysis applies more to DID than other disorders. The skeptics never dismiss any other disorder on these grounds.

2. *Skeptics Overgeneralize from Biased Samples.*

This error is epidemic in the skeptical literature: The skeptic encounters a few iatrogenic or factitious cases and concludes that no cases are valid.

3. *DID Is Not Valid because Its Treatment Has Not Been Proven Effective.*

This statement would be laughed at as absurd if made about other disorders, yet it gets published repeatedly in critiques of DID. Are AIDS, cancer of the pancreas, and Alzheimer's disease dismissed as unreal because they are untreatable? By this logic, there would have been very few diseases in existence prior to the twentieth century. Efficacy of treatment is irrelevant to diagnostic reliability and validity.

4. *DID Is Not a Disease because It Is Influenced by Culture.*

This argument is an artifact of biomedical reductionism. It rests on the assumption that real psychiatric diseases such as schizophrenia and depression are biomedical and endogenous, and not significantly influenced by culture except in trivial symptom content. This bioreductionist theory has never been proven about any psychiatric disorder and rests on pseudoscience (Ross & Pam, 1995). By the criterion of pure culture-free symptom expression, depression and schizophrenia are not legitimate diagnoses either.

No research evidence is ever presented that DID is more influenced by culture than schizophrenia, panic disorder, or bulimia. Like many skeptical arguments, this proposition is tautological: the fact that DID is an artifact of hypnotizability and culture proves it is an artifact of hypnotizability and culture. The "argument" mounted by the skeptics is simply insistence, like someone trying to get a point across to a foreigner by speaking louder and louder.

5. *The Absence of Cases Outside North America Proves DID Is a North American Artifact.*

This argument is faulty because the absence of cases outside North America is neutral with respect to whether DID is a North American artifact. All the absence of cases tells us is that clinicians outside North America do not make the diagnosis as often as those inside North America. Whether this is because cases are being missed elsewhere or created iatrogenically in North America cannot be determined from the differential rates of diagnosis. Only systematic epidemiological studies with standardized measures can provide evidence one way or the other. This is another example of an argument skeptics would never use for any other disorder.

6. *The Increase in Diagnosis of DID in the 1980s Is Evidence of Its Artifactual Nature.*

This argument is logically fallacious because the increased rate of diagnosis is neutral concerning the validity of the disorder, for the same reasons as apply to the differential rate of diagnosis in North America. I mention it separately only because it is launched as a separate argument by the skeptics.

7. *DID Was Rarely Diagnosed in the Nineteenth Century.*

This is an extension of the North American artifact argument backward in time instead of outward in geography. Diagnoses that were never made at all in the nineteenth century include schizophrenia, panic disorder, bipolar mood disorder, and AIDS.

8. *Skeptics Make Appeals to Authority.*

Skeptics frequently argue that DID is not real because they and their friends don't believe in it. This is similar to the process by which homosexuality was removed from the list of psychiatric disorders between *DSM-III* and *DSM-IV*: It is a purely political process. DID believers also often make the appeal to authority, which does not advance the field.

9. *Validity Can Be Inferred from Anecdotal Short-Term Treatment Outcome.*

The skeptics say that DID is not valid because of the absence of adequate outcome studies, which is a logical error. At the same time, they frequently use their own anecdotal outcome observations to prove that DID is not valid. They say that in their experience, ignoring the alters makes the DID melt away quickly. In the skeptic's universe, DID can be proven to be invalid by anecdotal observations of the skeptics, and at the same time it is not valid because the believers have not done adequate outcome studies. The threshold of scientific outcome studies the skeptics require of themselves to prove their position is set far lower than the standard they demand of believers: This allows them to prove that DID is not valid due to its outcome in the absence of valid outcome studies.

In fact, in the absence of adequate outcome studies, neither side can claim victory in this micro-pseudo-debate, which is based on a logical fallacy that diagnostic validity depends on treatment outcome.

10. *Bad Therapeutic Practices Call the Validity of DID into Question.*

This logical fallacy is a permutation of the error about treatment outcome. Skeptics frequently rail about examples of bad therapy, then use these as an argument against the validity of DID. This is equivalent to arguing that leeching proves congestive heart failure is not real, or laetrile proves cancer is not valid. Such arguments would never be used elsewhere in medicine or psychiatry, and their erroneous logical foundations would be immediately apparent to all physicians. This proves that the use of such arguments against DID is not based solely on intellectual incompetence, and must have political and personal motives.

11. *Diagnostic Criteria for DID Are Vague, Therefore DID Is Not Valid.*

This argument is a logical fallacy for several reasons. For one, it confuses reliability with validity. Vagueness of diagnostic criteria is primarily a problem for reliability—if criteria are too vague, reliability will be impossible to establish, and validity will therefore be unattainable. This is because validity depends on reliability, which in turn depends on nonvagueness of criteria sets. Second, the vagueness of diagnostic criteria cannot be established merely by talking about the wording in *DSM-IV*: The criteria must be subjected to formal interrater reliability studies before any conclusion can be reached. Otherwise, no diagnoses in *DSM-IV* would be considered valid, since semantic objections can be mounted against all of them.

For example, in *DSM-IV* (1994a), the diagnosis of alcohol intoxication requires the presence of "Clinically significant maladaptive behavioral or psychological changes (e.g., inappropriate sexual or aggressive behavior, mood lability, impaired judgment, impaired social or occupational functioning) that developed during, or shortly after, alcohol ingestion" (p. 197).

Following the logic of the DID skeptics, I could say that no psychiatrist can diagnose alcohol intoxication in a valid fashion because "Clinically significant maladaptive," "inappropriate," and "impaired" are all subjective, inadequately defined, prone to observer bias, and can be applied by a moralizing teetotaler (the analog of the DID enthusiast) to anyone who has had a couple of drinks.

A similar argument could be made about any diagnostic criterion set in *DSM-IV*. The skeptics mounting this argument about DID never reference or discuss the reliability literature. They also claim that the vagueness of the DID diagnostic criteria results in vast overinclusiveness by enthusiasts, but ignore the literature on the epidemiology of DID in clinical populations.

12. *Unproven Etiology Invalidates DID.*

This argument can equally as well be applied against schizophrenia, which has no proven etiology. Many diagnostically reliable and valid surgical diagnoses can be treated with complete success in the absence of any proven etiology. This a common paradox in the skeptical position: Skeptics claim to be mainstream, conservative, sensible, and medical, but make antimedical arguments that would be laughed at if mounted in internal medicine or surgery. The skeptics have no medical sense.

13. *Lack of Proven Physiological Differences between Alters Invalidates DID.*

This argument could be used to invalidate all psychiatric diagnoses in which a clear, pathophysiologcally relevant, replicable, and specific physiological difference between the disease state and normal has not been demonstrated, which is all diagnoses in the *DSM-IV,* except for a few that are trivially and tautologically related to specific lab findings, such as elevated blood alcohol levels in alcohol intoxication.

14. *The Validity of DID Can Be Disproven by Accumulating Examples of False-Positive Diagnoses.*

Most psychiatrists have probably rediagnosed a schizophrenic as bipolar and then noted a good response to lithium. Have any concluded as a result that schizophrenia is not real? Anecdotal accumulation of false-positive cases contributes nothing to the debate, and is based on the assumption that scientific questions can be solved by a war of tally-keepers. All valid medical diagnostic categories generate false-positive diagnoses.

15. *If Repression Is Not Proven, DID Is Not Real.*

This argument rests on the fallacy that the validity of DID hinges on Freudian repression theory, which it does not. There are also Freudian theories of depression, panic disorder, obsessive-compulsive disorder, schizophrenia, and transvestic fetishism, but this is irrelevant to whether those diagnostic categories are valid. The word *repression* does not appear in the *DSM-IV* diagnostic criteria for DID, or in the accompanying text. Nor does it appear in the *DSM-IV* index, glossary of technical terms, or anywhere in the dissociative disorders section.

This is another form of *straw man argument.* In fact, dissociation theory is distinct from repression theory, and the former was abandoned by Freud for the latter. This argument against DID doesn't even make sense from a Freudian point of view.

The memories recovered by DID patients in therapy could be 100% false in all cases, and this would not invalidate the diagnosis—false recovered memories could then become a diagnostic criterion. The skeptics have not grasped the basic rules of the DSM system: The system was modified in *DSM-III* to be atheoretical and phenomenological in all its sections including the dissociative disorders. The skeptics are functioning by pre-*DSM-III* logic.

16. *The Diagnosis of DID Encourages Irresponsible Behavior.*

This is yet another straw man argument. Whether or not DID provides a license for irresponsibility is a political and legal question, and has nothing to do with the medical validity of the diagnosis. If a diagnosis of cancer of the pancreas provided one with a license to kill in our society, would the skeptics solve the problem by canceling the diagnosis? This is what they advocate for DID, thereby providing another example of medicine being overridden by politics. In any case, the argument is irrelevant because the treatment guidelines for DID of the International Society for the Study of Dissociation (1994), this text, and all other authoritative writings in the field specifically state that patients should be held accountable for their behavior.

17. *Multiples Are Really Just Borderlines.*

This statement is refuted by the published data reviewed in Chapter Eight: in various studies, 56% to 70% of DID subjects meet criteria for borderline personality disorder, meaning that 30% to 44% do not. The interrater reliability for DID is higher than that for borderline personality disorder, and borderline personality disorder cannot be reliably differentiated from its neighboring diagnoses in Axis II Cluster B, whereas DID can be reliably differentiated from DDNOS. Therefore skeptics who dismiss multiples as "really just borderlines" are using noise to explain a signal, which violates the basic logic of science.

Claims that iatrogenic cases are really just examples of bulimia, depression, or other disorders amplified into DID are variations of the borderline error; even if the skeptic is correct about specific iatrogenic cases, he overgeneralizes to all cases.

18. *DID Is an Artifact of Suggestibility in Highly Hypnotizable Individuals.*

All existing research data shows that the correlations between measures of hypnotizability and measures of dissociation are modest, and this has been known for over half a decade (Carlson, 1989). Hypnotizability can explain only a modest amount of the variance in levels of dissociation. Hypnotizability has subcomponents, of which suggestibility is only one, and this is never taken into account by the skeptics. Nor do the skeptics ever address which of the three DES factors correlate with hypnotizability scores. If the correlation, which is modest to begin with, is mostly with the absorption/imaginative involvement factor of the DES, then the relationship between hypnotizability and pathological dissociation is further weakened. The skeptics never approach this level of analysis.

19. *It Is Impossible to Have More Than One Personality in the Same Body.*

This objection is purely a straw man argument. No leading expert in DID endorses this proposition: I specifically and repeatedly stated that I did not in the 1989 edition of this book. The proposition is irrelevant to the question of whether DID is a valid diagnosis, because DID can be valid even if the proposition is correct. The skeptics are arguing that delirium tremens is not a valid diagnosis because it is impossible for pink elephants to be on a detox unit.

20. *A Few Clinicians Are Making All the Diagnoses.*

As analyzed earlier, this common error is refuted by the skeptics' own data. It is an argument that is out of date by over a decade, although it was accurate epidemiologically in the early 1980s. My 1989 series of 236 cases, for example, was reported to me by 203 clinicians who had jointly seen 1,807 cases: This series represented the experience of much more than a small clique. This argument is a good example of ones which can be made only by ignoring the published literature; it is erroneous for both logical and epidemiological reasons.

21. *Incorrect References Are Indicative of Careless Research in Skeptical Literature.*

The sloppy scholarship in the skeptical literature takes several forms: citations that are incorrect; citations that do not support the point being made; ignoring relevant major literature; citing substandard work by other skeptics as authoritative; and claiming to have reviewed the literature when major work has been ignored. Papers with these features get published in leading psychiatry journals, when they would be rejected by reviewers if the subject was schizophrenia or depression.

There is a two-by-two table governing standards for publishing papers on DID in many psychiatry journals: One can publish supportive papers of high scholarly quality on schizophrenia but not DID; one can publish hostile papers of low scholarly quality on DID but not schizophrenia.

22. *DID Has Been Created Experimentally, Which Proves It Is Not Valid.*

This logic defies all reasoning in the rest of medicine. Medical scientists learn as undergraduates that a laboratory model of a disease is a boon to research, and great effort is expended to develop such models. All research in psychopharmacology depends on animal models for predicting whether a compound will have psychopharmacological efficacy in humans. For no other disorder in medicine is a laboratory model viewed as evidence against the validity of the disorder. The skeptics compound this error by stating that DID has been created in college students when it has not, and by ignoring the creation of something approaching closer to enduring DID by G. H. Estabrooks.

The analogs of DID created in college students would not meet the DDIS or SCID-D profile of DID; none of the subjects have completed the DES or other standard measures; none of the subjects report childhood trauma histories; none of the role enactments of DID persisted outside the laboratory; none of the student subjects has ever required treatment for their DID; and the experimenters would be sued for unethical conduct if they actually created DID.

23. *DID Must Be Completely Unconscious to Be Genuine.*

This error is based on a simpleminded misapplication of Freudian theory. Nowhere in the DID literature is it stated that all behavior by DID patients must be completely unconscious to be genuine. This is another straw man argument. It is obvious to any experienced clinician that DID patients often use their symptoms for secondary gain, however, this does not differentiate them from people with schizophrenia who abuse anticholinergics, or terminal cancer patients who manipulate their families. The straw man criterion of complete unconsciousness is set up, then evidence of conscious elaboration of symptoms or secondary gain is used to prove that no cases are real.

There are no data showing that psychiatrists can reliably differentiate between conscious and unconscious symptom motives.

24. *If Satanic Ritual Abuse and Alien Abductions Are Not Real, Neither Is DID.*

According to this argument, Satanic ritual abuse and alien abductions are not real, therefore DID is discredited. Stated differently, the logic of this argument is, a high school classmate of yours is in jail, therefore you are a criminal. DID is condemned through guilt by association. The argument is meaningless, setting aside its logical flaw, because the accuracy of DID memories is irrelevant to the validity of DID, as pointed out in Error 15.

The skeptics fail to account for several facts: (a) alien abductions are more prominently featured in Hollywood movies and on television, by far, than are Satanic cults, (b) the ratio of DID patients claiming participation in Satanic human sacrifice to those claiming alien abduction is 100:1, and, (c) the vast majority of alien abductees do not have DID. The differential absorption of these two cultural myths by DID patients is not addressed by the skeptics, though DID patients are characterized by the skeptics as uncritical sponges for whatever is suggested to them by their therapists or culture.

That some DID patients have Satanic ritual abuse memories is irrelevant to a discussion of diagnostic validity because it does not account for the majority who do not have such memories, nor does it account for individuals who retract their Satanism but continue to have DID. There is no memory content criterion in the *DSM-IV* text or the diagnostic criteria set for DID.

Having AIDS makes one susceptible to bacterial infections: Having DID makes one susceptible to "infections" of memory, which are called false memories. Does anyone argue that a complication of AIDS invalidates the diagnosis? Only the DID skeptics make this argument in the entire history of medicine.

25. *The Extreme Case Escalation Tactic Creates a Perception of Extremism.*

I encountered this tactic several dozen times in a three-hour conversation with a prominent skeptic. Whenever the opponent is trying to establish common ground, and make a preliminary point that is conservative and potentially can be agreed upon, the tactitian escalates to the extreme case, and uses the extreme case to invalidate the point being made about the modal case. This maintains a polarized opposition between the debating partners, and entrenches the perception of the opponent as an extremist in the mind of the tactitian.

THE SKEPTICS CONSIDERED ONE BY ONE

In 1992, George Fraser and I debated Harold Merskey and Francois Mai concerning the validity of DID at the Canadian Psychiatric Association Annual Meeting in Montreal. I subsequently debated Merskey again at a meeting that resulted in the book by Cohen, Berzoff, and Elin (1995). I spent about three hours talking with Richard Ofshe and Ethan Watters at a meeting jointly sponsored by Johns Hopkins Department of Psychiatry and the False Memory Syndrome Foundation in Baltimore in December 1994. August Piper and I exchanged correspondence in the *Canadian Journal of Psychiatry* (Piper, 1990; Ross, 1990d) and the *American Journal of Psychotherapy* (Piper, 1994a, 1995b; Ross, 1995e), and Allan Seltzer and I exchanged correspondence in the *Canadian Journal of Psychiatry* (Ross, 1995f; Seltzer, 1995). I also debated Michael Weissberg about DID at the Hospital and Community Psychiatry Annual Meeting in Los Angeles in 1991. I mention these encounters as evidence that I have attempted to participate in a debate, and know the skeptics well.

The 12 DID skeptics discussed here include 7 psychiatrists, one clinical psychologist, one experimental psychologist, one journalist, one philosophy professor, and one social psychologist.

Harold Merskey

Harold Merskey (1994, 1995) is a psychiatrist who has written on hysteria and conversion disorder in the past. Merskey's (1995) major paper on DID was originally published in the *British Journal of Psychiatry,* and generated much correspondence, which is also reprinted in the Cohen, Berzoff, and Elin (1995) book.

Merskey says that 100% of cases of DID occurring since 1980 are artifactual, the only question being whether they were caused generally by the culture or by therapy. He says that cases cannot arise in an uncontaminated fashion now because DID is too well known in the culture at large: "no later case probably since Prince, but at least since the film *The Three Faces of Eve,* can be taken to be veridical since none is likely to emerge without prior knowledge of the idea" (Merskey, 1995, p. 25). He makes Errors 1–12, 14, 16–21, and 25.

An analogous argument is that since the movie *Rain Man,* all cases of autism are media artifacts. Merskey does not make this argument because he would be ridiculed by his colleagues for it, and because he has decided a priori that autism is a legitimate disorder. His argument about DID is simply the reciprocal tautology; DID is an artifact because it is an artifact, while autism (and depression and schizophrenia) is genuine because it is genuine. The core cognitive errors here are 1, 4, and 18.

Merskey makes Error 23 when he states (1995, p. 24) that patients, "Hawksworth, Milligan, Sybil, Christina and Gloria consciously used their alternate roles for emotional relief, or social advantage." On page 23, Merskey (1995) says of Billy Milligan, "At one time he wanted to play with his baby sister, but his mother said he could not do so. When bored, he went to sleep and when he woke he had the identity of Christene, who could play with the baby. It is not clear if this was an unconscious switch. By the age of 9, he had six other imaginary identities, seemingly often conscious." What other possible functions could DID have besides emotional relief and social advantage? That is the whole point of DID.

Merskey rediagnoses Mary Reynolds as having bipolar mood disorder when her symptom course is completely unlike any case in the mood disorder literature, thereby committing Error 17 but compounding it with an implausible alternative diagnosis.

Merskey's sentences often do not follow in a logical sequence; for example (1995, p. 3), "The earlier cases involved amnesia, striking fluctuations in mood, and sometimes cerebral organic disorder. The secondary personalities frequently appeared with hypnosis. Several amnesic patients were trained with new identities. Others showed overt iatrogeneis. No report fully excluded the possibility of artificial production. This indicates that the concept has been elaborated from the study of consciousness and its relation to the idea of the self."

The final sentence in the quotation has no logical relation to the preceding sentences, yet is stated as if it is a conclusion proven by those sentences. This is typical of Merskey logic throughout.

Merskey (Freeland, Manchanda, Chiu, Sharma, & Merskey, 1993) presents four case histories of alleged false-positive DID that do not contain adequate information to rule in or out any *DSM-IV* diagnosis.

Francois Mai

Mai, a psychiatrist, (1995) was discussed earlier. In the 1992 debate at the Canadian Psychiatric Association Annual Meeting, he prefaced his remarks by stating that he was going to take an epidemiological approach to the problem. He then proceeded to cite a number of general population surveys that detected no cases of DID. My rebuttal comment was that the structured interviews used in these surveys do not inquire about dissociative symptoms or make dissociative diagnoses. Mai appeared not to have read my epidemiological paper published 12 months earlier (Ross, 1991a). Mai commits Errors 1, 2, 5, 6, 8, 9, 11, 14, 17, 18, 20, and 21.

Allan Seltzer

Allan Seltzer, a psychiatrist, (1994, 1995) described five cases of alleged iatrogenic DID. The problem with his paper is that none of the case descriptions provide enough information to rule in or out any *DSM-IV* diagnosis. His appeal to authority for his conclusions is solipsistic. Although

Seltzer claims to be free of bias, and to have imposed no demands on the five patients to conform to his expectations, he says of Case 5 (Seltzer, 1994, p. 444): "She has improved on chlomipramine 200 mg at bedtime but continued to hear the voice of one former alter with some insight into its implantation by the therapist."

It is quite possible that I might agree with Seltzer that all five of his cases are iatrogenic if I examined them, but there is no way to tell from his paper. How is the reader to decide whether Patient 5 is in denial that her DID was iatrogenic, or is refusing to conform to Seltzer's demands? Serotonergic antidepressants can shut down DID personality systems in patients who are not clinically depressed: How is the reader to rule out this possibility? The pre-DID diagnosis history in Case 5 that Seltzer agrees was genuine includes "a brutal, physically abusive father who was alcoholic" and "amnesic spells."

Seltzer referenced Ross and Gahan (1989a) when he was talking about Ross (1991c); says that DID patients have high IQs while referencing a Coons, Bowman, and Milstein (1988) study which disproves that; says that DID is discouraged by *ICD-10* when it is not; cites as authority for the opinion that DID can be diagnosed in anyone by enthusiasts a paper by Putnam, Loewenstein, Silberman, & Post (1984) in which 3 cases of DID were identified in a sample of about 225 inpatients; incorrectly references Freeland, Manchanda, Chiu, Sharma, and Merskey (1993) as Freeland, Manchanda, Sharma et al.; and cites an article in the *London Free Press* as authority for claiming, "The patients wish to please the therapists who in turn desire to uncover sexual abuse."

Seltzer commits Errors 1–6, 8–12, 16–18, 20, and 21.

Nicholas Spanos

Spanos, an experimental psychologist, provides the major example of Error 22 (Spanos, Burgess, & Burgess, 1995; Spanos, Weekes, & Bertrand, 1985; Spanos, Weekes, Menary, & Bertrand, 1986). He also commits Error 24. Spanos, who died in an airplane crash in 1994, never interviewed a DID patient and was unfamiliar with the clinical profile of DID, but considered these deficiencies irrelevant to his critique of DID and the design of his research (Kluft, 1995).

Spanos is reporting in a scientific journal that he has created a rhinoceros through crossbreeding of experimental caribou in Alaska, although he has never seen a rhinoceros, can't give a description of one, and has not read the relevant literature. Other DID skeptics hail this work as brilliant and definitive.

Spanos is the chief representative of the social constructionist dismissal of DID. This is an absurd argument because the English language, psychiatry, social psychology, the social constructionist perspective, scientific journals, bridges, toothpaste, Spanos's experiments, and the praise of his colleagues are all socially constructed. The whole point about DID is that it is socially constructed, on all four pathways: That is why it is treatable with psychotherapy. Errors 1 and 4 are implicit in the cognitive error that a social constructionist analysis can discredit DID, which is impossible. The Spanos argument doesn't even make sense from a social constructionist perspective.

Spanos commits Errors 1, 2, 4, 8, 10, 12, 14, 15, 18, 21, 22, 24, and 25.

Ian Hacking

Hacking (1991, 1995) is a philosophy professor. His analysis of the British tradition of double consciousness and its differentiation from the French emphasis on hysterical symptoms is valuable to me personally, and to the field. Hacking believes that DID is real and that Merskey's position is untenable. He has other opinions that are cognitive errors, however.

Hacking sets up a tautology in which it is impossible for DID researchers ever to demonstrate that DID exists outside North America, because any such demonstration is defined as an artifact of contamination (Hacking, 1995, p. 108): "We can well imagine that if multiple practitioners trained by Ross were to take over a South African hospital, they would find that 5% of patients admitted were multiples."

In a sense I agree with Hacking: The key research project is for Michael Simpson, who lives in South Africa, to administer the DES, DDIS, and SCID-D to a sample of inpatients at his hospital, record the structured interviews on video, analyze past records for undiagnosed dissociative disorders, interview collateral historians, and then bring me over to interview subjects positive and negative for DID on structured interview. The problem is that the skeptics never actually participate in any research. Such a study could be done for a modest amount of money if recorded telephone interviews by me were substituted for in-person interviews.

I predict the following findings from such a study: at least 15% of Simpson's inpatients score over 30 on the DES; at least 5% meet structured interview criteria for DID but do not claim to have it; DID can be easily suspected from prior medical records in some cases; long-standing secondary features of DID can be confirmed by many collateral historians; some DID trauma histories can be externally corroborated on aggressive seeking of collateral confirmation; and kappa for the rate of agreement between the DDIS and myself for the presence or absence of DID will be above 0.90.

Until the skeptics actually conduct and publish such research, their arguments can have only limited weight even if free from the 25 cognitive errors.

Hacking cannot read the DID research literature fluently, as evidenced by this comment (1995, p. 110):

> When the DES is used as a screening instrument, a high enough score is taken to indicate multiple personality. Carlson et al. urge a cutoff point of 30, and the DES says you are multiple. . . . Carlson et al. use a base rate of 5%, which means that 1

in 20 psychiatric patients is a multiple. They do not state where this figure comes from. This is the figure Ross expected and Fernando found preposterous. On the basis of *this* figure the probability of a psychiatric patient's being multiple, given a score above 30 on the DES is 17%. The remaining 83 patients picked as multiples are not multiples.

This is a complete misreading of the paper in question, on which I am third author (Carlson et al., 1993). In this paper, we stated the following: that the DES is a screening not a diagnostic instrument; that 17% of subjects scoring above 30 on the DES in the sample of 1,051 patients had DID, and 83% did not; that our receiver operating characteristic analysis provided data on the trade-offs for sensitivity and specificity at different cutoff scores; and that cutoff score utilities are a function of the base rate of the target disorder in the population sampled. A base rate of 5% did not enter into our calculations concerning the sample of 1,051 clinical subjects.

On page 276, Hacking says, speaking of the DID movement, "Movement writers do not cite Hilgard, one of the great students of experimental hypnosis, but it is not clear that his work much influenced them." One of Hacking's references is the first edition of this book (Ross, 1989), which contained a section heading entitled, "Hilgard's Neodissociaton Theory of Divided Consciousness," and four Hilgard references. On page 69 of the first edition, I say of Hilgard's (1977) book: "His book single-handedly revives the serious study of dissociation." There are 22 separate citations of me in Hacking's index, and 14 references in his bibliography, but he does not appear to have read my book, thereby committing Error 21.

Hacking does not appear to be aware that David Spiegel, a movement writer he cites five times in his index and references twice, appointed Ernest Hilgard to the *DSM-IV* committee for dissociative disorders: all the other movement writers Hacking cites also sat on this committee.

Hacking commits Errors 1, 5, 6, 8, 12, 18, and 21. He is the only one of the 12 skeptics discussed here who has made a positive contribution to the field.

Michael Simpson

Michael Simpson (1995) is a South African psychiatrist. He provides the most witty critique of any of the skeptics, though the humor is all ridicule and sarcasm. He commits Errors 1–6, 8–22, and 25. He adds variants of errors 5–7 by saying that the gender ratio and socioeconomic profile of DID patients calls the diagnosis into question. Simpson sets up a straw man he calls *the immaculate perception,* as do other skeptics, and characterizes DID believers as believing that their perceptions are uninfluenced by all social-psychological variables, which is an absurd mischaracterization.

In the false memory debate, a related tactic is employed: DID therapists are characterized as believing simplistically in a video recorder model of memory, as opposed to a constructionist view held by contemporary cognitive psychologists: The false memory camp forgets to mention that the video recorder model of memory was the orthodox model of academic cognitive psychology two decades ago.

Simpson uses two strategies common among skeptics: He insults DID therapists then makes negative characterological attributions about them when they take offense; and he quotes DID writers as "admitting" a point he then uses against them, as if the writers have slipped up or betrayed the orthodoxy, when in fact the point is central to the writer's view of DID, and Simpson agrees with it. This rhetorical strategy traps the opponent in a tautology: Whenever the opponent makes a sensible statement, the statement is characterized as an anomaly and used against the opponent thereby preserving the view of the opposition as a foolish orthodoxy.

Alan Siegel

Siegel (1995) presents a composite mismanaged case as evidence against the diagnostic validity of DID. The case, as presented, was clearly mismanaged: The complications flow from the mismanagement, not the diagnosis, do not occur in properly managed DID cases, and would also occur in mismanaged therapies of borderline personality disorder. Siegel's argument follows this logic: A surgeon amputated the wrong leg, therefore osteosarcoma is not a valid diagnosis. Siegel commits Errors 1, 2, and 10.

August Piper

August Piper (1990, 1994a, 1994b, 1995a, 1995b) is a psychiatrist who has been committing various of the 25 errors for five years. He is the skeptical psychiatrist most likely to listen to reason, and seems interested in improving the standards of care for DID. His tone is rude when he writes in the *Newsletter of the False Memory Syndrome Foundation.*

Piper (1994a, 1995a) is the leading exponent of Error 11: in his chapter in the Cohen, Berzoff, and Elin book (Piper, 1995a), he sequentially makes Errors 11, 6, 10, 12, 16, 10 again, and 18 in his topic headings.

Theodore Sarbin

Sarbin (1995), a psychiatrist, makes the most naive variant of Error 19 I have read. He also states Error 23 repeatedly, as on page 163: "In reviewing the history of multiple personality and the writings of current advocates, it becomes clear that contemporary users of the multiple personality disorder diagnosis participate in a subculture with its own set of myths, one of which is the autonomous actions of mental faculties." The autonomous action of mental faculties does not appear to be a subcultural myth to me: Examples include simple phobia, perception of color, startle responses, dreaming, delirium, perception of the passage of time, proprioception, and pain. Sarbin also heavily emphasizes the fallacy that a social constructionist perspective can invalidate DID.

Sarbin and Spanos are both interested in DID as grist for an ideological mill, and use their error-ridden analysis of it to support a polarized position in an academic pseudodebate. The two polarized positions in the debate are summarized by Sarbin as, "The absence of agency implied in the conventional use of the terms *dissociation* and *repressed memories* follows from an outdated and discredited theoretical claim that the mainsprings of action are in the mental faculties." According to the pseudodebate, the only two options are that all aspects of DID are intrapsychic, unconscious, and autonomous, or all are determined by the laws of social psychology. DID must be attacked by Sarbin because those who treat it are misperceived as a polarized adherents to the opposing ideology.

Sarbin makes Errors 1–8, 10–12, 15, 16, 18–21, 23, and 24.

Paul McHugh

Paul McHugh (1995) is a psychiatrist. He is the main exponent of Error 9, which he combined with Error 2 in his published commentary and in his talk at the False Memory Syndrome Foundation Meeting in Baltimore in December 1994. Other errors made by McHugh include 1, 3, 4, 10, 12, 14, 16, 17, 18, 20, and 24.

McHugh states, "Babinski was bringing the null hypothesis to Charcot and with it, not a rejection of these women as legitimate victims of some problem, but an appreciation that behaving as if epileptic obscured reality and made helping their actual problem different" (p. 958).

McHugh is claiming, in effect, that Babinski said to Charcot, "There is no real neurological difference between the patients without pseudoseizures and those with pseudoseizures. With adequate analysis you will be unable to reject this null hypothesis." McHugh is using Charcot's failure to reject the null hypothesis as an argument by analogy to support his claim that DID can be treated with benign neglect and behavioral extinction. He is saying that the patients are hysterics, and don't have real seizures or real DID.

If I was Charcot, my reply would be, "You are correct, however that is not the null hypothesis I am testing. I am testing the null hypothesis that there is no observable behavioral difference between the two groups. You, Babinski, have not rejected a null hypothesis I propose to you: One hundred years from now, systematic treatment outcome studies will fail to differentiate the treatment methods of Ross and McHugh for DID."

Richard Ofshe and Ethan Watters

Ofshe and Watters (1994) are the most inflammatory of the DID skeptics. As a rhetorical strategy, their exaggerated prose style ensures that opponents in the debate will not hear what they have to say. This strategy reinforces polarization and entrenches the skeptics' position of moral outrage.

While trashing me in various locations in their book as incompetent and unscientific, Ofshe and Watters make curious use of one of my papers (Ross, Heber, Norton, & Anderson, 1989a, p. 72):

> Once adjusted for this error, Pope and Hudson found the significantly different rate of abuse in the eating disorder group disappeared. In other words, sexual abuse was no more likely in the life histories of eating disorder patients than it was in the histories of other patients.
>
> Remarkably, a second study that compared patients diagnosed with eating disorders to three groups of patients with panic disorders, schizophrenia, and multiple personality disorder, respectively, made the same mistake. By not ensuring that the control groups were matched for gender, the slight increased rate of sexual-abuse histories among the bulimic and anorexic subjects became meaningless.

Ofshe and Watters place this paragraph in a section of their book devoted to a critique of recovered memory therapists as overestimating the rate of childhood sexual abuse in patients with eating disorders.

The paper of mine they cite was in fact focused on DID, and the eating disorder patients were a comparison group: The paper's title is, "Differences between Multiple Personality Disorder and Other Diagnostic Groups on Structured Interview." Ofshe and Watters turn this around and make the DID, panic, and schizophrenia subjects the controls. They make it sound as if the paper failed to find a significant increase in rates of childhood sexual abuse among eating disorder subjects, when the point was that the rate was significantly lower in the three other groups, which did not differ from each other, than in DID. They state that the controls for the eating disorder group were not matched for gender when the only group that differed on gender from the other three was the schizophrenics.

Most curious of all, Ofshe and Watters cite a paper by Pope and Hudson (1992) which reviewed and tabulated the literature on childhood sexual abuse in eating disorders, and concluded that there was no evidence for an elevated rate. The table in Pope and Hudson's paper includes my paper on differentiating DID from other diagnostic groups! Ofshe and Watters do not mention that the paper they criticize is by me. They have thereby constructed a double bind: My paper supports their position in one paragraph and is an example of unscientific therapist error in the next.

This kind of rhetoric cannot be dealt with by the usual rules of debate and intellectual discourse. Ofshe and Watters make Errors 1–12, and 14–25.

CONCLUSION

I doubt that work of such low intellectual and scholarly standards can be found anywhere else in the current medical literature. It wouldn't be tolerated and couldn't pass peer review if applied to any other disorder. Although the skeptical critique can be refuted on logical grounds, I actually agree with much of what the skeptics say. It is true that iatrogenic cases of DID are a serious problem; it is true that memory is reconstructive, error-prone, and highly influenced by social-psychological variables; it is true that DID is socially constructed (how else could it be?); it is true that DID patients can construct elaborate and detailed false memories; it is true that DID can be used for secondary gain; it is true that incompetent therapists are practicing in the field (I have acted as expert witness against them); and so on. The skeptics need to be cured of their excesses so that therapists can hear what they have to say.

Treatment of Dissociative Identity Disorder

The treatment of dissociative identity disorder is complex, difficult, and rewarding. Part Three deals with treatment outcome, general principles of treatment, and specific techniques. The techniques are described in detail. The core treatment of DID is individual psychotherapy, but many adjunctive interventions including hospitalization, medication, working with social agencies, and group therapy can be used. The treatment must be embedded in sound general principles of psychotherapy and must have a foundation of trust, safety, good boundaries, and a solid treatment alliance. These are all conflicted issues for the victim of severe child abuse.

The techniques are suitable for both inpatient and outpatient psychotherapy. They can be used by therapists of any professional background working in any setting. Only a small part of the discussion focuses on hospitalization, medication, physical restraint, and other interventions not available to the community-based nonmedical therapist. DID can be treated to stable integration without hospitalization, although some hospital-based treatment is required in most cases.

There are treatment techniques and issues unique to DID, but I want to emphasize the need for therapy to be based on good general skills. The work is best thought of as regular psychotherapy with a number of special techniques blended into it. It is technically eclectic but is guided by an understanding of the nature and function of the personality system. The DID patient has used dissociation in a complex way to cope with childhood trauma; in therapy she must integrate the conflicts, feelings, and memories arising from the abuse.

The DID patient needs to learn how to be a single person. This involves unlearning an overreliance on dissociation and acquiring a new set of flexible, adaptive coping strategies. Most of the treatment in the late and postintegration phases of therapy is no different from the therapy of an adult victim of child abuse who never developed DID. This work is less technically challenging but is as important as the earlier phases.

DID is the most severe psychiatric disorder that can be cured with psychotherapy. It is also the only diagnosis for which managed care will certify inpatient treatment based on a primary treatment modality of psychotherapy. The cognitive-behavioral treatment of panic disorder can result in long-term remission, but DID is much more complex than panic disorder, therefore the treatment takes longer. There is no psychiatric disorder of comparable severity that carries such a good prognosis. The prognosis depends, however, on the availability of specific intensive psychotherapy for the disorder.

The purpose of Part Three is to describe the techniques and principles of DID psychotherapy in sufficient detail that the reader can begin using them. The discussion focuses on the treatment of the childhood trauma pathways to DID.

— *CHAPTER ELEVEN* —

Treatment Outcome of Dissociative Identity Disorder

Strictly speaking, there are no treatment outcome data for dissociative identity disorder (DID) in the literature. There have been no randomized controlled trials of any method of treatment for DID. Nor have there been studies of the treatment of one of the comorbid diagnoses of DID, such as depression. It would be possible, for instance, to conduct a standard study of the efficacy of serotonin re-uptake blockers in treating the depressive symptoms of DID patients.

An adequate study of the psychotherapy of DID would involve a number of measures, not all of which are available. There would have to be valid and reliable diagnostic assessment with standardized instruments at the beginning of the study. The DDIS and DES would be satisfactory for this purpose. There would have to be good measures of the target symptoms; These would have to be sensitive enough to track treatment response. It would be necessary to have a well-defined treatment protocol and to demonstrate that the therapists in the study were in fact delivering the protocol. There would need to be a comparison group. These are requirements of a definitive psychotherapy outcome study for any disorder. They sound straightforward, but they present major logistical and measurement problems for investigators.

Although there are no outcome data according to these strict criteria, we do know quite a bit about the treatment of DID and its outcome. There is a large body of collective clinical experience accumulated in North America, and an uncertain number of therapists have treated the disorder to stable integration. I would estimate the number of therapists in North America who have treated DID to stable integration at greater than 500.

Richard Kluft has provided virtually all of the literature on treatment outcome, based on careful observation of his own caseload (Kluft, 1982, 1983, 1984a, 1984c, 1985a, 1985b, 1985c, 1985d, 1985e, 1985f, 1986a, 1986b, 1987a, 1988d, 1988e). In this chapter, I will review the requirements for the first multicenter treatment outcome study of DID, review Kluft's treatment outcome data, discuss childhood DID and its treatment outcome, and conclude by describing the treatment results we have obtained.

REQUIREMENTS FOR A MULTICENTER TREATMENT OUTCOME STUDY

A multicenter treatment outcome study is required for a number of reasons. We know anecdotally that the treatment of DID is often highly effective, and we have a basic outline of what needs to be done in therapy. There are two kinds of research: the first is a bookkeeping kind of research in which you demonstrate what you already know in order to convince others that you are correct. An example of this would be doing a systematic study to determine whether child personalities often hold abuse memories. This is something that everyone who works with DID knows, so there isn't much intellectual excitement in documenting it. However, it would be useful to be able to say that in a series of 100 cases of DID, there were so many child alters, x percentage held abuse memories, and y percentage of other types of alters held abuse memories.

In practice, the logistical effort required to produce such data is so large compared to the payoff that researchers are unlikely to devote scarce time and resources to that particular piece of work. The other kind of research involves finding out what is going on when you really don't know. An example of this is the study we did to find out how clearly DID can be differentiated from temporal lobe epilepsy with the DDIS and DES (Ross, Heber, Anderson, et al., 1989). We really didn't know what we would find in this study and weren't predicting results as clean and unequivocal as those we got.

DID treatment outcome studies are necessary to establish scientifically the efficacy of a therapy we already know anecdotally is highly cost-effective. This is in turn necessary to legitimize the field and to ensure that treatment will be paid for by third-party insurers. There is no reason that third-party insurers should continue to fund expensive treatments indefinitely in the absence of solid outcome data. The history of medicine is replete with examples of officially sanctioned ineffective treatments.

A multicenter treatment outcome study would be very challenging and interesting to conduct. There would be numerous problems demanding innovative and creative solutions, ranging from logistic to psychometric, to transference-management issues. The first step would be to assemble a sufficient number of therapists who were willing to commit themselves to the paperwork involved. The study would last at least ten years if subject enrollment took six months, treatment five years, and follow-up five years. Because each therapist could enroll only a small number of subjects during the six months, several hundred therapists would need to be involved.

It is standard procedure in any treatment study to start off with pilot projects which do not involve randomization or control groups. In study of a new medication the first stage, called Phase I, involves animal experimentation and administration of the drug to healthy human volunteers to ensure safety. Phase II involves dose-finding studies and uncontrolled, nonblinded investigations that provide initial data on efficacy, followed by the first double-blind studies. Phase III involves full-scale, multicenter randomized, double-blind placebo-controlled studies in a number of different countries. The data from the first three phases are required to get permission to market the drug. In Phase IV, which occurs after permission to market the drug has been obtained from a particular government, further studies of possible new indications and applications, new preparations, and so on are conducted.

Generally, to move a new drug from discovery in the test tube to market takes ten years and 100 million dollars. This development of new medications illustrates the minute amount of time and money society is investing in the treatment of DID. The treatment of DID, though, is actually in Phase II despite the lack of resources, and we are only twelve years out from the major burst of publications in 1984.

At intake into a multicenter DID treatment outcome study, at least 75 percent of subjects should score above 20 on the DES. All should meet DSM-IV criteria for DID clinically, all should have histories of childhood physical and/or sexual abuse, and therapists must have contacted alter personalities directly. In addition, at least 75 percent of subjects should fit the full DDIS profile for DID with somatic symptoms, substance abuse, depression, Schneiderian and borderline symptoms, secondary features of DID, and ESP experiences.

The DDIS cutoff values for enrollment in the study could be: somatic symptoms—5; Schneiderian symptoms—3; secondary features of DID—6; positive borderline criteria—3; ESP experiences—2. These values would require that 75 percent of subjects be not more than one standard deviation below the mean for DID on their DDIS symptom profile and DES scores (Ross, Miller, Reagor, et al., 1990). This would ensure that the sample was not biased in favor of mild cases.

Concurrent schizophrenia, organic brain syndrome, serious medical illness, ongoing current victimization or perpetration of abuse, pending criminal charges, and lack of a stable fixed address should also be exclusion criteria. These items are all necessary to provide a reasonably stable setting for therapy free of confounding variables and secondary gain. It doesn't matter whether the victimization and perpetration are corroborated or not, because false memories or factitious claims of either should not be exclusion criteria.

All subjects should pay for their treatment in accordance with the standard billing practices of the individual therapists. This is necessary to maintain a realistic treatment frame, and to maintain a positive countertransference in the therapists, who cannot reasonably be expected to work for free. Subjects dropping out of treatment for financial reasons would be part of the outcome data. All therapists should have read this book, Putnam (1989), and the Treatment Guidelines of the International Society for the Study of Dissociation (1994). Sessions should be a minimum of once a week and should not exceed three sessions a week with the primary therapist except for time-limited periods of crisis. This is necessary for standardization and to approximate usual clinical practice. There is no use in demonstrating the efficacy of a treatment if 14 hours a week of therapist time are required for each patient.

The next requirement is measures of treatment response. These will include the DES, DDIS, Beck Mood Inventory, SCL-90, Beck Hopelessness Scale, Beck Suicide Scale, SCID, and MCMI. Therapists will tabulate number of sessions, inpatient and partial hospitalization days, and all other forms of psychiatric health care utilization, and tabulate a cost for these. They will measure employment status and monthly income of subjects. A reliable measure of overall psychosocial function should also be administered. All measures should be done annually, and the self-report measures monthly.

In terms of measurement of treatment process, besides using the Therapist Dissociative Checklist (see Appendix B), I would employ Kluft's (1994) Dimensions of Therapeutic Movement Instrument (DTMI). This is a promising measure with 12 items that yields an overall score ranging from 0 to 60. Lower scores on the DTMI indicate more impairment and less productive work being accomplished in therapy, and the DTMI appears to be a good predictor of prognosis. Prognosis is predicted by a combination of how low the starting score is, and how quickly the score increases during treatment.

The problems of randomization and control groups would have to be addressed. I doubt that a randomized controlled study of the psychotherapy of DID will ever be conducted. The ethical and logistical problems of randomization and controlled treatment are insurmountable because of the long duration of treatment, its efficacy, and the morbidity experienced by untreated patients. It would be inhumane and unethical to assign a DID patient to a waiting list or placebo control for five years. In fact, it would be technically unethical because no university ethics or human subjects committee would approve randomization to placebo treatment for five years given the Dallas outcome data reviewed later in this chapter.

My solution to this problem is to compare competing treatment protocols, say the treatment recommended in this book with that recommended by McHugh (1995). Different schools of thought on the treatment of DID need to compete with each other, not ideologically, but through adequately designed systematic prospective treatment protocols. The burden of proof is on each school to demonstrate the superiority of its approach. Subjects admitted into the competing studies would have to be clearly described according to which of the four pathways they were on, otherwise differential outcome results could be an artifact of differential pathway representation in the samples.

Comparing subjects who enter treatment with those who decline would be worthwhile, but would not provide definitive data because those who decline may be quite different from those who accept. Because the treatment lasts years, is complex, and involves many, many variables, it will be impossible to follow initial multicenter studies with attempts to dissect out the active and inactive components of the different treatment packages, by controlling individual variables in subsequent studies. This can be done economically for treatment regimes that last 10 or 20 sessions, but not for a treatment that requires years. I think, though, that rigorous enough studies can be done to convince all reasonable persons of the efficacy and cost-effectiveness of the treatment of DID within the next six or seven years.

It is vitally important for the subspecialty of dissociative disorders, for psychiatry in general, and especially for patients, that multicenter treatment outcome studies be started within the next few years. Such studies, along with other research, and continued vigor in the life of the ISSD, are essential if dissociation is to be firmly established in the mainstream. It is still possible that dissociation could fall into obscurity again, as it did early in the twentieth century.

One of my goals is to begin an unfunded multicenter DID treatment outcome study within the next two years by recruiting participating therapists through the ISSD newsletter and requiring them to fund the psychometric and mailing costs of their participation.

TREATMENT OUTCOME DATA OF RICHARD KLUFT

Treatment outcome data on DID are provided entirely by Kluft except for one paper by Coons (1986d). All other outcome data consist of single case studies (Carlson, 1984; Cutler & Reed, 1975; Hall, LeCann, & Schoolar, 1978; Lipton & Kezur, 1948; Rosenbaum & Weaver, 1980; Sizemore & Pittillo, 1977). I mentioned treatment outcome in three cases (Ross, 1987). Coons (1986d) reported on a series of 20 cases of DID followed for a mean of 39 months after intake. He found that 5 (25%) were integrated, while 2 had achieved unstable integration prior to redissociating, and 2 were partially integrated.

In addition, Coons reported that 100% of the 20 patients had accepted their diagnosis, and 77% had developed coconsciousness. He devotes most of his attention to events within the therapy, describing transference, countertransference, and therapeutic modalities in detail. Kluft has been publishing detailed studies of his caseload for much of the 1980s, and has described by far the largest individual caseload of any investigator.

Kluft (1982, 1984c) has provided an operationalized definition of integration that could be used in treatment outcome studies. He defines fusion or integration as requiring the presence of three stable months of:

1. Continuity of contemporary memory.
2. Absence of overt behavioral signs of multiplicity.
3. Subjective sense of unity.
4. Absence of alter personalities on hypnotic reexploration.
5. Modification of transference phenomena consistent with the bringing together of personalities.
6. Clinical evidence that the unified patient's self-representation included acknowledgment of attitudes and awareness previously segregated in separate personalities.

I fully endorse these criteria except for the fifth one, which I would retain as a clinical criterion but drop as a research criterion. The transference criterion is insufficiently operationalized, depends too much on the observer's ideology, and would have little or no interrater reliability for use in formal research. A therapist might want to retain this criterion in his own practice, but it could not be part of a scientific study unless it was operationalized.

Kluft's (1984c) outcome data are based on 171 cases he saw over a period of a decade. Of these, he treated 117, and in addition he was able to monitor the treatment of another 6 patients who reached integration, making a total of 123. Of the 123, 20 were still in treatment, 10 had interrupted treatment, and 10 cases were unsuccessful, leaving 83 cases (67.5%) treated to stable integration. Based on these data, one can say that two thirds of DID patients entering treatment should reach stable integration.

Kluft, however, excluded 50 of the 83 patients from his final report for a variety of reasons: 7 were excluded because the full protocol for demonstrating stable integration (Kluft, 1985g) was not used, or the therapists were inexperienced in treating DID; 16 had not been stable for long enough; 20 were lost to follow-up or had not yet been followed up; 2 patients were of questionable reliability; 4 had partially relapsed or shown dissociative features after integration; and one had died.

The remaining 33 patients met more rigorous criteria of 27 months of stable integration (two years following the initial 3 months). The 33 patients consisted of 25 females (75.8%), had a mean age of 36.1 years at fusion, a mean of 13.9 personalities, and an average duration of treatment of 21.6 months. Putnam et al. (1986), analyzing these data, found that the number of personalities correlated with the time to reach integration at $p < .004$.

This figure of 21.6 months to reach integration is one of the key pieces of information in the field. It means that DID is a treatable disorder in the majority of cases and that the duration of treatment is reasonable given the amount of work to do: in only 8 cases (24.2%) was the length of treatment longer than 30 months. This means that three quarters of Kluft's DID patients were treated to integration in less than 2½ years. Of the 33 patients, only two (6.1%) took longer than 3½ years to reach integration.

The 21.6 months is not representative of the current treatment of DID across North America for several reasons. Most important, no other therapists have the experience of Kluft, so few if any will have his level of skill to offer. In addition, Kluft's patients are not as sick as the average North American patient with DID. Kluft (1982) reported that of his first 70 patients treated to integration, only 22.8% "had strong borderline features." In comparison, 56% to 70% of cases in other series met *DSM-III* or *DSM-III-R* criteria for borderline personality. In addition, only 45.5% of Kluft's (1984c) 33 integrated cases had been hospitalized prior to diagnosis, while 6 were hospitalized during treatment: Kluft does not report whether these patients overlap. Of the 236 cases reported to us, 74.6% of 236 had been hospitalized. Kluft's patients were treated in private practice, while those of other practitioners are seen in state mental health clinics, hospitals, prisons, and a variety of other settings serving more impaired populations. The patients described by Kluft in the 1980s are not representative even of Kluft's caseload in the 1990s (Kluft, 1994).

In the 1980s, I noticed an unexpected negative therapeutic reaction in patients who were told by me that the average duration of treatment to integration is 21.6 months. Patients who did not make the deadline became discouraged, thought of themselves as failures, and blamed themselves for not getting better on schedule. Having seen this a couple of times, I now tell patients that with hard work the duration of therapy may be in the range of three to five years, but that it could be longer.

It is important to understand that 21.6 months was arrived at by one therapist with one caseload. The length of time to integration is affected by the skill of the therapist, difficulty of the case, availability of social supports, life stage and situation of the patient, amount of treatment delivered per week, luck, and probably a host of unrecognized factors. Therapists should not become preoccupied with their "stats." For example, we treated the polyfragmented woman mentioned in earlier chapters to stable integration in less than 21.6 months, but more than half of the first year was inpatient work. This patient received more than 500 hours of psychotherapy from myself, my cotherapists, and ward nurses in a year. Without that, she might have taken five years to integrate. There is no way that a solo outpatient psychotherapist could treat such a case to integration in less than two years.

Treating DID to stable integration is a bit like running a marathon. There is only so fast you can go. I could run 100 miles a week for a year and still not reach a 2:30 marathon: my physiological endowment limits me to a maximum life goal of sneaking in under three hours, if I ever get the training time. Similarly, in the psychotherapy of DID, the most skillful therapist in the world could not take the patient faster than her maximum rate. It is humanly impossible to deal with so much trauma in a brief psychotherapy. In fact, if you go too fast, you end up going more slowly because the patient creates symptoms and resistance to put on the brakes.

Multicenter treatment outcome studies will confirm Kluft's finding that the majority of DID patients can be treated to integration, but not within two or three years. I say this with some confidence because a growing number of therapists throughout North America have treated DID successfully. The treatment delivered by Kluft has not been described in sufficient detail to attempt a replication of his methods, but he has described its general principles and many of its techniques. Most successful therapists probably have at least 80% of their interventions in common because they practice good generic psychotherapy, and because there are certain things, such as negotiation between alters, that you just have to do in treating DID.

TREATMENT OUTCOME OF CHILDHOOD DID

Like the literature on adult treatment outcome, most of the work on childhood DID has been done by Richard Kluft (1984b, 1985b, 1985c, 1986e). In a review of the literature, Vincent and Pickering (1988) identified 12 reported cases of childhood DID: Of these, one was reported in the nineteenth century by Despine (Fine, 1988), 4 are cases of "incipient DID" (Fagan & McMahon, 1984) and 5 are Kluft's cases. An additional case in a 3-year-old was reported by Riley and Mead (1988). This means that of 8 modern cases of full DID in childhood reported up until 1990, 5 (62.5%) are reported by Kluft, while Malenbaum and Russell (1987) report 1, Weiss, Sutton, and Utecht (1985) 1, and Riley and Mead (1988) 1.

Since 1990, articles and chapters by Hornstein and Tyson (1991), Peterson (1990, 1991), McMahon and Fagan (1993), Peterson and Putnam (1994), Putnam and Peterson (1994), and Benjamin and Benjamin (1993) have added to our understanding. A special issue of *Child and Adolescent Psychiatric Clinics of North America* published in April, 1996 adds to our knowledge and inventory of cases. Nevertheless, the total number of reported cases of childhood DID is still under 100 as of early 1996: in comparison, I have published three independent series of adult DID cases totaling 441 patients.

This is a very unusual situation in the history of a childhood psychiatric disorder. There are a number of probable reasons so few childhood cases have been identified. For one thing, most DID specialists are adult mental health professionals. DID is less well developed in childhood, and doesn't present with a 20-year history of chronic psychopathology, secondary features of DID, somatic symptoms, extrasensory experiences, and other features that raise the diagnostician's index of suspicion. Kluft has pointed out that the external behavioral manifestations of DID are more muted in childhood because children don't have the finances, mobility, or independence to develop alters with different sets of friends, clothes, and interests. Many of the secondary features arising from the activities of alters may therefore not be present.

As well, it may be difficult to differentiate switches of personalities from developmentally normal discontinuities of state that occur in children. Kluft (1985b) has listed seven reasons for the difficulty of identifying childhood DID. These are, in summarized form:

1. There is no index of suspicion by professionals.
2. Symptoms suggest some other disorder.
3. Fluctuation of symptoms suggests other disorders.
4. Other explanations for behavior are invoked, such as lying.
5. Child is unaware of his or her circumstances and/or condition.
6. Child withholds data.
7. Childhood DID has different features.

As Dell (1988a, 1988b) has pointed out, professional skepticism about DID is often extreme to the point of overt hostility. It may manifest itself as "malicious harassment, contemptuous ridicule, and deliberate interference in the medical care of the patient" and it may be "uninformed, instantaneous, reactive, and unyielding" (Dell, 1988a, p. 537). Such not uncommon responses go far beyond the limits of reasonable skepticism defined by Bliss (1988), Hilgard (1988), and Spiegel (1988) in discussion of Dell's paper. Cases of childhood DID may evoke such extreme reactions more commonly because there is less literature on childhood DID, and because the abuse is more likely to be ongoing.

Despite the limited database, predictors of childhood DID have been developed and are referenced in Chapter Seven. Many of the items on the measures also occur in adult DID, including intermittent depression, trance states, voices, Schneiderian passivity experiences, disavowed behavior, and fluctuating mood and behavior. Since I have little direct experience with full DID in childhood, and because the literature is so sparse, I am not going to say anymore about the phenomenology of childhood DID, except to emphasize that cases can present with the full classical features of the adult form.

What is most important to understand is the treatment outcome in childhood DID. Childhood DID seems to be treatable to long-term stable remission with short-term psychotherapy in a substantial number of cases. This probably means permanent cure. For this to happen, the abuse must stop. It is unethical to try to treat childhood DID in the face of ongoing abuse, because the treatment would rob the child of his or her way of coping. The data on the treatment of DID suggest that primary prevention of the disorder is possible.

This is the most important goal of the field, to identify and cure DID in childhood. If that could be done on a large scale, huge savings in dollars and suffering would result. There would be a major interruption of the transmission of abuse to future generations. If as much money was allocated to DID research and treatment as for AIDS, we could diagnose and treat tens of thousands of children to stable integration in North America, if not more. I am not suggesting that DID is a more important public health problem than AIDS; it definitely isn't. But a budget of hundreds of millions of dollars could be spent effectively on the diagnosis and treatment of DID in North America.

The treatment of childhood DID to stable integration takes 5 to 10 sessions in many cases. The longest treatment in the literature consists of 30 sessions over 5 months. The shortest took one session. It would be hard to imagine a more cost-effective preventive intervention in all of medicine, other than vaccinations. The ease of treatment of childhood DID, compared with the painful and arduous course of adult treatment, is evidence that DID is entrenched and reinforced in an extremely powerful way by physical, sexual, and emotional abuse, and other experience, including therapy in badly managed cases.

The preliminary data on the treatment of childhood DID is so important that it *must* be followed up with good research and clinical investigation. No other disorder in psychiatry could be prevented on such a scale with methods already available.

FINANCIAL TREATMENT OUTCOME DATA FROM WINNIPEG

I am going to review my experience in treating DID prior to moving to Texas in 1991 by summarizing a financial analysis I did there (Ross & Dua, 1993). I diagnosed my first case of DID in 1979 as a medical student, my second in 1982 as a resident, and my third in 1985 as a staff psychiatrist. At that time, in 1985, I couldn't comprehend how Kluft, Braun, Caul, Bliss, and others could accumulate so many cases. Before leaving Winnipeg, I saw about 80 cases of DID; since then, we have admitted over 500 patients to our program at Charter Behavioral Health System of Dallas, for a total of over 1,000 admissions, and I have been the attending physician on 165 admissions.

In conversations with colleagues, my experience has been confirmed by others: Many therapists find DID to be treatable to stable integration, with a marked reduction in health care utilization and improvement in function.

This leads to a paradox: DID is both the most terrible and the most hopeful mental disorder to have. No other group of patients has anything approaching the degree of trauma to remember and work through. But, unlike lithium-nonresponsive manic-depressives, schizophrenics, persons afflicted with delusional disorders, and many other mental patients, the person with DID can escape from the mental health system. DID can be cured.

In our financial paper (Ross & Dua, 1993), we reviewed all medical records at all hospitals in Winnipeg on 15 women with DID admitted under my care at St. Boniface Hospital. This was obviously a highly biased and nonrandom sample. We tabulated all psychiatric health care services delivered to these 15 women including inpatient, outpatient, and day hospital treatment, emergency department visits, consultations, and intensive care unit admissions, and costed these out in 1989 dollars using the fee codes of the Manitoba health care system. We divided these costs into those incurred prior to the diagnosis of DID and those incurred afterward.

The 15 women had been in the psychiatric system for an average of 8.1 years (98.77 months) each prior to diagnosis, at an average cost of $1,688.64 per month, or a total of $166,786.97 each. Some women had been in treatment for 20 years or more before diagnosis of their DID at a total cost of over $500,000. These figures are probably representative of DID patients circulating through university departments of psychiatry in Canada.

There was great heterogeneity in the sample, which markedly limits its generalizablity. Some patients had modest prediagnosis costs; for some, costs escalated dramatically after diagnosis, whereas for others the costs dropped precipitously after diagnosis. The average length of time in treatment for DID was 2.6 years (31.53 months) up until the cutoff point of the study on September 1, 1989.

To calculate the potential savings due to the diagnosis and treatment of the DID, I made an assumption that the average duration of DID therapy would be 4 years, and that patients would exit from the psychiatric health care system at that point, an assumption warranted by the course of these subjects in informal follow-up until 1996. To my knowledge, none of these subjects have been chronic consumers of inpatient services in the past 5 years.

I then compared the cost of 4 years of DID therapy, based on the cost for the 2.6 years actually tabulated, to baseline costs projected forward for 10 years. There was no indication of any reduction in consumption of services during the 8.1 years of baseline treatment. The projected saving per case over 10 years was $84,899.44. If one reduced the prediagnosis baseline in the system from an average of 8.1 years to one year, and instituted four years of therapy at that point, savings per case would be in the order of $250,000.

The total tabulated lifetime psychiatric health care costs for these 15 women in 1989 dollars up until September 1, 1989, was $4.1 million. Given the extensive social services consumed in Canada by DID patients, in the form of medical care for psychosomatic symptoms, legal aid, homemaker support, education, child care, and job training, a reasonable estimate of the total lifetime cost of these 15 women to the Canadian taxpayer is about $10 million.

Given the Dallas clinical treatment outcome data to be reviewed in the following section, and the psychiatric health care costs of undiagnosed DID calculated in Canada, the need for formal treatment outcome studies is apparent. I believe that the treatment of DID is the most cost-effective intervention in psychiatry and that this can be demonstrated convincingly with research to be accomplished in the next decade. One of the most interesting pieces of information that will flow from this research is the predictors of poor treatment outcome.

PROSPECTIVE TREATMENT OUTCOME DATA FROM DALLAS

In 1992 and 1993, we assessed 103 DID patients admitted to our Dissociative Disorders Unit at Charter Behavioral Health System of Dallas with a battery of measures. All patients had clear clinical evidence of alter personalities; however, we did not assign the patients to one of the four pathways to DID. The patients were at various stages of treatment at the time of assessment and were referred and followed up by therapists all over the United States. Their treatment progress samples a wide range of different therapists and geographic locations.

Two years later, we were able to contact and readminister the assessment battery to 54 subjects; these 54 follow-up subjects did not differ demographically or on clinical measures from the 49 who did not participate in follow-up, therefore they appear to be representative of the entire 103 patients interviewed at baseline. At follow-up, 12 patients had reached stable integration by Kluft's criteria, as established by interviewing their therapists; these 12 subjects did not differ at baseline from the 42 who had not yet reached integration except that their baseline depression was a bit milder.

At follow-up the overall group was taking fewer medications in lower dosages than at baseline. As well, the integrated patients were taking less medication than the nonintegrated patients at follow-up, and less medication than they had themselves at baseline. Clinical improvement therefore cannot be attributed to medication.

The follow-up group was 88.9% female; had an average age of 39.3 years; was 33.3% married; and 44.4% employed; and had an average of 1.3 children. The clinical treatment data concerning the entire follow-up group are presented in Tables 11.1 through 11.4: the number of subjects varies because not all subjects completed all measures. The data concerning the integrated patients are presented in Tables 11.5 through 11.7.

It is evident from the tables that these 54 DID patients made significant progress in two years: the improvement in the overall group is statistically significant, as is the difference between integrated and nonintegrated subjects at follow-up.

Table 11.1.   Dissociative Identity Disorder Two-Year Follow-up Study: Current
Diagnoses on the Structured Clinical Interview for DSM-III-R (SCID) (N = 44)

Diagnosis	1993 (%)	1995 (%)	Chi Square	p
Schizoaffective	56.8	20.5	10.7	.01
Psychotic disorder NOS	2.3	20.5	8.0	.01
Major depression	77.3	47.7	8.9	.01
Social phobia	50.0	22.7	7.2	.01
Simple phobia	38.6	13.6	7.1	.01
Obsessive-compulsive disorder	65.9	40.9	5.8	.05
Somatization disorder	43.2	18.2	8.1	.01
Pain disorder	27.3	6.8	7.4	.01

Table 11.2.   Dissociative Identity Disorder Two-Year
Follow-up Study: Mood and Dissociative Symptoms (N = 54)

Measure	1993	1995	t	p
DES	52.4	33.0	6.5	.00001
Beck	33.4	23.2	4.7	.00001
Ham-D	43.4	28.4	6.5	.00001
SCL-90-R	2.15	1.53	3.9	.0004

*DES = Dissociative Experiences Scale; Beck = Beck Mood Inventory; Ham-D = Hamilton Depression Scale; SCL-90-R = Hopkins Symptom Checklist-90.

Table 11.3.   Dissociative Identity Disorder Two-Year
Follow-up Study: Dissociative Disorders Interview Schedule
(DDIS) Profile (N = 54)

Symptom Cluster	1993	1995	t	p
Schneiderian symptoms	6.8	4.2	2.6	.00001
Borderline features	5.5	3.7	1.9	.00001
Secondary features of DID	11.5	8.6	5.3	.00001
Amnesia items	4.7	3.9	0.8	.0003
Somatic symptoms	17.2	10.8	5.6	.00001
ESP experiences	6.5	3.2	3.3	.00001

Table 11.4.   Dissociative Identity Disorder Two-Year
Follow-up Study: Positive and Negative Syndrome Scale
(PANNS) Profile (N = 43)

Symptom Cluster	1993	1995	t	p
General psychopathology	50.6	39.0	7.5	.00001
Positive symptoms	24.2	16.3	9.0	.00001
Negative symptoms	17.5	13.4	6.5	.00001
Composite score	6.7	13.4	3.2	.003

Table 11.5. Dissociative Identity Disorder Two-Year Follow-up Study: Self-Report and Structured Clinical Interview for DSM-III-R (SCID) Profile of Patients Treated to Integration

Symptom Measure	N	1993	1995	t	p
DES	11	50.5	15.4	8.0	.00001
Beck	9	27.9	9.7	4.0	.004
Ham-D	12	36.5	16.0	4.2	.001
SCID I & II	8	11.5	1.9	7.6	.0001
SCID I	8	7.8	1.3	10.9	.00001
SCID II	9	3.6	0.7	3.0	.01

*DES = Dissociative Experiences Scale; Beck = Beck Mood Inventory; Ham-D = Hamilton Depression Scale; SCID I = Structured Clinical Inventory for *DSM-III-R*–Axis I; SCID II = Axis II. SCID figures are the average number of positive diagnoses.

Table 11.6. Dissociative Identity Disorder Two-Year Follow-up Study: Dissociative Disorders Interview Schedule (DDIS) Profile of Patients Treated to Integration (N = 12)

Symptom Cluster	1993	1995	t	p
Schneiderian symptoms	6.2	1.4	5.7	.0001
Borderline features	5.9	1.7	7.0	.00001
Secondary features of DID	11.7	4.1	6.4	.0001
Amnesia items	4.8	2.3	4.6	.0008
Somatic symptoms	14.3	4.3	5.8	.0001
ESP experiences	5.8	1.9	4.6	.0008

Table 11.7. Dissociative Identity Disorder Two-Year Follow-up Study: Positive and Negative Syndrome Scale (PANSS) Profile of Patients Treated to Integration (N = 9)

Symptom Cluster	1993	1995	t	p
General psychopathology	46.7	31.8	5.8	.0004
Positive symptoms	24.9	12.8	11.6	.00001
Negative symptoms	14.1	9.7	4.9	.001
Composite score	10.8	3.6	12.1	.00001

Table 11.1 shows that the subjects developed more psychotic disorder not otherwise specified at follow-up than they had at baseline. Our explanation for this is that subjects stopped meeting criteria for more severe psychotic disorders, and dropped into the less severe NOS category as a result of improving: Very few if any DID patients who have reached stable integration meet criteria for any psychotic disorder.

One criticism we often receive from skeptics is that we do not treat our patients' chemical dependency problems aggressively enough; the data show remarkable improvement on this dimension, with complete abstinence in all integrated patients. These outcome data are as good as or better than those achieved by chemical dependency programs. At the same time, using the diagnostic rules of the SCID, we have successfully treated a lot of psychosis with psychotherapy. None of the integrated patients were taking antipsychotic medication, and four were taking no psychotropics of any kind at follow-up.

MCMI data on eight integrated subjects showed complete normalization of the MCMI profiles compared with markedly pathological profiles at baseline (Ellason & Ross, 1996).

If outcome data of this sort are obtained in the proposed multicenter study, the findings will present a problem for competing schools: There is no room for a clinically significant greater degree of improvement. The only way a competing school could show superior outcomes, assuming that representation of the four pathways to DID was controlled for, would be by obtaining the same results more quickly and/or more cheaply. The scores of the integrated patients on the DES, MCMI, and Beck Mood Inventory, for instance, are within one standard deviation of the mean for the general population, even though the baseline scores were two standard deviations above the mean.

The 1995 scores of the integrated patients on items such as secondary features of DID are elevated in part because the subjects were reporting on their overall experience for the previous year, and some had been integrated for less than one year. At four- and six-year follow-up we anticipate that there will be further improvement in overall group scores; further improvement in the scores of patients integrated by first follow-up at year two; and more patients treated to stable integration.

A typical patient requires no further inpatient treatment postintegration, little or no day-hospital treatment, a reduced amount of outpatient psychotherapy, less psychotropic medication, and less phone call support, makes no psychiatric visits to emergency departments, is self-supporting, and experiences a dramatic improvement in the quality and quantity of her personal relationships. Much of this improvement is evident by the late preintegration phase of therapy.

The sample of 54 DID patients is probably reasonably representative of those in treatment in North America. At baseline, they had a typical DID profile on the DES and DDIS, and typical demographics. They were not treated by therapists who were obviously unrepresentative of the field in any way, and all were severely enough impaired to require inpatient treatment. They were motivated enough to travel considerable distances to our Program in many cases, but this degree of motivation is common in DID patients. There is no clinical or research reason for me to conclude that this group of patients was unusually easy to treat.

As far as I am aware, these data represent more systematic prospective treatment outcome research than has been generated by classical psycho-analysis and long-term psychoanalytic psychotherapy in 100 years.

DISSOCIATIVE DISORDERS PROGRAM PROFILE, CHARTER BEHAVIORAL HEALTH SYSTEM OF DALLAS

In addition to the outcome data just presented, I am going to describe our overall experience in Dallas with the inpatient treatment of DID. It is the in-patient component of psychiatry that generates by far the most costs, and requires the most control by managed care. About half the patients are on Medicare, 40% have managed policies, and 10% have indemnity policies or are self-pay; about half are from outside Texas, and about half of those from Texas are from outside the Dallas-Fort Worth area. Our average inpatient census for 1992 to 1995 was 17 patients. Almost all the patients are already in treatment for DID at the time of first admission to our Program.

In a survey of 452 DID patient records for the period 1992 to 1995, we found that 181 (40.0%) had been readmitted. The total number of readmissions subsequent to the 452 index admissions was 387, making an average of 0.9 readmissions per patient. The average length of stay was 17.4 days, and the median was 13.0 days. The average total inpatient days per patient over the three-year period was 33.1 days, and no single admission was as long as 100 days.

Of the 181 patients readmitted, 51.4% had a shorter length of stay than on their index admission, and only 21.1% showed a clear pattern of in-creasing lengths of stay. Patients with 10 or more psychiatric admissions prior to their first admission to our Program are common in our population. The number of nursing incidents, which includes self-destructive behavior, and seriously volatile or unstable behavior requiring some sort of specific nursing intervention, did not differ per patient day from the rate in the rest of the hospital in 1994 and 1995.

To our knowledge, of over 500 patients admitted to our Program from 1991 to early 1996, only four have completed suicide postdischarge. This is a lower rate than one would expect for a general adult inpatient population, and lower than one would expect for schizophrenia, depression, and bor-derline personality disorder. It is not unusual for our patients to have self-mutilated themselves severely enough to leave scars dozens of times prior to diagnosis of their DID and prior to first admission to our Program.

During this period, the Program and the hospital were inspected repeat-edly by Medicare, the Texas Department of Health, and the Joint Commis-sion on Accreditation of Health Care Organizations. The Dissociative Disorders Program was never sanctioned, restricted, or in any way nega-tively regulated by these bodies. Patients with managed policies are regu-larly referred to us from other states, and I am consulted by managed care companies for whom I am not a provider. Two of the physicians working on our Unit have reviewed for managed care.

These data show that we are able to manage a highly disturbed and self-destructive population with good outcomes, in a reasonable period of time, with good management of financial resources. We have seen too many patients whose DID has just been diagnosed but who have only 20 lifetime freestanding psychiatric inpatient days left on their Medicare policies.

Based on the field's cumulative clinical and research experience, I conclude that most committed, motivated DID patients can be treated to stable integration if they stay focused and maintain a working treatment alliance. Such patients can be treated within an insurance policy that provides for 100 days of inpatient treatment, with inpatient days flexible to partial hospitalization on a 1:2 ratio basis (that is, each inpatient day can be exchanged for 2 partial hospitalization days), and 500 hours of individual outpatient psychotherapy. At current managed care rates, this means treatment to stable integration within a policy capped at $100,000 lifetime, a figure that should be compared with the lifetime healthcare costs of renal failure, diabetes, rheumatoid arthritis, multiple myeloma, stroke, and multiple sclerosis.

When making healthcare cost comparisons with these other disorders, analysts should bear in mind the age of DID subjects, their future economic productivity, and the fact that many can be cured. The treatment also does a great deal to interrupt the transmission of childhood trauma to future generations.

CONCLUSION

All existing evidence indicates that the treatment of DID, as described in this book and its references, is effective clinically and can be delivered in a fiscally responsible manner. Healthcare costs can always be reduced by denial of service, but a properly managed policy capped at $100,000 lifetime should be sufficient for the treatment of most cases of DID to stable integration. I recommend that this figure be reduced by instituting co-payment provisions after the first $50,000 has been expended. Patients who require further care after they reach their lifetime cap should go onto some form of disability.

These conclusions are probably not generalizable to people with DID who are homeless, in prison, currently victimized by pimps or battering spouses, or unable to control extreme substance abuse. Setting aside these extreme populations, which may be untreatable or require additional specialized care, DID appears to be the most treatable severe psychiatric disorder. Successful treatment of DID appears to resolve the extensive comorbidity that characterizes the condition, or at least reduce it to manageable proportions. Definitive prospective treatment outcome studies are required to verify these conclusions.

— CHAPTER TWELVE ——————————————

General Principles of Treatment

The basic principle of the treatment of dissociative identity disorder (DID) is that it is the treatment of a person. Technical wizardry, creative ingenuity, accurate empathy, extrication from double binds, these and other interventions are worth nothing if the *person* does not get better, and live better. The operation was a success but the patient died—that saying describes a potential error in the treatment of DID.

The goal of the treatment of DID is not palliation: It is cure. Lesser outcomes may be all that is possible in certain cases, but they are not cures. It takes an artistic temperament to treat DID successfully, and it also takes spiritual discipline. The treatment is prolonged and difficult, and many subtle traps lie in wait for the therapist (Chu, 1988). This makes the treatment of DID challenging and rewarding work.

The treatment of DID can be medical when medications and an inpatient unit are used. Except for these two components, an MD confers no advantage or special expertise in the treatment. The psychotherapy of DID can be done by any qualified psychotherapist, of any professional background (Lego, 1988). The physician need not be the primary therapist and can play an adjunctive role even in cases that require medication and admission.

In this chapter, I am going to describe the broad general principles of treatment. There are principles that apply to any psychotherapy, and to DID in an overall way; for example, contracting is done in many forms of treatment, including behavioral containment of psychotic behavior, but contracting with alter personalities is unique to DID. The unique elements of the treatment are the techniques, interventions, and strategies that form the microcosm of therapy.

AN OVERVIEW OF TREATMENT

In some residency programs, future obstetricians are required to do a year of general surgery in order to learn basic principles and techniques of surgery. Similarly in psychotherapy, all therapists must possess certain skills. No one should treat a DID patient as their first training case, because the treatment requires general skills and experience. Robert Mayer (1988) eloquently describes the uncertainties of starting to work with MPD patients in a hostile and unsupportive environment.

One of the reasons I am writing this book is to contribute to a literature that will help therapists who find themselves with a case of DID, and no prior experience. The DID patient will test, test, test, and retest the therapist. It is impossible to treat severely borderline multiples without getting angry at them, wishing they would die, and dreading coming to work at times. I think it is also impossible to work with such patients and not act out against them a little bit once in a while, at a minimum. That doesn't mean such acting out is okay, and it certainly needs to be minimized. But it is, I believe, humanly impossible never to act out in therapy. If you don't have a basic positive feeling for the person you are treating, I don't think you will be able to tolerate the projective identification pressure the patient exerts, and will therefore not be a good therapist.

Trying to work effectively with a DID patient you don't like must be a bit like trying to spend six months in the biosphere with someone you can't stand. One consequence of this reality of human social contracts is that hateful patients are less likely to get good treatment, or any treatment. The DID therapist must be able to tolerate uncertainty, and strong "unacceptable" countertransference feelings including hate and erotic arousal, all admixed with plenty of hysteria. Psychiatric jargon supplies ample terminology for covert expression of the hostile countertransference aroused by DID patients.

The main thing to ask oneself is, "Who wouldn't be like this, with that childhood?" Defining the patient's bad behavior as "characterological" reinforces negative feelings in the therapist, because it attributes causality to the patient's character, rather than to the abuse. This raises the next trap, which is displacement of negative countertransference onto the abuser. Many fathers of DID patients are hateful, or at least their abusive alters are, and the therapist can't help but feel angry. In the end, the therapist just has to be able to handle the intense feelings that are part of therapy, without acting out in any direction.

It is essential to have supportive colleagues and administration. Running a Dissociative Disorders Program is like running a heart transplant service: There is a lot of stress involved. Having to deal with acting-out colleagues in the absence of supportive administration makes the work too difficult to bear.

A final general caution: You shouldn't treat DID if you have an empty, lonely personal life or if you are married to someone with a severe personality disorder, or unresolved chronic trauma. It just isn't possible to do the work at work, then come home and have to do it at home. You will be a bad therapist and a bad spouse. If your life is empty, the drive to fill it with overinvolvement in therapy will be too great. Although no one in late twentieth-century urban North America is truly healthy, the DID therapist must "have it all together" to a reasonable extent. This is so because the patients don't.

GENERAL CONSIDERATIONS

General principles of treatment have been enunciated by Braun (1986a) and Kluft (1985f). These build on earlier statements by Bowers et al. (1971) and Allison (1974), as well as collective experience and the DID literature as a whole. The main recommendation of Bowers and his co-authors was that the therapist should stay within the limits of his competence. Although this is true, it is only part of the truth. Even expert therapists will be stumped at times: Everyone will make some mistakes, no matter how experienced.

There should be a balance between intimidating beginning therapists with the need for "expertise" and an anything-goes attitude. I am particularly mindful of the first error, having met psychiatrists who misuse countertransference comments on trainees for power, intimidation, and control. Experts in the treatment of DID should not erect false criteria of expertise for the purpose of establishing themselves as gurus.

George Greaves (1988) has written with great restraint about some of the incredible therapeutic errors he has encountered as a DID consultant. When I talk about the inevitability of making errors, I am referring to "small potatoes" mistakes compared with breast-feeding a patient, or taking a patient on holidays as a baby-sitter. There is a hierarchy of severity of errors: The most extreme example Greaves cites is a therapist who allegedly treated a DID patient by day and abused her in a cult by night. Such behavior is so pathological that it can't be classified as an error. Until I read Greaves's paper, it never even occurred to me that therapists might breast-feed their patients' child alters under the title of reparenting. I have since consulted as an expert witness on such a case myself.

Bowers enunciates 12 principles of treatment that Kluft (1985f) says have "stood the test of time." These are, restated in my words:

1. The treatment goal is integration.
2. Help each alter personality to understand that she is one part of a whole person.
3. Use the alters' names as convenient labels, not licenses for irresponsible autonomy.
4. Treat all alters fairly and empathetically.
5. Encourage empathy and cooperation between personalities.
6. Be gentle and supportive. Remember the severity of the trauma.
7. ECT is contraindicated.
8. Stay within the limits of your competence.
9. Use hypnosis judiciously.
10. Treat the person in her social context, and intervene systemically when necessary.
11. Group therapy may help.
12. Do not dramatize symptoms such as amnesia.

These are sound principles of therapy. The problem is, given these principles, what do you actually do? The therapy of DID is a problem-solving, practical therapy, requiring countless specific interventions.

Consistent with recent trends in psychiatry and psychotherapy research, Braun (1986a) has provided a more operationalized set of guidelines than those of Bowers. Braun's 13 steps are roughly sequential and have the feeling of chapter headings in a treatment manual:

1. Developing trust.
2. Making and sharing the diagnosis.
3. Communicating with each personality state.
4. Contracting.
5. Gathering history.
6. Working with each personality state's problems.
7. Undertaking special procedures.
8. Developing interpersonality communication.
9. Achieving resolution/integration.
10. Developing new behaviors and coping skills.
11. Networking and using social support systems.
12. Solidifying gains.
13. Following up.

The linear sequence of these steps exists only as an abstract outline of therapy. In practice, much like the stages of dying, all the issues are worked and reworked throughout therapy. For example, trust remains a major issue even after the system is completely mapped.

I don't think that this outline of the treatment of complex DID in late twentieth-century North America can be improved on: It can only be elaborated. A century from now major modifications may be required if the phenomenology of DID has changed significantly, and modified protocols might be required in other cultures. I think, though, that these are sound principles of treatment for therapists throughout the world.

It is important to bear in mind an observation of Braun (cited in Kluft, 1985f) that therapists of different schools do similar work with DID patients, despite their differences in vocabulary and theory. Effective treatment of DID seems to demand a common set of techniques and interventions, based on the patient's symptoms, conflicts, and needs. No matter what your theoretical orientation, for example, you will have to negotiate between alters because they will get into destructive, disruptive arguments.

In the remainder of this chapter, I am going to discuss inclusion and exclusion criteria for treatment, limit-setting and boundaries, and informed consent and memory, before going on to the core techniques and strategies in the next chapters.

INCLUSION AND EXCLUSION CRITERIA FOR TREATMENT

Inclusion and exclusion criteria apply to both client and therapist. They are broad and based on common sense. The patient must want therapy and must give informed consent to it. This means she must be aware of the goal and the difficulties of treatment. An immediate problem arises: How many alters should agree to treatment? The host *must,* and beyond that the more the better is a good rule of thumb. The presence of initially hostile alters is common and not a contraindication.

If the patient is willing to work hard, appears genuinely motivated, and can stay within the treatment contract, that is really all that is required. These principles alone are insufficient, though, because they don't help one decide who to treat and who to refer back to the referral source. The problem with the further guidelines I will provide is that none are based on good data, and all are contradicted by my own clinical experience.

You would think that a history of chronic involvement with the mental health system, welfare, the courts, drug abuse, and prostitution would be a contraindication to treatment. But I have treated such patients with good results. Long-term treatment with injectable antipsychotic medication, and first psychiatric hospitalization in childhood might suggest a difficult case, but such patients can be treated to integration. Actually it is hard to define good exclusion criteria.

The ones I use hinge on the severity of the trauma and any history of violence by the patient. Patients who have witnessed multiple murders, and those who have committed murders are difficult. This is true whether or not the memories are accurate. For example, one patient referred to us claimed that he used to masturbate his mother intravaginally with a loaded gun during his early adolescence, following which she would perform fellatio on him. He said that he had been sexually abused by nuns and priests, had witnessed murder, and had dreams and flashbacks containing large amounts of blood. He described a male alter whose sole sense of masculinity was derived from pounding his penis with a brick. Society just doesn't provide therapists the security or resources to work safely with such a man. The treatment would be too dangerous and traumatic for the therapist, let alone the patient. This is true whether the events actually occurred, or are a measure of the pathology of the man's fantasy life.

Another exclusion criterion is the patient whose function is precarious but whose world might be destroyed by therapy. Mental health professionals with DID sometimes belong to this group. Such people are probably best served by a slow-paced supportive therapy with very gradual engagement of alters and abuse memories (Kluft, 1994). Anyone starting to treat a mental health professional must be careful about confidentiality.

I spent a number of sessions with an articulate professional person (she is not in a mental health or medical field) deciding whether to start therapy. The final, correct decision was that at her stage of life, and in her life situation, her total amnesia for experience before age 12 was best left intact. The alters I spoke with all agreed on this point, and made the decision in consultation with me: This case is described in *The Osiris Complex* (Ross, 1994b).

Similarly, a separated mother with a major depressive episode could not remember anything before age 14. She was not a professional but was stretched to the limit coping with her current stresses. I left her amnesia barrier intact and referred her back to her social worker without a word about any dissociative disorder. She has never had any secondary features of DID, but even if she had I would have made the same decision. Recent involvement in major crime is a contraindication for therapists not already involved in forensic work. I think it would be a mistake to leap into a forensic case while working in a system that does not otherwise handle forensic patients, just because the patient has DID. Involvement in such a case would require prior consultation with administration and colleagues, at a minimum.

Another group of patients are the ultrasevere borderlines who have been in the system as borderlines for years. Such patients are known to every psychiatry resident, emergency room, and inpatient ward. There is no need to become a masochistic dumping ground for untreatable borderlines who have been caught up in the system for years. As ambassadors for DID in the profession, it would be a coup to take over and cure such patients, but the likelihood of success is low. Failure would only reinforce uninformed hostility toward DID and its treatment: Making "heroic" efforts with untreatable patients is bad medicine, not heroism. It deprives other more treatable patients of valuable finite resources. On the other hand, one must remember that "bad borderline" multiples can often make substantial treatment gains.

Related to this consideration, patients should not be accepted primarily because of pressure from colleagues to take over their most troublesome cases. The pressure can take many forms.

In deciding whether or not to take a case, the therapist must weigh all of these factors using clinical judgment. The availability of other therapists comes into the equation. It is also important to time treatment intakes in relation to the progress of patients already in treatment. You can't have all your patients in the intense midphase of treatment at the same time and therefore can't admit too many patients at one time. This means that some people have to wait for others to get better. The patients already in treatment figure this out, which becomes an added complication. Dealing with a patient's guilt about not getting better fast enough, or her desire to take a flight into health, is slightly compounded by the fact of a waiting list.

Because the treatment is long-term, even sabbaticals and possible pregnancies must be considered. If there are therapists at an institution who do not have permanent positions that adds another problem. Because we have an inpatient unit with skilled DID nurses, we can accept patients from out of state. Experience has taught us that they must have a therapist at home who is willing to follow them. Lack of such a therapist is a relative contraindication to admission because we otherwise get ourselves in the position of trying to function as long-distance telephone therapists, which doesn't work. We have felt our way into these guidelines by trial and error, reading, consultation, and attending conferences.

Whatever the guidelines suitable for a particular setting, it is important to think carefully about whom you are going to treat and why; this will become more crucial as more mental health professionals diagnose more cases. The number of diagnosed cases suitable for treatment is going to run ahead of the available treatment slots over the next five years.

We work in a setting in which we can be primary therapists for our local patients on an inpatient and outpatient basis. We treat some difficult patients as cotherapists, with no one seeing the patient on a sole basis much of the time. The isolated therapist with no supportive colleagues will have to apply all the exclusion criteria more stringently.

LIMIT-SETTING AND BOUNDARIES

An organism that cannot establish boundaries and set limits will die. This is true of amoeba, which must maintain a balance between rigidity and fluidity in their cell walls. If the membrane is too rigid and impermeable, the organism will die. Similarly, if the membrane is too permeable, the amoeba cannot maintain its integrity. If this happens at an organ level within a human being, death may occur at all hierarchical levels in the system from cells to the whole person. This in turn will have a harmful effect outside the person in broader systems. The point is that limit-setting is not an optional aspect of therapy. The only questions are what limits, and how many?

Problems with boundaries are by far the largest cause of iatrogenic complications in the dissociative disorders field, and tightening up of boundaries is the number one change required of therapists. My analysis of therapist boundary problems is that they are based what I call *the reenactment of the incest family dynamic in the dissociative disorders field.*

Reenactment of the Incest Family Dynamic in the Dissociative Disorders Field

As described in *Satanic Ritual Abuse,* most DID therapists are women, and in one survey I conducted at a DID conference, 60% of 310 female therapists reported a history of childhood sexual abuse, compared with 35% of 69 male therapists. This means that about half of DID therapists are themselves victims of childhood sexual abuse. The data showed that many of the therapists were uncertain about the identities of their perpetrators and the specific acts of sexual abuse perpetrated on them. The female therapists were most uncertain about female perpetrators. This is a troublesome situation.

On the one hand, I know highly competent and ethical therapists currently in treatment for dissociative disorders, in addition to individuals with DID working as physicians, senior executives, university professors, and researchers. Many of these people show no evidence of impairment in the workplace. On the other hand, the potential for acting out, overidentification with clients, and premature closure in favor of certainty about the accuracy of recovered memories, is high (Kluft, 1995). I believe that many therapists take the "believer" position and a rigid, absolute stance concerning client memories, in part because they cannot tolerate uncertainty about their own childhood abuse histories.

Another dynamic I see at work in therapists is *reaction formation,* which means adopting a feeling and attitude as a defense against a more deeply held opposite feeling and attitude. This occurs in therapists who are dealing with the positive pole of their ambivalent attachment to their childhood perpetrators by encouraging counterperpetration on their clients' perpetrators. This occurs through ill-considered confrontations, accusatory letters, and disconnection from the family of origin, all rationalized in the name of healing and safety. These therapists are too angry at *the perps,* and it is too clear who is the therapist's enemy (the client's father) and who is the client's friend (the therapist). I will describe these dynamics in more detail in Chapter Thirteen.

The structural norm of the dissociative disorders field, at least in Texas in the first half of the 1990s, is a reenactment of the incest family dynamic, as represented in Figure 12.1. The reenactment occurs in a thousand casual little ways, as well as through major boundary violations. In one case, for example, a therapist admitted living with a client for half a decade, having sex with her, involving the client in the therapist's personal life, exchanging domestic labor for therapy, using the client as a consultant in other therapies, participating in therapy with the client as a coclient, and having ceremonial ritualized sex with specific alter personalities in order to convert them from Satanism to allegiance to the therapist. I judged this to be a pure iatrogenic pathway DID case. This case is the only example I have seen of documented ritual sexual abuse, including candles, symbols, chanting, saying key words backward, elicitation of specific alters for sex, a highly developed ideology justifying the abuse, and ritualized sexual practices.

Most reenactments are more subtle and involve violations of confidentiality during supervision, idle gossip, dual relationships that are not highly pathological, minor overinvolvement with the client, and similar errors.

Figure 12.1 represents this milder level of reenactment. A group supervision leader provides group supervision to a number of different therapists; one of these therapists has a former roommate who is a former roommate of a sister of one of the other therapists; the former roommate is the lover of a woman who is the former lover of another woman, who in turn once had an affair with one of the other therapists; and so on. In this social system, some people know sexual secrets about other people that they aren't supposed to know, while others in the system are ignorant of these involvements; some people talk about the sex, others do not;

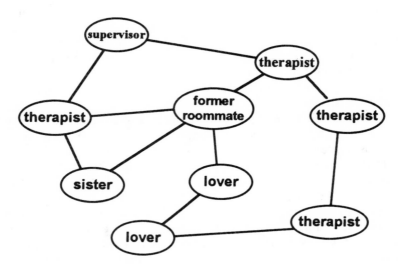

Figure 12.1. Reenactment of the Incest Family Dynamic in the Dissociative Disorders Field

relationship boundaries and confidentiality barriers are violated without consent in supervision and in social relationships among therapists, who talk shop informally; and clients end up knowing things about therapists' sex lives that they shouldn't.

All of this re-creates the dynamics of the incest family, and embeds the client in an unhealthy social network that she has likely already re-created in her personal life prior to coming to therapy. The therapy thereby repeats what should be cured. Dual-track relationships are common in this social field and include friend-friend and therapist-client; colleague-colleague and copatient-copatient; colleague-colleague and therapist-client; and many other permutations. I have interviewed therapists with corroborated five- and six-track relationships including being the client, friend, employee, colleague, business partner, and supervisee of the same person. Sexual involvement with clients is far from rare. This reenactment is not peculiar to therapists and can commonly be observed in psychiatrists and nonpsychiatric physicians.

These problems in the field give rise to the need for clear boundary rules.

Boundary Rules

Despite the need for flexible boundaries, the following rules should be adhered to by therapists and clients:

1. No sexual contact between therapist and client.
2. No weapons brought into sessions.
3. No threats against the therapist's family.
4. The client does not enter the therapist's home (unless the therapist's office is at home).
5. Excessive numbers of phone calls are not permissible (the definition of "excessive" varies widely).
6. The client is not given the therapist's home phone number.
7. The therapist's personal life is not discussed, except perhaps in the most general manner to illustrate some point being made in therapy.
8. Therapist and client do not socialize outside therapy.
9. The client does not know the therapist's family members' names.
10. Therapy usually does not exceed three hours per week, except during periods of crisis or in cases where this can be done without fostering dependency or regression.

If these 10 rules were followed, the majority of damage done to clients by therapists would be prevented.

There are other limits. Patients can't barge in on other people's sessions, and I rarely see an outpatient more than twice a week. The therapist should rarely take phone calls during sessions, and only for true therapeutic emergencies or pressing business or personal reasons. There are many such commonsense rules, most of which are logistically based and don't have to be mentioned to the patient.

Combined with these rigid boundaries is permeability in others. A reasonable amount of asexual hugging is fine, as are small gifts, and going for walks in sessions; these can become problems when they are too frequent, however. Generally, I am willing to express my thoughts and feelings about the therapy, the patient's life, transference, and countertransference in an open manner. I think it's important to discuss the sickness of social systems, including the healthcare system, in therapy, and I am prepared to discuss my analysis of these systems if my views are directly relevant to therapy. I wouldn't talk about U.S. foreign policy in therapy because it isn't relevant, but I might discuss the prevalence of clitorectomy in the Middle East.

One thing I don't set limits on is what the patients call me. Some call me "Colin," some "Dr. Ross," others "the doctor," "doc," "my shrink," "my head shrinker," or "my psychiatrist," and I have also been referred to as "the Ross man" and "Mr. Dr. Ross" by alters of various ages, not to mention colleagues. All of these are fine with me. I don't see any reason to make a big deal about what the patients call me. Some patients call me "Dr. Ross" sometimes and "Colin" other times.

I regularly set limits on my availability, the amount of ownership of the patient's problem I am willing to undertake, the length and number of sessions, the duration, frequency, and intensity of abreaction's, the amount of written material I can review (very little), and a host of other issues.

The balance between being a friend, parent, and therapist often requires limit-setting. I think it devalues the meaning of friendship to pretend to be a patient's friend, and it also reduces therapy to rent-a-friend, which is distasteful. I didn't go to school for 10 years after high school to be a rent-a-friend. I prefer the role of expert consultant on DID and general consultant on life path strategies. This doesn't preclude fondness for the patient, without which therapy might not be as effective.

It helps to like the patient in order to do three or five years of intense work with her. But it is not necessary to be the patient's friend. I tell patients when I find them irritating and advise them that such behavior is likely to drive away anyone but the most dedicated masochist. Patients have to accept that the relationship is limited to the therapy and that this makes it an artificial, largely one-way relationship. We discuss this.

Therapists working with their first case or two often get into trouble because of insufficient limit-setting. To some extent, this is unavoidable because the patients are so interesting and needy. I doubt that there is a single DID therapist who hasn't gotten overinvolved in some way or another at some point. It's easy to spot overinvolvement with hindsight, but not so easy when the patient is hurting badly and in crisis. Criticism of insufficient limit-setting is difficult for therapists to accept, but if acted on is always very helpful. The main thing to remember is that the client, at some level, feels stifled by the overinvolvement and is relieved when healthier limits are set and maintained.

Limits are more important in inpatient work than in an outpatient setting because powerful regressive forces are activated by an inpatient admission, both within and outside the patient. Limits also have to be set on colleagues and social institutions. It is important not to think of limits as punitive measures directed at the patient, because they keep the therapy alive and well. There is no formula for limit-setting, not counting the absolute rules. The main thing is to view limits as necessary and positive aspects of therapy that increase the effectiveness, efficiency, and humanity of the treatment. It is not kind to allow a disturbed patient to be all over the map. Lack of limits can result in deterioration into an iatrogenic psychosis.

INFORMED CONSENT AND MEMORY

A major change in the dissociative disorders field since the 1989 first edition of this book has been spearheaded by the False Memory Syndrome Foundation (FMSF), which was formed in 1992. Many of the skeptics reviewed in Chapter Ten are active in the FMSF, and I have been vilified in the *FMSF Newsletter,* nevertheless I agree that false memories and iatrogenic DID are serious problems in North America. In the mid-1990s, it became much more necessary to pay careful attention to the error-proneness of memory in therapy and to obtain informed consent concerning memory-retrieval processes. A sample informed consent for memory retrieval with hypnosis is provided by Hammond et al. (1994) in the guidelines issued by the American Society of Clinical Hypnosis.

In this section, I am going to talk about memory and informed consent as an ongoing matter that must be discussed throughout therapy, rather than in terms of a consent form. In individual therapy and in group therapy at Charter Behavioral Health System of Dallas, I do a good deal of direct teaching about the reconstructive nature of memory, the impossibility of differentiating accurate from false memories on clinical grounds alone, the need to think carefully before making any major decisions based on memories alone, and the possibility that any given memory, no matter how detailed and subjectively compelling, may never have happened in the external world. I have also discussed the four pathways to DID and the characteristics of a destructive psychotherapy cult in group.

I do very little "memory work" as such. Treatment as I provide it does not focus on the content of the memories, and healing occurs at the level of process and structure. No patient of mine has ever sued her perpetrator, and I have never recommended that a patient of mine sever contact with her family of origin. I have had cordial and productive family meetings with parents accused of ritual abuse and military mind control involvement, without this content ever being brought up, and I have treated patients with major false memories to integration. I have also been an expert witness for the plaintiff in false memory/iatrogenic DID cases.

Therapy cannot be conducted successfully based on "believing the client" or similar principles. The patient is always ambivalent about her attachment to her perpetrators, even if the abuse is all false memory, and is always harmed when the therapist overidentifies with one or the other pole of the ambivalence. The therapist's job is to be neutral with regard to the reality of the memories, and to act as a consultant to the client on her analysis of her childhood. It is true that a therapist cannot tell scientifically that a given memory is true. It is equally true, however, that a therapist cannot tell that a given memory is false without external evidence, unless the memory is impossible.

DID therapists need to stay informed about memory: Good places to start are the Guidelines of the American Society of Clinical Hypnosis, *Clinical Hypnosis and Memory: Guidelines for Clinicians and for Forensic Hypnosis* (Hammond et al., 1994); the October 1995 issue of the *Journal of Traumatic Stress;* the September/December 1994 issue of *Consciousness and Cognition;* and the October 1994 and April 1995 issues of the *International Journal of Clinical and Experimental Hypnosis.* I deal with specific strategies for handling the problem of false memories in *Satanic Ritual Abuse* (Ross, 1995a).

THE PROBLEM OF HOST RESISTANCE

Over the past few years, *the problem of host resistance* has come into clearer focus in my clinical work. Previously, I tended to think of the alters as the problem, and worked with the host to solve the trouble being caused by the alters. As I will describe in more detail in Chapter Thirteen, I was taking the rescuer position and putting the host in the victim position. Gradually, the patients taught me the error I was making, which was obvious all along: The alters can't be the problem, because they were created to solve the host personality's problem, which was the trauma in a childhood onset case. This is still true in a factitious or iatrogenic case, only the age at onset and motives are different.

The host personality will often take the victim position, experience her persecutor alters as, not surprisingly, persecutors, and ask the therapist for help and protection. The more tearful, helpless, and pathetic the host is in this regard, the more likely the problem is host resistance. In some systems, the host plays the role of dutiful, conscientious therapy client, and laments that her system will not communicate with her; the host frames this as a technical problem that needs to be solved by the therapist. In fact, though, the host is delivering a double message to her system, because although she wants to "remember," anytime an alter does give back a memory, the host decompensates and devalues and rejects the alter. The underlying message not to communicate is heard clearly by the alters, who withdraw and/or counter act out against the host. The host is covering her resistance to the work of therapy with reaction formation, and is actually avoiding any serious engagement in treatment.

Such resistance must be analyzed and confronted in a direct manner. The therapist must talk through to the system in the course of this confrontation in order to establish a preliminary treatment alliance with the alters, who likely feel frustrated, angry, hurt, and rejected. I always tell the host that she is defining the problem as technical in nature when in fact she needs to make a decision: Does she want to talk to her system or not? Does she want to remember or not? Does she want to consider the possibility that her alters have something positive to contribute, or not? Unless the answer to these questions is affirmative, there is nothing the therapist can do. The therapist takes a position of impotence to empower the host, who is already in control, which paradoxically is the most powerful possible therapeutic intervention.

One inpatient taught me something about host resistance when she was working in cognitive therapy group on the problem of an alter seizing executive control and acting out by head-banging. As I asked the host to describe the sequence of events leading up to the head-banging in more detail, the behavioral precipitant and interpersonal strategy of the acting out became clear, and the host casually remarked, almost under her breath, that she let the alter out. This permutation of host resistance is *host collusion with the alters.* The host takes the helpless victim position but in fact covertly allows switching to take place and internally reinforces the acting out of the alters. The problem is not that the alters come out, but that the host decides to let them out.

This analysis should not be overgeneralized and does not apply to all switching or acting out. It is only one kind of system dynamic among many, but it is common. The key corrective is to point out to the host that she is in charge, that the alters were created to help her, and that they are still doing so—their job is to protect her from things she doesn't want to deal with, which is the basic rationale of DID. The alters are acting out primarily because of host resistance, not because they are bad, and if the host wants the acting out to stop, she must take the lead and make the necessary changes in the way she relates to the system. When the host makes a serious commitment and actually follows up on listening to the alters, they are usually very thankful and deescalate their behavior, though they may take a while to let go of the tough guy role.

Whenever the client is stuck and making less progress than would be expected from the apparent effort being expended, the therapist should always consider the problem of host resistance. Often, the host needs to stop harassing her alters to give her back memories, and admit that she does not want them. Therapist, host, and alters can then set up a desensitization hierarchy and contract for slow, tolerable memory processing. Host resistance can also be a source of false memories: The alters give her increasingly horrendous and extravagant false memories to distract her from the real work of therapy, which may have little to do with memories of any kind. The host and the therapist may go off on a long mutual excursion into virtual reality primarily so the host doesn't have to deal with actual reality. In this scenario, the paradox is that the more system information given out, the more internal worlds, layers, and subsystems entered, the less is known about the real problems and conflicts.

Host resistance is not intrinsically bad. It needs to be done in a reasonable and balanced fashion, and can be excessive or deficient. The host who is blamed for being too resistant will withdraw from the work of therapy into shame. A better tack for the therapist to take is to act as a consultant to the host on a cost-benefit analysis of her resistance, and an analysis of its mechanisms and logic. A deficiency in host resistance occurs in the client whose child alters are out too much in the outside world: This is often paired with a strategy of sending the kids out during therapy in order that the host does not have to work. The same phenomenon of too much executive control by child alters can be due to insufficient host resistance to switching in one context, and host collusion with switching driven by excessive host resistance in another. This kind of complexity makes the treatment of DID strategically challenging for the therapist.

CONCLUSION

The main point of this chapter, which I will repeat again, is that good DID therapy is good generic therapy. The patient is a person, not a diagnosis, not a group of people in one body, and not a diversion for the therapist. Complex DID patients challenge all the skills, staying power, and self-discipline of the therapist. At the same time they have the most to teach and are the most rewarding, by far, of any patients I have worked with. I have met many people with DID who impressed me as human beings with great courage and faith in life.

CHAPTER THIRTEEN

The Problem of Attachment to the Perpetrator and the Locus of Control Shift

The major development in my thinking about treatment since the 1989 edition of this book centers on *the problem of attachment to the perpetrator* and *the locus of control shift*. I invented these terms to capture the core conflicts in dissociative identity disorder (DID), which are now the primary target of my treatment plans. Intertwined with these two principles is the victim-rescuer-perpetrator triangle, which is widely understood among trauma therapists.

In this chapter, I will explain the thinking behind these three fundamental principles of therapy and illustrate them with clinical examples. The principles can be used in the psychotherapy of trauma survivors without DID as easily as those with, and are designed to shift the therapy of DID further in the direction of generic trauma therapy. As well, this method of therapy does not hinge on an estimate of the accuracy of the trauma memories: the same interventions are used no matter what percentage of the memories are real. The content of the memories is symbolic of the core conflicts whether the events ever happened in the external world or not.

A young DID patient taught me that even reality is symbolic. She was in a crowded outdoor public place accompanied by reliable witnesses who later confirmed her story, when an old man collapsed on the ground in cardiac arrest. The patient did mouth-to-mouth resuscitation on the man, but he died. The next day, the young woman had to be readmitted to the inpatient unit overnight for exacerbation of her PTSD symptoms—the most traumatic aspect of the event, for her, was that the old man died alone with no one who knew him at his side. The patient was very disturbed that the old man had lived his final years in isolation and loneliness.

It was not in fact true that the old man died alone, as confirmed by independent reliable witnesses on the scene. It was true that the DID patient was there and administered mouth-to-mouth resuscitation, and the man did die; however, a woman who knew him was on the scene and she confirmed at the time that he was married and living with his wife. It became evident quickly that the old man's loneliness was a projection onto him of the loneliness of some of the patient's alter personalities. The exacerbation of her PTSD was guilt-driven, and based on the host personality's conflicts about neglecting her alters. The internal myth was that the alters were going to die of neglect, and this was a reenactment of childhood fears arising from parental neglect.

This case taught me that even objective, verified, accurately recalled traumatic events can be traumatic primarily for symbolic reasons. The problem that must be solved in therapy has nothing to do with the information content of the memory; the information about what transpired is useful therapeutically only because it allows one to analyze the system conflicts, cognitive errors, reenactments, and dysfunctional defenses at work. These are the target of therapy, not the memory.

THE VICTIM-RESCUER-PERPETRATOR TRIANGLE

Although the therapy I do looks and feels more like cognitive therapy than psychoanalysis, much of it can be conceptualized in analytical terms. Analysis of the victim-rescuer-perpetrator triangle, for example, from an analytical point of view, is really analysis of the classical transference triad. It involves the therapeutic transference; the original relationships with significant others, usually the parents, in the past; and current transference acting out in the world. I use the victim-rescuer-perpetrator triangle as a framework because it lends itself more easily to the strategic-systemic aspects of therapy, because it is accepted vocabulary in the sexual trauma field, and because it makes sense to the patients. The triangle is shown in Figure 13.1.

The host personalities of DID patients are usually in the victim role. The persecutor personalities are in the perpetrator role, based on identification with the aggressor, and the protectors are in the rescuer role. All three points of the triangle are located internally in the personality system in this scenario. The problem is that there are dozens of triangles, they are not stable, and they oscillate at varying frequencies. For example, in another

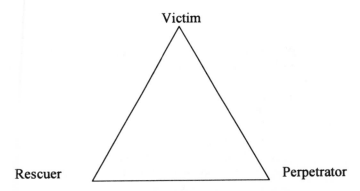

Figure 13.1. Victim–Rescuer–Perpetrator Triangle

permutation, the incest father is the perpetrator, the patient is the victim, and the therapist is the rescuer.

In another variant, a child personality is the victim, a persecutor is the perpetrator, and the therapist is the rescuer. In yet another, the therapist is the victim, the host personality is the rescuer, and another patient is the perpetrator. The therapist's responsibility is to maintain neutrality, not to get fixated at one corner of the triangle, and not to act out any one of the three roles. In analytical terms, this requires the analysis of powerful projective identification pressures.

The most common countertransference error made by DID therapists is to get into the rescuer role. When this happens, there is always simultaneously an overidentification with the victim role in the patient: The therapist is rescuing the child in herself, who was not loved enough by her parents, by projecting the child into the patient, who then melds into the patient's host personality or one of the child alters. These dynamics result in the therapist losing neutrality and looking at the patient's problems from a vantage point inside the patient's personality system.

The patient's inner world was created using the magical properties of a little girl's mind, and it still works this way. The therapist who identifies with a child alter tends to perceive the inner world from the perspective of a child alter—the inside and outside perpetrators then look very big, scary, and bad, and patient and therapist huddle together in a mutual victim-rescuer dyad. It becomes unclear who is the client and who is the therapist.

Such countertransference errors can occur to a mild degree, in which case there are technical problems in the therapy, or can be acted out at the level of negligence and malpractice. The extreme cases on which I have acted as an expert witness illustrate the general principles most graphically. In audio-taped sessions, the therapist can be heard crying repeatedly, talking in detail about his marriages and sex life, receiving support and soothing from the client, and joining with the client in condemnation of the client's family. In cases where the therapist has also sexually victimized the client, the triangle has flipped over so that the therapist becomes the incest father, the client is daddy's special princess, and, once a lawsuit is filed, the plaintiff's lawyer is the rescuer. The client filing the lawsuit then has to deal with internal pressure to flip the triangle again, such that she becomes the perpetrator of a malicious legal action, the therapist the victim, and the defendant's lawyer the rescuer.

Tracking the ambivalence resulting from these simultaneously activated triangles is an important aspect of the therapeutic work. In patients who are currently being battered by their spouses, the victim-perpetrator dyad has overridden all others, and it can be very difficult for the therapist, police, or social service agencies to effectively get into the rescuer role. In these situations, the patient's drive to maintain her attachment to her perpetrator is being acted out in a fixed, rigid attachment to a current perpetrator.

The therapist's role is to map out and analyze the permutations of the triangle, then to consult to the patient on strategies for better managing the conflicts, with a focus on both the inside and outside worlds. I regularly tell patients that they are acting out of the victim role; this intervention has been made more effective over the past two or three years by a general disidentification with the victim role in our society. I am particularly inclined to confront victim-role behavior when the patient is seeking secondary gain from the patient role, which is common on inpatient units.

The reason that therapists recommend confronting the perpetrator, disconnecting from the family of origin, and launching lawsuits against the incest father, is not because they mistakenly believe in the reality of false memories, as alleged by the False Memory movement. Taking these actions does not flow inevitably or necessarily from believing in the memories. For these actions to be taken, one of two things must be true: The actions are warranted, or they are not. If the actions are not warranted (if they are acting out), they are not driven solely by believing in the memories.

The best analogy to clarify this point is with enzymatically augmented biochemical cascades. It is common for biochemical pathways, such as the synthesis of adrenaline, to have a series of steps: Each step is sped up by a specific enzyme. In the synthesis of adrenaline, the conversion of dopamine to adrenaline by the enzyme dopamine decarboxylase must be preceded by a prior step. Tyrosine must first be converted to dopamine by tyrosine hydroxylase. In the absence of tyrosine hydroxylase, no adrenaline will be made.

The existence of adrenaline cannot be blamed solely on tyrosine hydroxylase, because the synthesis of adrenaline will not occur in the absence of dopamine decarboxylase. The prior step, conversion of tyrosine to dopamine, is a necessary but not sufficient condition for the manufacture of adrenaline.

Similarly, believing in the reality of false memories is a precondition but not a complete explanation of rescuer acting out by therapists. If the therapist is not intrapsychically driven to act out, believing the memories will not result in lawsuits against the father. Reducing the legal and psychological damages to falsely accused perpetrators and their families depends on understanding all the steps in the biochemical cascade. Simply shutting off false memories will not suffice, because the drive to disconnect from the perpetrator father will then be rationalized on other grounds. The impaired therapist will find some other way to fixate himself in the rescuer role, the patient in the victim role, and the father in the perpetrator role. It is true, of course, that without the false memories, the father cannot be falsely accused of incest. However, he can still be vilified and disconnected from his daughter.

How do these triangles get started? What keeps them going? To understand that, one must grasp the problem of attachment to the perpetrator. The problem of attachment to the perpetrator is the core conflict; understanding it prevents the therapist from getting lost in endless permutations of the victim-rescuer-perpetrator triangle.

THE PROBLEM OF ATTACHMENT TO THE PERPETRATOR

The core conflict in childhood-onset DID arises from the structure of the abusive and neglectful family, and is embedded in everything we know about mammalian attachment. The abused child with DID is like the young monkeys experimentally abused by having cloth or wire mothers (van der Kolk, 1987). The Harlow monkey experiments can be understood as studies of the psychobiology of child abuse, using an animal model.

Children are different from monkeys in that, even by age four, they are already little sociologists. The abused child walks around in her family with a clipboard and a pencil, making sociological field notes, and constructing a theory to explain and order her observations. Being four years old, this junior sociologist does not use the vocabulary or thought processes of the graduate student, however. She uses developmentally normal principles of child cognition, and devises *the locus of control shift* as her overriding sociological theory. I will expand on this later in this chapter.

The abused child is trapped in her family. She cannot run away from home and live on the street, move away to college, take drugs, or get married to escape from the family. She cannot get the abuse to stop, cannot predict it, and cannot control it. If she tries to tell anyone outside the family, she is not believed, or she is so overwhelmed by threats, intimidation, and mind control tactics, that she does not try to tell. The reality of her situation is that she is trapped, helpless, and overwhelmed.

The child has an additional problem. She must attach to her perpetrators. The child is biologically driven to form attachments to her primary caretakers, just like the ducklings who imprinted on Konrad Lorenz (an animal model of transference). She is biologically dependent on adult caretakers for

physical survival. More than that, the child has no choice spiritually or emotionally—she must love her parents, and must want to be loved by them. The
child cannot exercise an option of no love.

If the child does not attach to her parents, she will fail to thrive, and in extreme cases, her brain will not develop normally, or she will die. She must
also attach to her parents for her spiritual and emotional growth, or she will
have failure to thrive in those spheres. In a reasonably normal family, this all
works out reasonably well. In an abusive family, the child has a problem with
no good solution: She must love the people who hurt her, or die.

This is the core problem in DID, and the primary driver of the dissociation. I used to think that the most painful material to be dealt with in therapy was the specific events of sexual abuse. It followed from this model
that once all the memories were recovered and processed, the most painful
work was over. This was a pure Janetian model. Experience showed me that
Janet was not correct. The deepest pain is processed *after* there are no more
memories to recover, in the late preintegration phase of therapy.

The deepest pain arises from the overall *gestalt* of the person's childhood.
It is not so much that Dad did this on this day, or that on that day, it is more
just the whole reality of life in that family, all the denial, the hurtful things
said, the secrets, the betrayal, the lies, and the endless insoluble double
binds. This is what hits the patients the hardest. The deepest pain is not
event-specific, and does not depend on the accuracy of any given set of
memories.

When I explain this to the patients, I state directly that what Dad did in
the bedroom, or in the cult, is not what hurts the most. I make it clear that
ritual abuse memories are not the most painful or traumatic material,
thereby diverting attention from them, whether they are true or false. Once
the focus is shifted to the problem of attachment to the perpetrator, the preoccupation with ritual abuse content melts away.

The primary drive to dissociation, in this model, is the need for the
abused child to keep her attachment systems up and running. The modules of
the mind that maintain attachment behavior must be disconnected from
those taking in the traumatic information from the outside world. The basic
purpose and motive is not to solve intrapsychic conflicts, or deal with feelings, but to maintain attachment. An advantage of this model is that it embeds dissociation in a large body of science about mammalian attachment,
learned helplessness, and the biology of stress. It is irrefutable that the child
must keep her attachment systems up and running in order to thrive, that
there is a biological imperative at work, and that dissociation is required to
prevent reactive shutdown of the attachment systems.

The child's only other option, besides death, is permanent trance, depersonalization, or catatonia.

The elaboration of separate identities as a means of maintaining attachment is an epiphenomenon of the core dissociation. The inescapable reality
with which the child must deal, is that she cannot survive in the world

alone. She needs Daddy, to put a roof over her head, feed her, and clothe her: The child is very little, and the world is very big. The problem is that Daddy is also the one who is hurting her. The solution is dissociation.

There are now two realities, which are split apart from each other: Daddy is big and safe and kind; and Daddy is an incest perpetrator. Now, the child can safely attach to her perpetrator, keep her attachment systems up and running, and thrive. Everything is all right. The abuse is happening to that other little girl, not me, to that other little body, not mine. I don't need to shut down when Daddy comes near, because that's not my daddy who is doing that, it's that other little girl's daddy. Come to think of it, I don't have to worry, because I don't even remember what happened to that other little girl.

Still, in the back of her mind, the child asks, "Why doesn't Mommy come and save me?" The need for a rescuer is structurally built into the situation. The rescuer could be a good daddy, one who never comes, and the trauma could be an absent father, without overt sexual abuse. The attachment figure could be the idealized biological mother of an adopted child, or it could be a fantasy-replacement for an emotionally absent depressed mother. All of these are permutations of the theme of traumatic attachment.

There must be somebody to love. If there is no one on the outside, then create one on the inside, is the motto of the DID mind. Part of the drive to the delusional separateness of the alters is the need to have secure attachment figures. I have framed the problem in terms of stereotypical parent roles to illustrate the principles. In fact, there are often memories, real or false, of overt maternal sexual abuse.

This is how the victim-rescuer-perpetrator triangle is created in childhood, according to my treatment model. The problem of attachment to the perpetrator can be acted out in myriad ways throughout life. The paradox is that the child feels safe only when the perpetrator is nearby. Setting aside the social, financial, political, and economic factors that keep women trapped in battering relationships, the battered spouse is maintaining her attachment to her spouse in order to feel safe. She is trapped in the logic of her childhood, and is still making the locus of control shift. She is too little, helpless, and scared to live alone.

It is simultaneously true that the victim wants to be rescued, wants the abuse to stop, and wants to get as far away from the perpetrator as possible. The extreme example on this side of the equation is the woman who goes into a ritual abuse underground, moves out of state, and changes her identity. That is a futile strategy because an alter somewhere inside will recontact "the cult" in order to maintain attachment to the perpetrator, whether or not the cult actually exists. In most situations, either the problem of attachment to the perpetrator has been solved, in which case there is no need to go underground, or going underground is futile. In some cases, however, when the attachment ambivalence has been sufficiently resolved, but the perpetrator is stalking the victim, the underground option would make sense.

A common therapeutic error is to identify only with the negative pole of the ambivalent attachment, ignoring the positive attachment. Few parents are all bad. The mere fact that the client is in treatment shows that there must have been something positive about the parents, and something there for the child to bond with. Otherwise psychotherapy would be impossible. This mistake can be stated as a cognitive error: *To accurately perceive the negative, I must deny the positive.*

A patient's alter told me that therapy was bullshit and recovery was impossible, because if you don't feel bad, then the abuse never happened. The alter believed that recovery would mean buying into the family's denial system. My response was to say that I agreed with the alter: Given the rules of her universe, it is better to feel bad and maintain one's integrity. However, she had failed to consider another option, to step outside the family system rules altogether. In fact, she was still inside the family system rules, and was simply taking a reactive opposite position.

The alter was living by the linked equations: *happy = phoney and in denial; miserable = authentic and not playing the game.* The other option, not yet considered by the alter, was: *happy and not in denial.* The linkage of the two equations was reinforced for the alter because other alters in the system tended to escape from bad feelings through overwork, dissociation, and denial. The alter's cognitive errors could be traced back to the original problem of attachment to the perpetrator.

Alters holding the bad memories and negative feelings usually believe that no positive feelings about the father are allowed. They make a related cognitive error: *If I loved Daddy, I wanted the abuse.* The primary treatment for this cognitive error is to explain the problem of attachment to the perpetrator. Once a patient arrives in the late preintegration phase of therapy, most of the hard work of processing specific traumatic memories is completed, and she now must mourn the loss of the parents she never had.

THE LOCUS OF CONTROL SHIFT

The final element of the model is the locus of control shift, shown in Figure 13.2. The four-year-old sociologist mentioned earlier reads and rereads her field notes, and tries to make sense of the crazy-making transactional patterns in her family. Why do Mom and Dad hurt me, she asks herself? The cognitive machinery employed by the child to solve this problem is consistent with her stage of development: Now the model is embedded in everything that is known about developmental psychology. The child uses self-centered, magical thinking to analyze her world.

One might object that dissociation has been used to cause amnesia for the trauma, therefore there is no need for the child to explain to herself why the abuse is happening. This objection is based on an assumption of *total amnesia,* which is rarely observed clinically. The child can use

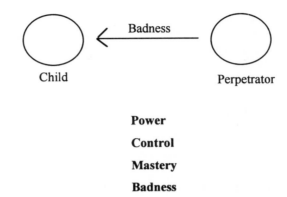

Power

Control

Mastery

Badness

Figure 13.2.   The Locus of Control Shift

event-specific dissociation to block out the memory of any given act of abuse, but blocking out a few hours here and a few hours there does not solve a more pervasive and fundamental problem: The world is dangerous, arbitrary, unpredictable, and uncontrollable.

It is the overwhelming sense of powerlessness, helplessness, and victimization which requires the locus of control shift. The helpless and overwhelmed child cannot escape; the only way to cope is in the mind, since nothing can be done in the outside world. At this point, using developmentally normal thought processes, the child identifies with the aggressor, and shifts the locus of control inside herself: Here the model rests on a foundation composed of the literature on coercive persuasion, brainwashing, mind control, and thought reform.

Now, it isn't the perpetrator who is causing the abuse to happen, it is the child. She has power, mastery, and control over the situation. She is big and strong like the perpetrator, and she is calling the shots. Like the perpetrator, she is bad. But it is good to be bad, because the badness is what causes the abuse. If the badness is inside me, then I can potentially control the abuse, because I can control myself. I can figure out how to be good, then Daddy won't hurt me anymore. This gives me hope.

The bad feelings that are caused by the abuse prove to the child that she is in fact bad, and reinforce the locus of control shift. Simultaneously, the shift preserves the idealized good parent, thereby allowing the attachment systems to stay up and running. Any normal physiological arousal caused by the abuse, or any positive feelings arising from the attention, prove that the child wanted the abuse, which proves she is bad, which proves it is her fault, which proves she is not helpless and overwhelmed, and is in control. To stay in control, however, she must stay bad. It is good to be bad.

Sometimes children forget that they are bad, and need to be reminded—this job is taken on by the persecutor alters, who cut, burn, threaten, and harass the host personality. They do this for a number of motives, one being to keep expectations as close to zero as possible in order to minimize disappointment. If someone in your head tells you are bad and ugly every day, you are less likely to take the risk of dating, and therefore are less likely to be reabused or disappointed. Also, dating is a sexual betrayal of the incest father, to which he might react by withdrawal of attachment. When the father is inside as an introject alter, the bind has been internalized and becomes self-perpetuating in a positive feedback loop.

When little girls grow up, they sometimes need daddies on the outside to remind them that they are bad. This is called being a battered spouse. In order not to be abandoned, the victim of domestic abuse maintains her negative self-evaluation and refuses to blame her husband. She is looking at the world from the perspective of a dependent child because she is locked in the logic of the past. The victim's rationalizations of her abuser's behavior as her fault reinforce the locus of control shift. The spousal abuse might stop if she cooks better, loses weight, participates in more bizarre sex acts, or keeps the house cleaner.

The illusion of control created in the child's mind is developmentally protective. It is a clever strategy created in a desperate situation. Stating to the patient that it was smart to be bad is paradoxical: it tells the persecutor alters that they are good and intelligent, which is true. The problem with the locus of control shift, in the adult patient, is that it does not match the outside reality of the adult world. What was an excellent strategy in childhood is now self-defeating. It isn't necessary to be bad anymore. To let go of being bad, however, one must solve the problem of attachment to the perpetrator.

When the illusion of power and control is broken, the truth can be seen, and with it come the feelings that have been defended against for decades. Now, in the late preintegration stage of therapy, a more generic yet deeper pain must be processed, false memories must be recanted, long-standing patterns must be broken, and life starts anew. Integration cannot be reached without passing through this stage.

One of the purposes of false memories of Satanic ritual abuse is to defend against the positive pole of the ambivalent attachment to the perpetrator through reaction formation. If Dad is all bad, the conflict about also loving him disappears. That is why the process of trauma therapy is similar to classical psychoanalytical mourning and melancholia: Using object relations terms, one must resolve ambivalent attachment to an introjected parent in both instances.

Another function of false memories of Satanic ritual abuse is to provide a myth that gives some sort of meaning and grandeur to the abuse. Otherwise it is just grubby, petty, and meaningless.

I chose the term *locus of control shift* because it has a technical ring to it, and because it evokes a scientifically grounded literature on internal versus external locus of control. The overall strategy is to ground the treatment model in science—in mammalian biology, cognitive psychology, social psychology, and the psychobiology of trauma.

CONCLUSION

The target of treatment in DID is not the content of the memories. Rather it is the problem of attachment to the perpetrator, the locus of control shift, the set of cognitive errors characteristic of the disorder, the permutations of the victim-rescuer-perpetrator triangle, and the systemic conflicts in the personality system. The locus of control shift and the problem of attachment to the perpetrator are also core considerations in the psychotherapy of non-DID trauma survivors.

The major evolution of the treatment model since the 1989 edition of this book is the material in this chapter.

CHAPTER FOURTEEN

Specific Techniques of Treatment: The Initial Phase of Therapy

The treatment of dissociative identity disorder (DID) must be based on good general principles of psychotherapy. This poses a problem for psychiatry because of the current swing of the pendulum away from psychotherapy training, and toward diagnosis and medication as the special expertise of the psychiatrist. In some residency programs in North America, trainees are not receiving adequate instruction in psychotherapy. This means that many young psychiatrists will not have the general skills and experience to treat DID successfully.

The psychiatrist who is going to treat DID must be a diagnostician, physician, and psychotherapist. This is especially the case if inpatient work is going to be done. Of the triad, physician is the least important, although medications can be helpful during the middle phase of therapy in many cases. Medical training provides an advantage, though, in assessing the physical complaints of the DID patient, which can be complex. As for any psychotherapy patient, an adequate physical assessment is necessary, but the same person rarely does both the therapy and the physical examination.

Most DID patients will not receive their psychotherapy from physicians. Therefore the emphasis in psychotherapy training should be on social work, psychology, and nursing students. It simply isn't realistic or cost-effective to expect psychiatrists to do most of the work. Nor is there anything about medical or psychiatric training that uniquely prepares one to be a DID psychotherapist.

For psychiatrists to be an optimally effective component of the treatment team, however, they must be skilled psychotherapists as well as diagnosticians and prescribers of medication. This is how our team works: Nonmedical therapists can treat DID to integration, but they can't prescribe medications and aren't trained in the differential diagnosis of mental disorders.

Many patients are best treated as clients in community-based agencies staffed entirely by nonmedical personnel. This is particularly true for DID clients who have had abusive treatment from hospital-based psychiatry, in the form of misdiagnosis and mismanagement. As I explained in the Introduction, I am referring to people with DID alternatively as patients and clients in this book and have adopted a convention of the patient usually being female and the therapist male. This is because I am a male physician who treats mostly females, and because the female:male ratio in clinical series of DID is 9:1. I am aware of the political, legal, social, philosophical, and economic aspects of the terms *client* and *patient*. The social context of the treatment has a strong effect on the tone of the therapy, and on the nature of the therapeutic alliance.

The special techniques I am going to describe can be used by any therapist of any background. Techniques that require an inpatient setting or medical training will be discussed as such under separate headings. I want to emphasize again though, that most of the work is good general psychotherapy. It involves supportively helping the patient to live in a way that is not self-destructive. The psychotherapy of DID is an *empowering* therapy in the feminist sense.

The reason I am going to describe the techniques in detail is because they are not described fully in the literature, or are not set in a broad and general context. Reading the literature, the practitioner doesn't get a grip on what to do, beyond general principles. In this regard, I take two texts on cognitive therapy as my model (Beck & Emery, 1985; Beck et al., 1979). A person cannot instantly become a fully-trained cognitive therapist just by reading these two books, but they provide detailed strategies and techniques that the clinician can actually implement.

It is important to provide a similar catalog for DID treatment because there are far more patients than therapists. Therapists who already have good general skills should be able to learn the special techniques of DID work without too much difficulty. The danger in describing these techniques in detail is that inadequately trained therapists will start using them in therapies that are out of control. Ideally, all practitioners should have close supervision from an experienced therapist on at least their first case. Thereafter less intense consultation may be all that is required. This is so partly because one complex DID patient can teach you more than 20 nondissociative cases. You can become familiar and comfortable with most of the specialized techniques and principles of DID therapy in the course of taking one person to integration.

A fact of life in North America is that not all therapists will get adequate supervision on their first case of DID. Robert Mayer's (1988) experience will be repeated by others in years to come, though others are unlikely to describe it with such eloquence. This means that there must be a compromise between compelling patients to go without treatment because of the shortage of trained therapists and advocating that "anything goes."

Another consideration is that DID patients often get into treatment before they are diagnosed, and can't just be dropped. One patient was diagnosed after she spontaneously switched to a child alter: She was effectively instantaneously in therapy for DID since I had to deal directly with a frightened personality that feared I would assault her. Often, it just isn't feasible to "put a lid on it" and continue with supportive therapy. Often, the lid comes off and stays off: This may occur in reaction to stressful life events in the present. When the therapist has no prior experience, can't find adequate supervision, and can't transfer the case, there is a problem. I hope this book will be of some help to therapists who find themselves in this situation.

As a brief general outline of therapy, I think that the patient needs to resolve her core problems, integrate into one person, and learn how to live effectively without pathological dissociation. I don't think there's any need to get into hairsplitting arguments about how integrated a "normal" person is: Most people feel like they are one person most of the time, and so do integrated DID patients. It isn't necessary to advocate a mythic unity of self never attained by non-DID people. Nor does DID provide an earthshaking challenge to usual concepts of the self and individual responsibility (Braude, 1995). DID is a dissociative *disorder*. It is a dysfunctional adjustment that needs treatment.

It is important, I emphasize again, not to lose sight of general principles and common sense in the treatment of DID. The first intervention in the treatment is to say hello to the patient. The second is to introduce oneself. These simple acts set the context of therapy: The participants are human beings and therapy is a conversation. If it can begin as such, things are off to a good start.

The more DID therapy I do, the less I use specific techniques. At first I thought that I had discovered a gold mine. I thought that there would be no limit to the clever techniques, creative interventions, and tricky maneuvers I could come up with. I envisioned an endless series of papers on special techniques. Rather than being sadder but wiser, I am now happier and wiser. Special techniques are important, but not as important as general ones. Indeed, "techniques" can get in the way if they detract from the core reality, which is two human beings in conversation. The therapeutic conversation has a context, rules, and rituals that I will describe. So does talking with a bank teller, or any other human transaction.

In this chapter and in Chapter Fifteen, the special techniques of DID treatment are discussed under a number of headings, with techniques peculiar to inpatient work described separately in Chapter Sixteen. Chapter Fourteen focuses on techniques used predominantly in the initial phase of therapy.

THE OVERALL METHOD OF TREATMENT

Many models of psychotherapy are after-the-fact accounts of therapy dressed up in jargon. On the other hand, good therapy can't consist only of the application of techniques, with no overall sense of their purpose. What is DID therapy for and how does it work?

I practice a psychotherapy that is a mixture of psychodynamic, cognitive, and systems techniques and formulations. It is a pragmatic, active therapy in which I do a lot of talking. When people describe the work I do with DID patients as "long-term psychotherapy," I reply that that is not what I do. I do short-term therapy that goes on for a long time. The difference is important.

Long-term psychoanalytic psychotherapy is characterized by things I don't do, and I do many things that are not "allowed" in strict psychoanalytic psychotherapy. From an analytic point of view, there are more "parameters of treatment" in my work than treatment. I don't think of the things I say as "interpretations," I talk a lot, offer advice and personal opinions, make political comments and jokes, try to reduce the transference rather than augment it, prescribe medication, and bring cotherapists, students, and trainees into sessions (just as cotherapists bring me into sessions). I try hard not to be "deep" in the usual analytical sense because I deal primarily with observable behavior and cognitive errors stated by the patient. There is no need for "deep" exploration because the most important material is immediately available on the surface, though the surface is dissociated into separate compartments.

I remember a colleague saying to me that DID is important because it proves the existence of the unconscious. I take the opposite view. For me, DID demonstrates that the so-called unconscious is not unconscious at all—it is wide-awake and cognitive in nature, but dissociated. The unconscious no doubt exists, but I don't try to deal with it much in therapy. I interact with the alters and find that I can do the work of therapy by sticking to what they consciously know.

For example, a patient misses a session and is amnesic for two hours starting 10 minutes before the session was to have begun. The last thing she remembers is walking across the parking lot on the way to our session. To find out what happened, there is no need for months of exploration. An alter, if he or she agrees to come out and talk, will readily explain his or her motivation for taking executive control prior to the session, and ensuring that "she" missed it. The work of therapy is to understand the cognitive errors behind the alter's behavior, their dynamic origins in childhood abuse, and their current protective function, form a treatment alliance with the alter, and then negotiate an alternative strategy. The alternative strategy will usually be a step toward coconsciousness, cooperation, and eventual integration.

DID therapy is an "up-front" kind of therapy, as I practice it. I give the patient lots of feedback, am frank about what I am thinking, and encourage what the cognitive therapists call "collaborative empiricism." This involves patient and therapist working together in a pragmatic, hypothesis-testing, problem-solving fashion to reach the goals of treatment. My work is not strict cognitive therapy because it involves analysis of the systemic and intrapsychic functions of the cognitive errors, and replacing them with more adaptive strategies. Although what I do resembles strategic family therapy in many ways, it isn't family therapy because there is only one patient in the room, who has a "family" inside her head.

My model of therapy, which blends techniques from three different schools of thought, is no more than this: The patient has developed DID in response to childhood abuse; she needs to integrate; after integration she needs to learn how to function as an integrated person. The next three chapters are a set of guidelines and suggestions for helping the complex multiple reach that goal.

THE PHASES OF PSYCHOTHERAPY

The psychotherapy of DID can be divided into four phases; initial phase; middle phase; late phase; and postintegration work. Integration may occur anywhere from halfway to nearly at the end of therapy. I will describe postintegration work separately at the end of Chapter Sixteen.

Like the stages of death and dying, the phases of DID therapy are only a rough linear map of the work: There is much going back, reworking, premature going ahead, and simultaneous presence of more than one stage. Just as it is important not to reify the alters into people, it is important not to view the phases as more than rough guidelines. With that caution, certain tasks and techniques predominate in the different phases of therapy.

The initial phase is often preceded by a lengthy involvement in the mental health system. Often patients have worked for extended periods with other therapists. There are two ways to think about this previous work, which are not mutually exclusive. One is to belittle the previous therapist who did not make the diagnosis, and view the previous therapy as a waste of time.

Usually, however, I find that previous diagnostically nonspecific therapy has been essential preparation for the DID work. The previous therapist may have established a good treatment alliance, done extensive supportive work, involved appropriate services and agencies, helped in coping with friends, relatives, and children, shored up weak life skills, worked through some of the incest, and carried out other necessary tasks. Often the patient was not personally ready, or was not in a life situation, to do the intense definitive work. A medical analogy would be the internist who treats a number of metabolic and infectious illnesses in order to prepare a patient for surgery. Without the surgery, the patient would die, but without the preparation the surgery couldn't be done.

Sometimes the referral source is a therapist who has been doing good work and has a good treatment alliance. I sometimes suggest in consultation that the previous therapist continue his or her work, but gradually shift into DID therapy with ongoing consultation and supervision. Occasionally, I transfer a case from the referral source to a more experienced therapist, if the consultation includes a request to take over the case.

In such cases, I make a straightforward explanation to the patient: She is transferred to a new therapist for specific psychotherapy for DID because it is an area of subspecialty expertise. The transfer has the same rationale as transfer of the metabolically stabilized patient from internist to surgeon. In some cases, I may act as cotherapist with the referring person, which is analogous to the internist managing the diabetes during the surgical admission: Consultant and consultee function as a team.

The transfer of a patient can be rocky at times. In one case, a DID patient maintained a delusion that her previous therapist was dead for several months after transfer, lamented the loss of the "only good mother she had ever had," spoke of joining her previous therapist by suicide, and idealized and devalued both the new and old therapists. The delusion could have been rated correctly as a diagnostic criterion for a psychotic depression on a structured diagnostic interview, except that a major depressive episode was not present. The delusion responded to time, support, clear statements that the previous therapist was not dead, empathic discussion of the loss, formation of a positive transference with the new therapists, small doses of trifluoperazine, and psychotherapeutic work dealing with the patient's childhood. The only component of this multimodal treatment package for the delusion I would have felt comfortable about dropping was the antipsychotic medication.

In another case, the patient did not manage the transition to a new therapist well. The patient maintained the prior therapist in the rescuer position and cast the new therapist as the perpetrator. She was unable to resolve her ambivalence about which therapist deserved greater loyalty. The patient was acting out her problem of attachment to the perpetrator: To attach to the new therapist, the patient tried to get the new therapist to align with her against the prior therapist, in a victim-rescuer dyad, but this never worked. A great deal of projective identification pressure was exerted on the new therapist to perceive the prior therapist as bad, and the transition was slow, stormy, and difficult.

The initial phase of therapy begins with the first diagnostic assessment session. The major tasks of this phase include making the diagnosis; sharing the diagnosis with the patient; educating the patient about dissociation and abuse; proposing a treatment goal of full integration; negotiating a treatment contract; educating the alters about being in the same body in the present; forming an initial treatment alliance; and beginning to map the system. Because mapping involves contacting alters who are hostile, many of the techniques of the middle phase quickly come into play. The initial phase of therapy is best thought of as the preliminary phase of a stage that encompasses both it and the middle phase.

The middle phase of therapy includes the most painful recovery of childhood abuse memories. There is further mapping of the system, an increase in interpersonality communication and cooperation, extensive negotiation, dismantling of amnesia barriers, and sometimes several integrations or fusions of alters. This is the period of therapy during which specialized techniques are most required.

The late preintegration phase is less intense. It involves reworking, final negotiations between alters, development of new skills and relationships, and a lot of work that will be carried into the postintegration period. One can think that therapy is in late preintegration then discover another layer or group of personalities, and go through the stages of therapy all over with that layer. It is important to understand that different groups of alters may move through these stages nearly independently, and be integrated as groups. In the treatment of DID, nothing follows a simple linear progression.

After the final alter personality has been integrated, there is still a lot of work to do. Some patients just seem to be better and have no major difficulties postintegration. Others make a transition from multiple personality disorder to posttraumatic stress disorder in a single personality. Such patients may have intense flashbacks and continue to be suicidal, unstable in their mood, and self-destructive in their manner of living for a period of time postintegration. For some the outcome may be resolution of their DID with a residual untreatable personality disorder.

As a generalization, though, postintegration work is much less intense, requires few if any specialized techniques, and has a greater supportive component. Although progression through these stages is not linear in any simple way, one can see definite increments of progress throughout therapy. There are many milestones on the way from diagnosis, to the first partial removal of an amnesia barrier, through the first integration, to full resolution of the DID. I will go through the therapy describing the techniques in our Therapist Dissociative Checklist (see Appendix B).

ESTABLISHING TRUST AND SAFETY

These two items are closely linked. Both are issues throughout therapy and have to be reworked with newly encountered alters or groups of alters. The therapist establishes trust by being trustworthy. That may seem self-evident, but it is an example of the empirical approach I take, and it is what I recommend to the patient. It is important to remember that the complex

DID patient has had her trust in loved ones violently broken countless times. She has developed a complicated system of protectors, persecutors, and other personalities to deal with problems of trust and safety: The total personality system simply won't accept "caring" statements about how much the therapist can be trusted. There are often child or other alters who are dangerously naive and trusting and who have been ruthlessly exploited by a variety of people.

As always in DID, one must be alert for paradox and contradiction. There will be alters who are too trusting, and ones that don't trust enough. In his workshops and talks, Richard Kluft always emphasizes the need to treat all personalities in an "evenhanded" fashion. That is a correct and necessary principle. Being evenhanded, however, doesn't necessarily mean acting the same with all alters: I couldn't act the same with all alters even if I wanted to, anymore than I could act the same with children, colleagues, friends, and enemies.

To establish trust and safety with some frightened child alters, it is important to tell them in a gentle, straightforward manner that it is safe. I might say, "It's all right. You're safe now. I'm a doctor and I'm not going to do anything to hurt you. I just want to talk to you." The alter might reply, "You promise you're not going to hurt me?" I would then go on to explain that the bad things happened a long time ago, Daddy is far away now, and the nurses and doctors are going to help the alter to feel better. I might say, "I promise I'm not going to hurt you. I completely, completely promise. You can believe me and I wouldn't lie to you. You'll see. We'll just talk and everything will be okay."

When child alters are hiding in the corner, shaking, screaming, trying to bang their heads, or scratching themselves, physical restraint may be necessary. Usually very little force is required, and it is more a comforting, holding form of restraint, than an aggressive control or containment. A hand on the shoulder may help. When touching any alter, it is usually best to get permission first, unless it is an emergency situation, because some alters are very frightened by touch and perceive it as assaultive. With child alters, the therapist might explain, after getting permission, "I'm just going to hold your hand now to stop you from scratching yourself. We're not going to let anything bad happen to you here. You're not allowed to hurt yourself, and we won't let any of the others hurt you either."

Trust and safety are complicated in DID because the therapist has to protect some alters against persecutory attacks by others. Alters may take control of an arm to scratch, slash, hit, or otherwise hurt the patient. With an adolescent or adult alter, simple reassurance may only help a little bit at most, and may be ridiculed. With more cognitively advanced personalities, I often give a set speech about how it is smart not to trust people. This is similar to paradoxical interventions made by a family therapist.

I tell the alter that it is true that many people broke her trust in the past, and that there are many untrustworthy people in the world. I congratulate her for her "street smarts," her advocacy of a nontrusting position, and her wariness. This is an excellent and necessary survival strategy in our world, I say. If there is another alter who has repeatedly been exploited because of being too trusting, I agree with the protector that this is dangerous. But I then go on to say that, although she may not have met any, there are in fact many decent people in the world. Without being self-aggrandizing, I simply tell the patient that she can trust me, but that I don't expect her to believe this right away.

I then recommend an empirical test of the hypothesis that I am trustworthy. I tell the alter to keep an eye on me and see if I do anything abusive. More than that, I ask the alter to tell me right away if I am doing anything she doesn't like. I recruit untrusting, hostile, and persecutory alters as consultants on the therapy at the first opportunity and try to get their opinions on things. This technique for establishing trust delivers the following therapeutic messages that the patient is likely never to have received in a sustained consistent fashion: Your opinion is worth something; you have a right to protest; abusive behavior is not acceptable; you already have many positive skills; I can't solve all your problems, but I am willing to help; I would like to talk with you at length.

Some patients bring transitional objects with them to sessions. This is fine with me. Some alters would not be able to work if they did not have a teddy bear with them. Also, some patients benefit from a transitional object given to them by the therapist. Patients can be highly resourceful at securing transitional objects; for example, one patient kept her appointment slips under her pillow during the most difficult period of therapy. Such behavior might be abhorred as "regressive" by some therapists. It is just a temporary technique for one phase of therapy, and the patient will soon enough leave it behind. If she doesn't soon enough leave it behind, then that becomes a problem in its own right, which must be solved.

Being available for phone calls is another way of establishing trust and safety. I have an absolute policy of never giving my home phone number out to any patients, and I have an unlisted number. If any patient got my phone number and started abusing it, I would get a new phone number and deal with the transgression in therapy. A major part of creating safety is establishing limits. However I am available for phone calls at work during the day, although I tell patients that I can't get back to them immediately most of the time. For those who work at a teaching hospital, patients are covered by the on-call staff as a general departmental policy. In general, the more educated staff are about DID, the safer the environment for the patients. This is also true on the Dissociative Disorders Unit.

Creating trust and safety is something that is done by both therapist and patient. Child alters will often stake out a corner of the office, or a chair as their territory. They will feel safer there. As I do most of the time in therapy, I discuss trust and safety in a straightforward, open, problem-solving fashion. This will often involve joint strategy-making in consultation with a number of alters. Child alters may also make good use of inner safety techniques. They may simply leave, or they may seek out a protector inside to be close to them. One group of ritually abused children were safe if they could get to a tree in an inner landscape: There, the father-alter could not harm them.

Innumerable imaginative, magical forms of protection can be given to the patient, or may already have been created. One can mark alters with magical retrieval markers which will allow the therapist to retrieve them by calling their names. In the magical world of inner hypnotic reverie, anything is possible, but all is not fantasy, for there are terrible memories of real trauma hidden behind the amnesia barriers.

I will discuss hospitalization and limit setting under separate headings, although they are key tools for establishing safety. All the techniques overlap, interdigitate, and reinforce each other. I discuss them as if they were separable only for clarity.

If it came down to a choice between me dying or the patient dying, I would choose to live. The safety of the therapist must be protected, as well as that of the patient. Therapists who work with difficult DID patients know that the risks to the therapist are not theoretical. Safety for the therapist depends on limits and toughness. It is not kind to the patient, therapist, therapist's loved ones, other DID patients, or the institution, to allow the therapist to be harmed. Such events would only impede the treatment of other DID patients.

The first way to protect the therapist is not to accept patients with convictions for violent crimes except in a secure forensic or hospital setting that is able to handle non-DID forensic cases. That is simple. A more common problem is to uncover past or ongoing violence, witnessing of murder, severe physical and sexual abuse by pimps, and other violent acts during therapy. In this situation, the therapist has formed a treatment alliance, has taken the lid off, and would feel badly about dropping the patient. The patient would be at high risk of suicide, and would have difficulty trusting anyone in the future if termination of therapy was the response to disclosure of such violence.

If therapy is to continue with the previously violent patient, appointments should not be scheduled for evenings. There should be other professionals nearby. Sometimes two therapists will have to see the patient jointly. There must be a contract not to bring weapons to the sessions. If there is a suspicion that the patient is carrying weapons, she must consent to being escorted to the security station for a weapons search. Searches may be required prior to each session. If the patient persists in bringing weapons, therapy should be unilaterally terminated without arrangements for transfer to another therapist. These rules tell the patient that abuse is unacceptable, and that safety is going to be ensured for both participants in therapy.

If the therapist is nervous enough to be even faintly considering having a weapon of his own in the office because of a particular patient, consultation is *mandatory*. It is foolhardy and stupid to try to handle such cases without consultation. In some cases, contact with the police may be required, and if so, the safety of the therapist overrides patient confidentiality. That is a personal and therapeutic opinion of mine, not a legal or professional-ethics statement. I would rather be sued and alive than dead and a virtuous protector of patient confidentiality.

One useful technique for therapist safety is to implant a posthypnotic suggestion, and to periodically reinforce it hypnotically. David Caul told a story of freezing a patient in mid-air with a posthypnotic signal, as the patient was lunging at him with a knife. In one case, we used a posthypnotic suggestion to go into a catatonic trance whenever a staff member yelled, "Time out!" and made a time-out hand signal. A nervous evening nurse unnecessarily froze the patient in front of the nursing station one night, with no untoward effects on the patient. We were reassured by this impromptu test, and were able to treat the Evil One to stable integration, partly because of our own sense of safety.

There is nothing unprofessional about opening the door of the office and standing near the door if it seems necessary. One can ask the patient to sit on the floor, giving the therapist an escape advantage if a hostile alter cannot be contained. If such techniques are required more than a few times, hospitalization, termination, and consultation should all be considered. The basic principle is that you have to do what you have to do to stay safe.

A single threat against my family by any alter is grounds for immediate termination of therapy.

There are hundreds of thousands of individuals with DID in North America, and most of them can be treated with safety. DID therapists are a scarce resource and must be protected. Handling DID patients is often like handling misbehaving children: Limits, toughness, strict rules, and consistent enforcement are the kindest and most effective treatment. Not everyone agrees with that parenting approach, but the patients will eventually teach it to most therapists who are committed to effective, efficient treatment. Within such rules, DID therapy can be curative.

DEVELOPING A TREATMENT ALLIANCE AND DISCUSSING THE DIAGNOSIS

I have linked these two aspects of therapy because they depend on each other. In discussing the diagnosis, a balance must be struck between a matter-of-fact approach similar to that for any medical diagnosis, and traumatizing the patient with a flood of information. I set the grounds for the diagnosis by normalizing dissociation, then explaining the link between trauma and dissociative disorders. Some patients will already know their diagnosis and its etiology, but most will not. The way in which I discuss the diagnosis also depends on whether it is a diagnostic consultation or an early treatment session.

In consultation, I usually explain DID in a general way and give the patient the actual term dissociative identity disorder as a diagnosis. It is important to demystify the symptoms, put them in a framework, explain that they are common and treatable, and to emphasize that DID is not a form of insanity. I often use an educational metaphor, saying that treatment involves unlearning highly effective dissociative defenses used in childhood, which are now maladaptive, and learning new ones. I rarely use words like "defense, or transference" with patients. Instead of talking about defenses, I usually talk about strategies, ways of coping, or similar generic ideas.

I tell patients that DID is just a label we use for having other parts inside that are so separate they feel like different people. I state that they are not other people, that they are all parts of one person, and that the goal of therapy is integration. I think that integration is the best goal, and that you are cheating the patient if you don't try for it. This is analogous to striving for cure in all cases of childhood leukemia, while being prepared to abandon that goal in unresponsive cases for whom the treatment is worse than the illness.

I also talk about prognosis and the probable duration of therapy, being careful only to make ballpark estimates and to advise the patient that controlled studies have not been conducted. Overall, there isn't that much difference between the way I discuss etiology, diagnosis, treatment, and prognosis in panic disorder, schizophrenia, and DID. I review what is known, and what I recommend in each illness. When explaining schizophrenia to a patient or family, I make a point of clarifying that most psychiatrists view it as an illness of the brain, but that definitive research proof is still lacking. In panic disorder, I review a mixed biological-cognitive-behavioral model of etiology and treatment.

Discussing the diagnosis is not something that is done once or twice at the beginning of treatment, then dropped. Throughout therapy, the clinician will be educating the patient about her disorder, as more of its complexities unravel. Dissociation will have to be explained over and over with newly encountered alters. Like the emotions and memories, the cognitive information about the diagnosis has to be processed and reprocessed throughout therapy. The patient has to discover the meaning of DID for herself, which will have unique qualities and nuances. We call this "education and information processing" on our Therapist Checklist.

I am a strong advocate of diagnosis and differentiated treatment protocols. Some people view this approach as distastefully medical, but I see it as correct and humane. It is malpractice for a community-based psychotherapist capable of only one generic treatment modality to attempt to treat panic disorder, DID, and schizophrenia. I don't believe one model or school can account for all forms of emotional disorder. Without giving a formal lecture, I communicate a flexible, technically eclectic treatment plan to the patient and emphasize that treatment will be collaborative but not democratic. The patient is the patient and I am the doctor. We are not friends and I am the only one getting paid.

Some patients insist on being "equals" in a way that undermines therapy and is a resistance to getting on with the work. Patients are not "equals" in the social contract of therapy. Neither are they subordinates. In therapy, I expect patients to make their own decisions and be responsible for themselves, but at times they must defer to my greater experience and insight. This doesn't mean I am being paternal, it just means that I am a professional with skills. People don't get insulted or insist on being treated as "equals" when an architect makes decisions about structural details for their house. The same applies in psychotherapy.

The frame of psychotherapy in North America is often too personal, intimate, and private. The frame should be more like consulting an architect on house plans. It is the client's house and life; the architect has special skills; and the client can't design a house alone. In my architectural practice, I build whole selves in ongoing consultation and collaboration with my clients, who are called patients for sociological reasons extrinsic to the work. When the therapy contract is thought of in this way, the whole issue of being "equal" becomes irrelevant. That is the atmosphere I try to create in therapy, as a corrective to an excess of intimacy.

Of course, building a self is a far more important, difficult, and personal project than building a house. No effective therapy with an DID patient has ever been dry and technical. I think it's reasonable to say that creative work in architecture engages the architect in a direct, personal way, just as DID therapy does. The difficulty in advocating a more "professional" stance in therapy is that it will be perceived as cold and insensitive. In practice, nobody can treat a significant number of multiples in an overinvolved, overpersonalized way without hurting patients and burning out. Zen-like detachment is necessary. With these remarks, I am trying to convey a sense of the tone of the treatment alliance.

It is essential to establish a treatment alliance with as many alters as possible. With some, this will be very difficult. The host and rational adult personalities can be worked with on an adult level. With the child alters, a formal treatment contract doesn't have much meaning. With the children, the alliance may be closer to that of play therapy. Often it is necessary to do safe things with the children as a systematic desensitization to adult relationships: the patient sends out the children because she is afraid to be an adult. Reading books, playing cards, drawing, or going for walks may be necessary beginning steps.

These activities, described in more detail in Chapter Fifteen, are dangerous in that therapy may deteriorate into prolonged therapeutic play. The play is only a means to an end, which is integration. It is easy for the therapist to forget that he is treating an adult, and helping an adult to live better in the world. The therapist must also form a treatment alliance with the hostile alters, who will quickly dispel the illusion of delightful children.

As mentioned earlier, it is helpful to recruit the persecutors as consultants to the therapy. This may involve cognitive techniques aimed at challenging the destructive behavior. For example, attempts to kill the host through overdose or slashing are often viewed as helpful euthanasia by the persecutors. The first step in forming an alliance is to point out that both persecutor and therapist have the same goal: They only differ on means. Both want the suffering to end. I often make a little speech acknowledging that the treatment is increasing the host's suffering, but insisting that that is a necessary stage of therapy. I agree that if things could not improve, the therapy would be harmful and futile.

Persecutors are often very resentful of the therapist interfering and treading on their turf. They see therapy as implying that they are failures at taking care of "her." This cognitive error can be addressed directly. Simple statements to the effect that everyone needs a hand sometimes, can help. I acknowledge that the persecutor has far more knowledge of the system than I do, and ask for permission to draw on that expertise. A good strategy is to move quickly to a practical problem in which the persecutor can act as a protector. The therapist might ask the persecutor to come out in a predictable social situation in which some other aggressive or potentially abusive person has to be dealt with.

Alternatively, one layer of persecutors may be recruited as enforcers to keep another layer of hostile alters, who will not yet enter therapy, from harming vulnerable alters. Both internal and external tasks can be set. The most powerful way to form a treatment alliance with hostile alters is to divine their pain and sadness and comment on it. They too are suffering children and adolescents. One Evil One turned out to be a child who declared, "I don't want to hurt anybody" during her integration ritual. Most hostile alters act tough but want to be loved by the host personality.

Globally, the best way to form a treatment alliance is to know what you are doing and form a sensible plan of action. Patients can tell if you know what you are doing. The best way to undermine the treatment alliance is to fake expertise or certainty that isn't there. DID patients have received extensive training in detecting lies. I have found that DID patients are forgiving of therapist errors if the mistakes are acknowledged openly. It is also important not to promise what you can't deliver because such promises will come back to haunt you, and will weaken the alliance.

Usually forming a treatment alliance is not too difficult, although there will be strong resistance and hostile alters may provide protection for the system by acting out. Most patients are so relieved to meet a therapist who understands their disorder, and seems to know what to do, that a working relationship is readily established. The alliance is far from static, though. It varies from alter to alter, and fluctuates throughout therapy. With some patients, I have never gotten to first base therapeutically, and haven't been sure what went wrong. Some patients just don't seem to be ready to work, and sometimes the patient and I don't seem to click. It is important not to be personally offended if a patient can't work with you—sometimes they will come back later. I included some case examples of this type in *The Osiris Complex* (Ross, 1994b).

A STATED GOAL OF INTEGRATION

I am using a separate heading for this technique to emphasize its importance, having already discussed it. Although it is important to state this goal of therapy at the outset, and to contract for it at least informally with the host personality, overemphasizing integration can create unnecessary hostility in many of the alters. The alters view integration as dying. "You just want to get rid of us" is a statement I have heard many times. One of the ways to soften this resistance is to adopt the patient's metaphor of integration, rather than imposing one of your own.

For some patients, an explanation of integration in terms of computer circuitry seems to make sense. I say that the patient's mind is like a computer in which certain areas of the grid are disconnected from each other. These short circuits in the system impede the free flow of information and coordination of function. The goal of therapy is simply to repair the short circuits, not to remove or replace parts. Other patients may prefer an image of divided streams rejoining into one full, strong river. Leaves with their dividing veins and common stem, or trees, can provide a good metaphor, as can baking a cake, in which no ingredients are lost, and a new whole is created. Richard Kluft (1987e, Oct. 24) has a videotape of an integration ritual involving melting snows on a mountain flowing down to join together.

The essential principles of integration metaphors are that nothing is lost, all aspects of the self have their value and place, and a whole greater than the sum of its parts is created. I also include a statement at the beginning of therapy that for this particular patient full integration may not be a desirable goal. For example, one patient described in *The Osiris Complex* (Ross, 1994b) retired from her career unintegrated but felt that occasional blank spells were now tolerable, since the threat of losing her job, or publicly embarrassing herself was gone. For health and life-stage reasons, and because of the quiescence of most alters, she did not feel it would be beneficial to do the work required for full integration. Kluft (1988d) has described the need to go slowly in the older patient, and to be satisfied with a nonintegrated outcome in some cases.

Throughout therapy, integration is mentioned and discussed, but the work does not usually focus directly on it. One way to avoid unnecessary resistance to integration is to focus on the barriers between personalities, rather than on joining them together. If the amnesia is gradually dismantled, and feelings, attitudes, and memories are increasingly shared, the patient will approach integration without having to be talked into it. By the time every personality is aware of everything about everybody else, many will spontaneously consent to integration, or even integrate outside therapy. Movement toward integration should not be forced. Rather it should be viewed as the final outcome of work that deals directly with other issues. This approach sidesteps potential conflict between therapist and patient.

I often point out to resistant alters early in therapy that integration can only occur by consent; therefore it won't happen to them if they don't agree to it. They usually find this helpful.

CONTACTING ALTER PERSONALITIES

The idea of contacting alter personalities directly seems to "spook" many professionals, and make them leery of trying to treat DID. Actually contacting alters is usually fairly simple. The difficult part is figuring out what to do and say with them once they are out. In teaching beginning therapists about contacting alters I sometimes make a comparison with learning how to start IV's in medical school. In medical school, students are expected to start difficult IV's with minimal training. In fact when the IV nurse, who has started thousands of IV's, can't get one started, the medical student, who may have started 10 or 15, may be called. The same happens when the technicians can't draw blood: they may have been doing blood draws daily for years, but when they have trouble, the medical student gets called.

Most medical students get very anxious starting IV's at first, then become skilled and confident quite quickly. As a purely technical skill, calling out alters is easier and safer than starting IV's. A number of medical students doing two months of inpatient psychiatry on my ward in Canada called out alters. They watched me several times, did a few under direct supervision, then often carried on independently. To do this, they had to have a solid grip on the issues of therapy, and have specific limited therapeutic goals in mind. If there was any trouble, ward nurses who were experienced in DID work were available.

One medical student did supervised integrations of personalities as well. This young man had no previous experience in psychiatry and was not planning on going into psychiatry as far as I was aware. If medical students can learn this skill, I don't see why most mental health professionals can't. Calling out alter personalities is a skill that could be learned by all medical students in a two-month rotation if there was enough opportunity.

These remarks apply to reasonably straightforward calling out of alters. In some cases, there is greater technical difficulty. The point is that lack of experience with the technical aspects of DID work is only a minor barrier to the training of new therapists. Experiential workshops, videotape demonstrations, and limited direct experience would be sufficient training for most purposes.

As in much of the therapy, one good way to proceed is to ask the patient how her switching works. Some patients already know how to induce a switch, and can do so on request. In such cases, the therapist just asks to talk to a certain personality and the switch occurs readily. Virtually all patients learn how to switch on demand during therapy. When switching is well practiced, I just say, "Okay, could I talk to Mary now? Mary." This is followed immediately by a brief head nod, eye closing, and emergence of Mary. Naturally I make such requests in a context, with prior discussion, so that the timing makes sense to the patient.

I'm uneasy about making the calling out of personalities sound so simple, for fear that inexperienced therapists will call out hostile, frightened, or other alters they can't handle without adequate preparation of the patient, themselves, or the therapy. It may be simple to call out a screaming head-banging child, but not so easy to deal with her or get her to go back inside. Calling out of alters can be traumatic for both patient and therapist.

The first step in contacting alters may involve indirect methods described in the section on interviewing voices in Chapter Eight, in the discussion of schizophrenia. The first attempt at contacting alters is always based on some reason for suspecting their existence. Usually this is a history of blank spells, and this history is usually accompanied by voices and other secondary features of DID. The patient must be given a clear rationale for what is being done for what reason. Usually this will involve an explanation that the therapist is trying to help the patient recover missing memories.

After the necessary history-taking and an explanation that the missing memories may be recoverable, I might say the following:

> What I want to do is try to contact the part of your mind that knows what happens during the blank spells. To do this, I want you to be as relaxed as possible, so in a moment I'm going to ask you to close your eyes. This helps with the relaxation. You don't have to be worried, this is perfectly safe and nothing frightening will happen. All I am going to do is talk and help you try to relax, then I'll just ask to speak to the part of your mind that remembers what happens during the blank spells.

> I'd like you to close your eyes now, and sit as comfortably as possible in the chair. Good. Now I want you just to concentrate on my voice, trying not to think about other things. Just focus your mind on the sound of my voice. Simply by listening and concentrating on my voice, you will find that your body begins to become more and more relaxed and comfortable, just a pleasant, warm, natural sensation of relaxation and calmness as you listen to the sound of my voice.

> Now it will be as if a blank spell is starting. Just like when there is a blank spell in your life outside. You will find that the memories of the blank spells are coming forward so that I can talk with the part of the mind that holds them. That part of the mind will be here and be able to talk with me directly. While this is happening, your body will stay sitting in the chair, comfortable and relaxed. Everything will be perfectly safe and you will not get up out of the chair.

Now it's like Susan is starting to have a blank spell. The part of the mind that remembers will come forward and be able to talk with me. While that other part of the mind is talking, Susan can listen and be wide-awake if that is safe. She can remember as much as she is ready to remember. Or else Susan can be like she's asleep inside and not remember anything, just like during the blank spells. Susan will be able to hear and remember as much as she feels ready to, and it will be all right if she doesn't remember anything at all.

Now in a moment I want you to open your eyes, and when you do it will be that other part of the mind that is in control and talking to me, the part of the mind that remembers what happens during the blank spells. Open your eyes please, as soon as you are ready.

This procedure can have several outcomes. One is that nothing happens: the patient just opens her eyes and tells you nothing happened (if this is the end of the procedure, it is important to realize that the patient may nevertheless be in trance, so a suggestion to come out of trance must be given). With consent, one can next go on to a longer induction with heavier sleep and safety suggestions, and try again. If this is unsuccessful, one then goes to indirect techniques. A second outcome is that the patient talks lucidly in a hypnotic state, but there is no alter personality present. This is the case in simple psychogenic amnesia in which memories are recovered with hypnosis. The procedure can result in the recovery of memory without creation of alters in highly hypnotizable subjects.

Often a lucid, cooperative alter emerges, and one begins taking a history from it as will be described. Sometimes there is a brief switch of executive control, but the alter only stays out for a few seconds. Usually in such situations, a hostile alter tells the therapist to get lost. Sometimes the patient won't open her eyes, but a different voice will say, "There's no one here," or "We're not coming out." In such situations I might say:

I understand that you don't want to talk to me right now. That's fine. I'm certainly not going to try to force you to talk to me, because I don't want to do that. Anyway, I couldn't force you to talk even if I wanted to.

Let me explain why I would like to talk to you. I just want to get to know you a bit, and spend some time with you. I'm not going to try to get you to do anything you don't want to do. In fact, one reason I would like to talk to you is to get your opinion on things. Maybe there's something I'm doing that you don't like, that I could change if you told me about it.

What I was thinking was, maybe if you don't feel like talking with me, you could write me a note. Maybe when Susan is at home she could leave out a pad and pen for you. Then you could come out at home and write me a note, and Susan could bring it to the next session. Or there might be some other way you could communicate with me without coming out right here. I'd like you to think about it.

So let me ask again if there's anybody there, any other part of the mind, who would like to talk with me.

This approach can be used later in therapy when part of the system has been mapped, but there are alters who are reluctant to enter therapy. Depending on the degree of certainty as to whether alters are present, I will personify the absent part of the mind in my requests. If I am virtually certain that there is an unidentified alter, I will ask to speak to "someone I haven't talked to yet." If it appears to be a case of psychogenic amnesia, I will use generic referents such as "the part of the mind that remembers," or "the part of Susan's mind that holds the memories." This is done to avoid suggesting multiplicity when it is not present.

If an alter or alters will not come out, indirect conversation, ideomotor signals, inner conferences, automatic writing, and other techniques can be used. Often one just has to wait until the other personality states are ready. There are a number of different hints that an alter is nearly ready to take executive control, or of "someone being there," which can guide the therapist. Sometimes a given technique for calling out an alter seems to be working incompletely. In such cases, one can just try harder with the same technique, or try later, rather than switching techniques.

Often the host personality has a feeling of another personality being close to emerging. The host may feel anger, sadness, or another emotion rising to the surface, or just have an inner intuition of someone being there. She may hear a voice, or get bits of memory that seem to be coming from an alter. The patient may feel spaced out, "funny," depersonalized, or partially in trance. Or the host may feel herself starting to go inside, but the process stops.

The therapist may observe subtle facial changes. The patient may start to close her eyes, or nod her head. She may look tranced out. Or there may be a subtle change in facial gestalt that looks like the beginning of a switch. Sometimes the patient will enter a phase of uncontrolled trance switching without anyone taking executive control. The therapist may observe changing voice, face, and body language, without anything coherent being said, or any distinct entity taking executive control. The patient may toss her head, moan, or call out "Stop!" These episodes can sometimes reach a high level of drama.

Sometimes an alter will take control of a hand and arm and throw something, start scratching, or perform some other motor act. If the patient is holding a pad and pen for automatic writing, the hand may drop the pen when the therapist asks if there is anyone there. Alternatively, an alter may inflict pain on the host when the therapist touches on a delicate theme, or asks for a switch to occur. Sometimes the hostile alter in the background will cause a sudden headache, abdominal cramp, or other symptom that has been plaguing the patient for months. This is a handy demonstration of the psychogenic nature of the symptom, and allows the therapist to form initial hypotheses about its associated cognitions and dynamics.

As soon as such activity starts in sessions, the alters have declared themselves and are unwittingly in therapy. One can be confident that they will enter further into the work in a stepwise fashion. I might say at this point:

> I see that whoever is there can cause Susan to feel a lot of pain. It is clear that you have a lot of power to cause symptoms and that there's nothing Susan or I can do to stop that. So I'm not even going to try. If you're so powerful, it seems to me you should have nothing to fear from coming out and talking to me directly. But it seems you're scared to do that. I wonder why. If you are scared, let me point something out: If you did come out and talk to me, you could always go back inside anytime you felt like it. So there's no way I could do anything to you. You'd just disappear. But maybe you're too scared to try that.

This may be responded to with silence, increased headache, the arm and hand gesturing obscenely, or a switch of executive control. It is helpful to keep a sense of humor about all this and to share it with the patient. An alter may emerge, glare at the therapist, and declare, "I'm not scared of anybody." I always try to sidestep the power struggle, and confer control and power on the hostile alter. Like Janet (Ellenberger, 1970), I am willing to exploit the vanity of the demons.

It isn't necessary for an alter to be in executive control for it to be in therapy. One can talk through the personality in executive control to ones listening in the background at any stage of therapy. Sometimes uncontacted alters interact with the known personalities in dreams or inner hypnotic reveries, and sometimes these can be guided by the therapist. If all of the technical efforts to contact personalities directly, assuming it is a case of DID, are unsuccessful, the options left are a sodium amytal interview or waiting. I think of sodium amytal as a crude battering ram for entering an otherwise closed system and used it for that purpose in Canada. Once I was in, I proceeded psychotherapeutically much as I would without sodium amytal. I haven't done a sodium amytal interview since early 1992, but will discuss it further in Chapter Fifteen.

Contacting alters is only half the problem in therapy. The other half is getting alters to go back inside, which can sometimes be difficult. This is particularly the case in outpatient work, when the patient has to find her way home, go to school or work, or otherwise function outside the office. It may be near the end of a session, and a child who can't drive and doesn't know where she lives, may be refusing to go back inside. Or the alter may be abreacting, hostile, or intent on getting picked up after the session, taking drugs, or doing something else the therapist and host personality would not like.

Let me make a brief digression here, because of that last sentence. You can't treat complex DID in an acting-out patient by taking a morally neutral position. I tell patients that my treatment goals for them include getting off drugs, out of prostitution, and out of the mental health system. I tell them that I view prostitution, substance abuse, and wrist slashing as unhealthy and undesirable components of an unhappy life. Some people may think this means I am imposing my view of the universe on patients. I think it's impossible to do therapy without advocating a worldview. I feel fine about advocating that the patient get off the street. On the other hand, I rarely if ever talk with patients about my own religious beliefs.

The first step in trying to get a reluctant alter to go back inside, is to find out why she doesn't want to go away. There may be a simple misunderstanding or some finite issue that can be at least partially resolved. One can contract for a set amount of time out for that alter in the next session. If time is running short, or an agreement can't be reached, gentle force may be required. Remember that other parts of the system want the switch to occur, and that it is in the best interests of the whole patient. It is important not to get embroiled in disputes about alters' rights, and to keep the interests of the whole patient in focus.

It is countertherapeutic to allow alters to run amok, even in a pleasant childlike fashion. Sessions must come to an end in a reasonable time, and often on a predetermined schedule. If too many allowances or concessions are made, the rest of the therapist's caseload will suffer, the institutional system will start to act out against the DID patient, therapy will be out of control, burnout will begin, and the therapist's family will be unhappy. So the child must go back in.

This is where the hypnotizability of DID patients comes in handy. Usually the alter can be put to sleep. Once negotiation has failed, the therapist takes control and speaks in a firm but authoritative voice, giving repeated suggestions for sleep. Often these will be effective in a few seconds. Once the alter goes to sleep, it is useful to plant a posthypnotic suggestion for immediate switching in future sessions as soon as the therapist tells whoever is out to go to sleep. Then the host is called out.

If the physical setting allows, and it is safe, I sometimes leave the office if the patient refuses to leave. This only works if the setting is safe and if the therapist can outwait the patient. In such cases, I set the next appointment and tell the patient she can leave when she is ready. Or the patient might be able to wait elsewhere in the building till a switch occurs. The principle involved is that to preserve the therapy the therapist must find practical solutions for closing sessions. Like any problem in therapy, if this becomes persistent, it may be grounds for consultation. There is probably an unresolved conflict in the therapy.

The suggestion to go to sleep can be amplified with forehead touches or other cues. It is rare for this problem to get seriously out of control in a therapy which is otherwise proceeding reasonably well. Usually the alter agrees to go in or spontaneously switches in a reasonably short period.

Another problem is patients for whom the return of the host personality seems to be psychophysiologically difficult. Some host personalities just seem to have a harder time coming back. In such cases, the difficulty in switching seems to be a property of the system, and isn't linked to any particular alter, resistance, or dynamic. In such cases, you just have to work at it longer. Lengthy monologues by the therapist can help, as can physical touch, or holding a special object like a teddy bear, amulet, or diary.

With such patients, we give suggestions that the therapist's voice will pull the patient back. We give repeated instructions to focus on physical reality, and orient the host personality to where she is and who the therapist is, repeatedly. This can sometimes take 5 or 10 minutes. The worst that can happen, in our experience, is a longer delay than planned for.

A final problem is cases in which alters seem to shift rather than switch. In some patients, especially those on the border between DDNOS and DID, the personality system is not distinct and structured, or there may be structured and amorphous regions. Sometimes neither patient nor therapist is sure who is out, or who was just out. If nobody can tell, it may not matter much as long as there is coconsciousness. The only way to deal with this kind of fuzziness in a system is to ask for clarification and work with the parts that are clearest. Things may become clearer over time. Another observation of Janet (Binet, 1896/1977a, p. 147) may be helpful: Giving an alter a name may "crystallize" it and make it more distinct. This may be a therapeutic form of iatrogenic modification of the phenomenology if used sparingly.

In summary, the calling out of alter personalities, as an isolated technical intervention, is not the most difficult part of therapy. It can be learned easily by medical students and nurses. Most patients learn to manage their switches during therapy, so that alters can be called out with a simple request. When switching or lack of switching becomes a prolonged problem in therapy, this is usually an indicator of some other unresolved problem, rather than a purely technical difficulty. The therapist will have to keep the number of switches per session under control, to provide structure within sessions, and because too much switching is stressful for the patient.

The more experienced I become, the less I use formal techniques for facilitating switching. In fact, I rarely use them now. In my work, as I do it in the mid-1990s, switches occur spontaneously or by a simple request. Another technique I use more frequently now, is simply to talk through to an alter in the background, having obtained consent to do so from the host personality, and indirectly from the alter. I then ask the alter questions, the host relays the answers, and I give my response. After a couple of exchanges like this, it is common for the responses to shift from the third person to the first person. The patient looks confused when this occurs, and then it becomes evident that a full switch has taken place without my having requested it. I then carry on with the conversation.

As is generally true in therapy, the alters are not the problem: by definition they are the solution, and are holding things the host personality doesn't want to deal with. It follows from this principle, which I call *the problem of host resistance,* that technical difficulties with switching are usually due to host resistance. The solution to such problems focuses on the motives for resistance and the cost-benefit of the resistance, not on the switching itself.

ORIENTING ALTERS TO THE BODY AND THE YEAR

One of the most effective interventions in DID therapy, which I use over and over, is to orient alters to being in the same body in the present year. I often do this the first time I meet them, and I assign alters the job of repeating this teaching internally with other alters I haven't met yet. It is almost always the case that abreacting alters not yet engaged in therapy are locked in the past and have no idea what decade it is. Nor do they know that they are in a grown-up body.

The alters are in an emergency-activated state that matches the reality of 30 years ago, but not the reality of the present. When they abreact, they think the abuse is occurring now, and when they aren't abreacting they think it occurred last week, and therefore can occur again at any time. In outside reality, though, no abuse has happened for 20 years. The cognitive error about time keeps the level of PTSD symptoms much elevated.

For this intervention, it does not matter whether the memories are true or false; in fact, the efficacy of the intervention is probably amplified if the patient's belief in the reality of a false memory has not been challenged, because the subjective relief is greater, which in turn leads to a greater consolidation of the treatment alliance.

I teach the alters about their time distortion in a straightforward fashion by explaining the difference between inside reality and outside reality, and the fact that inside reality can be timeless. I have the alter look at her clothes, hands, general body size, and if necessary books and newspapers with dates on them. I explain who I am, what is going on, where we are, where the perpetrators are, when the abuse last happened, and the nature of the current external support system, if it is positive. I point out that no abuse has happened for 20 years, therefore it isn't necessary to be as frightened as the alter was when the body was 12 years old.

I also explain to the alter the age of the host personality now, her coping skills, and her commitment to keeping the alters safe. This information is almost always a great relief to the alter. Sometimes an alter will think this is a trick, but accumulating experience over a short period usually proves that what I am saying is true, especially if the alter is an outpatient and can look out through the host's eyes in public. The child alters are usually thankful that they are now in a bigger, stronger body.

When an alter objects that she has her own separate body, I explain that that is true, but her separate body exists in the inside world: In the outside world, everyone shares the same body. This strategy leaves the defensive delusion of separateness intact at a reduced level, and avoids triggering too much anxiety and resistance too fast. The alters can't agree instantly that they all have the same body because then the abuse would have happened to them, and they would have to deal directly with the problem of attachment to the perpetrator, rather than maintaining polarized attached or detached positions.

Always remember to go slowly in dismantling the defenses.

MAPPING THE PERSONALITY SYSTEM

It is impossible to treat DID without mapping the system. Mapping can be done formally with diagrams or informally, with the therapist constructing a mental map of the system as he goes along. I am going to talk about formal mapping because it illustrates the principles of both the formal and informal approaches. We draw diagrams in some but not all cases, and some but not all patients like to use maps in their diaries and treatment sessions.

Since the 1989 edition of this book, the main evolution in my practice concerning mapping is that I no longer request extensive written system maps early in therapy. Instead, I am more inclined to let the system unfold naturally, and I restrict my mapping to the key alters involved in the current pressing problems. This is a shift in degree and emphasis, not in category or basic method. The reason for the change is simply that complete maps lack any operational utility, and besides are never complete in the initial and middle phases of therapy.

Mapping and gathering a history of the personality system are intertwined and done at the same time. A full map includes the name, age, time of appearance, function, degree of amnesia, position in the system, internal alliances, and any other relevant traits of each known alter personality. Like most of the treatment, mapping is done in a straightforward way by asking the patient and consulting with the known alters.

The first step is to ask the amnesic host personality what she knows. Often this will be no more than a description of the voices, but the description can yield valuable information. The patient may know the sex of some voices, and can divide them into friendly and hostile voices. Collateral history of the patient's behavior during blank spells will yield clues as to the types of alters in the system, as will objects missing and present, and samples of unfamiliar handwriting: These can be important both in content and in penmanship.

An active DID diary will usually contain at least five or six different scripts. There will be hostile, furious scratchings with swear words and threats. A frightened childlike communication in block letters is common. There is often a microscopic script which may be an observer. Alters may identify themselves by name in the diary, and will reveal their conflicts and concerns. Such information is like an advance reconnaissance prior to the first guerrilla infiltration of the personality system by the therapist. Diaries in iatrogenic DID cases look much like those in childhood onset cases, so inspection does not establish which pathway the person is on. The key point is whether such a diary existed prior to therapy.

Some patients will describe with astonishment the out-of-character clothing they find in their closets and drawers. They may describe typical street prostitute garb. This always makes my heart sink a bit, because I know how hard the work is going to be. Others may find toys, teddies, or other items purchased for child alters in their home, and not know how they got there. Sometimes the patient "just has a feeling" that there is a little girl there, someone who's very angry, or someone who wants to help. The more prior information, the more specific and safe the first request for an alter will be.

Once the first alter emerges, it may be clear that it is an alter. There may be a dramatic shift in gestalt, and a charming child may announce with a smile, "Hi! I'm Susie." I then reply, "Hi, Susie. Nice to meet you. How are you?" Depending on how the child is feeling, and what she understands, I will then begin taking a history from her. As long as she is comfortable with this, I explain that I am going to ask a few questions, and that she is free not to answer any of them.

Soon after the emergence of a new alter, I ask who the alter is, and if she knows who I am. If it is unclear whether a switch has occurred, I may ask, "Can you tell me whom I'm talking to right now?" If the patient answers, "Susan," I then clarify that she knows who I am and ask, "Are you the same Susan that I was talking to before I asked you to close your eyes?" If she is, then I ask whether she remembers anything that she can't usually remember. If she can't, it is probably the host personality. Sometimes there will be a coconscious alter with the same name, or an alter behind an amnesia barrier with the same name, and these two possibilities must be inquired about directly.

The initial calling out of an alter and the questions after calling it out are the point in therapy at which iatrogenic creation of DID is most likely to occur. Therefore, therapists must take great care in a forensic assessment not to ask leading questions, suggest multiplicity, or create artifacts. The way of proceeding I have just outlined might have to be modified for forensic work. On the other hand, the questioner cannot be so indirect and nonsuggestive that the patient has no idea what is being asked. The therapist must avoid asking flagrantly leading questions in the absence of a history that supports such an inquiry.

If the alter is cooperative and comfortable, history taking proceeds much as in any psychiatric assessment. The assessor is serially interviewing members of a family about themselves and the family as a whole. Only in this family, some members know all about everybody, some know about only themselves, and others have varying combinations and degrees of amnesia. Mapping the system is like interviewing a family at its home. In a DID house, not all rooms connect to all others, some are connected by one-way mirrors, some by intercoms, some by open doorways, and some do not connect to anywhere but the outside world. The therapist has to find out who lives in what rooms, and what other rooms they can enter in what way.

Usually I ask the name and age of the alter early on. I then ask what the chronological age of the body was at the time of creation of the alter. If the alter knows about the host, I ask, "How old was Susan when you were first there?" Then I ask why the alter came at that time, and what she has been doing since. Next, I want to know how much time this alter has been in executive control since her creation, and how much she knows about what happens during the host's blank spells.

Having gathered this information, I then ask if there is anyone the alter talks to inside, or anyone else that she knows about. The answer to this may be, "There's Alice and Mary too," or "I'm not allowed to talk about that." Following the former response, I then find out everything that Susie knows about Alice and Mary, then ask if she thinks either of them would be willing to talk to me, and whether it would be safe. This may be followed by calling out Alice and repeating the sequence of questions with her. In a complex multiple, this process may be repeated many times throughout therapy, and the therapist may introduce himself to the patient numerous times.

A statement that an alter is not allowed to talk communicates important information. It is paradoxical because it reveals that there is an untrusting, hostile, controlling, persecutory alter in the background. This way of revealing hidden information is similar to a deep gruff voice announcing, "There's no one here." I usually tell the alter in control that I understand that she can't talk, and clarify that I'm not angry or disappointed. This is done to avoid making the alter feel guilty, and to avoid creating a tug-of-war between therapist and background alter, which the therapist will lose.

Mapping the system is not a cut-and-dried process. It takes place piecemeal over the entire preintegration phase of therapy. The mapping may proceed very slowly while abreactions occur, conflicts are resolved, and crises survived. The picture I have presented is accurate, but not for all personalities or all patients. It may take a great deal of finesse to learn why the frightened child alter can't talk, whom she is frightened of, and who could help protect her. Discontinuities in the mapping process often occur when an entire new layer of personalities is contacted: All the previously known personalities may be completely amnesic for the newly encountered layer, and the questioning must begin anew.

In complex DID, it is often necessary to write down the names of the personalities because there are too many to remember. This can get especially confusing when there are a number of complex multiples in the therapist's caseload. Different alters in different patients will have the same names, for one thing. As well, during the phases of therapy when alters are being fused, the products of the fusions may have new names or names compounded from previous alters, which will increase the mnemonic challenge to the therapist. Patients may be hurt and offended when the therapist gets mixed up about who is who.

Every system has its own structure, which must be recorded on the map. Different types of system are described in Chapter Six. Mapping is not an end in itself, and the diagrams are just helpful ways of remembering and filing information. It is easy to get overexcited about mapping and to see it as an interesting diversion in its own right: The therapist must focus on helping the patient get better and live better. When the therapist gets caught up in the phenomenology or in fascination with techniques, the therapy suffers.

TREATMENT CONTRACTS

As I mentioned earlier, with increasing experience I have gotten less gimmicky and technique-oriented in therapy. I now use formal contracting much less than I used to, and make written signed contracts only occasionally with the most behaviorally difficult patients. Therapy is not a love affair, an educational seminar, a spiritual journey, or a friendship. It is a specific type of collaborative work done within the boundaries of a social contract. In DID therapy its purpose is to cure the chronic trauma disorder and to help the patient live better. "Better" means more happily, more adaptively, at a higher level of function, more freely, and in a more whole and centered way. These are intrinsically worthwhile goals.

It is impossible to work without a contract, though the contract may be implicit and unconscious. There are two major contracts in therapy, of which the first is more informal. The first agreement is for a diagnostic assessment and a subsequent recommendation as to how to proceed. The following example illustrates this process.

A woman in her 20s was admitted to the hospital in the 1980s because of depression and suicidal ideation. She had been chronically depressed, met criteria for dysthymic disorder, and had a superimposed major depressive episode of several weeks' duration. She was completely amnesic for her life prior to age 15. Her retrograde amnesia extended backward in time from a point two or three days prior to a rape at age 15. She also had ongoing blank spells that lasted minutes or hours up until the present.

She denied auditory hallucinations. Positive secondary features of DID included objects present and being told of disremembered events. She said she had been raped by her stepfather at age 24, had a brief abusive marriage, and had a recent abusive heterosexual relationship. The stepfather had been on the scene since her childhood.

After taking the history, I outlined the decision tree of therapy with her, emphasizing that the goal was as short an admission as possible. There were three main problems: First was her depression, for which the treatment options were medication and/or psychosocial treatment. The second was her suicidal ideation, which made no passes outside hospital a necessary initial intervention. Treatment for suicidal ideation would also involve medication and/or psychosocial work. The third problem was her memory blanks.

Possible approaches to the memory blanks were to leave them alone, to try to recover some memory of the ongoing amnesia, or to go full-tilt at dismantling all the amnesia. The last option was presented to her only for completeness. She was told that this would be a long-term project, that the amnesia was probably highly protective, and that the work would likely involve recovering painful, difficult memories. I told her that such work might interfere with her function as a mother and student. I was advising her as to the possible benefits, risks, and side effects of all treatment options, in order that she could give informed consent.

She had fewer secondary features of DID than most undiagnosed DID patients and only scored 22.0 on the DES. The next step was to contract for an attempt to contact an alter, under the guise of "talking to the part of the mind that holds the memories of the blank spells." In this patient, this would be analogous to exploratory surgery under general anesthesia. If cancer was found, a decision as to its operability would have to be made, and further surgery, chemotherapy, or irradiation contracted for postoperatively. The alter would be contacted under the protective veil of hypnotic amnesia.

A hypnotic induction was contracted for, and it confirmed a diagnosis of psychogenic amnesia. In trance, the patient contracted for recovery of the memory of a number of recent blank spells, which occurred posthypnotically. The next step was to debrief the patient with a general explanation that additional memories were there, but that a decision would have to be made as to how to proceed. Next multidisciplinary discussions were held as to which therapists, counselors, and support persons might carry out which tasks. Other agencies were contacted and a tentative treatment plan was drawn up. This was then discussed in detail with the patient and a verbal contract was made for therapy that would leave the childhood amnesia intact, with a proviso that definitive work might be undertaken in the future if the patient's life situation permitted.

When a diagnosis of DID is made and the patient and therapist decide to go ahead with definitive treatment, a specific DID treatment contract is required. In outpatient work, this is usually a verbal contract, but for inpatient treatment the contract is always written and signed by the patient, myself, and at least one other team member. One or more alters may sign the contract. I will discuss written inpatient contracts since they embody all principles of contracting. Other aspects of hospitalization are discussed in Chapter Sixteen.

Inpatient admissions go much better if they are carefully planned. The more structure, the less acting out. The more operationalized and behaviorally defined the goals, the better. There is no use setting a treatment goal like "feeling better" since no specific plan follows from it, and the team will never be able to tell if the goal has been reached in a definable way.

I go into formal contracting meetings with an inpatient with a well-defined team consensus as to how to proceed. This is the first major intervention in controlling the splitting that will occur during the admission. Contracting is not a fully democratic process, and the patient does not have the last word. If the patient cannot agree to certain nonnegotiable terms, then there will be no admission.

During the contracting session, a full discussion of every point and its rationale is undertaken. Points are discussed until they reach a form acceptable to patient and staff. This process can get out of control and needs to be focused. Patients may digress into legalistic nitpicking, attempt a power confrontation on a side issue, or berate staff for their attitudes. The session has a defined goal of resulting in a signed treatment contract.

Contracts are more effective and therapeutic the simpler and clearer they are. Contracts with numerous subclauses and contingency plans quickly become unworkable. Convoluted contracts invite constitutional challenges by the patient that distract from the treatment goals. The following treatment contract from my work in Canada illustrates most of the principles of inpatient DID treatment plans:

Treatment Contract

The treatment contract is for Mary (including all her parts) and the staff of M3. The contract is in effect at the time of admission and throughout Mary's stay on M3.

The terms of the contract are as follows:

1. Mary's voluntary admission will be for approximately three weeks.

2. Mary will be seen in therapy by: Dr. Ross and Sharon Heber approximately 1-2 times per week, by Pam Gahan 1 hour per day, by her primary nurse and other nursing staff for a minimum of 15 minutes per shift on days and evenings.

3. Because of the angry and potentially aggressive part, "Fighting Mary," planned therapeutic sessions may be held in the seclusion room as deemed necessary by treatment staff and Mary. Mary may also request to go to the seclusion room if in need of a safe place.

4. Aggressive and threatening behavior is not acceptable on the unit (e.g., damaging or threatening to damage self, others, and/or property).

5. Consequences for such behavior will be dealt with as per unit guidelines; that is, Mary will be asked/ordered to go to the seclusion room for a time-out period voluntarily. If staff assess Mary's control to be minimal or absent, Mary will be physically assisted to the seclusion room and may need to be restrained for a period of time. In the seclusion room, the door will be locked, and Mary will remain in seclusion for 30 minutes. The last 15 minutes must be settled or additional periods of 15 minutes will be added until behavior is settled. Prn medication may be used as per Doctor's orders.

6. Angry Mary will notify a responsible person before acting on suicidal feelings.

7. All of Mary's personalities are expected to be honest and open and are encouraged to talk about feelings with the treatment team.

8. Mary is expected to follow general unit guidelines as outlined in the patient information booklet.

9. Mary requests that all staff give her space and do not touch her when her BACK OFF sign is posted in her room.

This contract is flexible and negotiable approximately once every week. The contract will be renegotiated by Mary and a core treatment team member.

Signed: _____   Date: _____

The contract is accompanied by general unit guidelines provided for all patients, including specific guidelines for use of the seclusion room.

The function of the contract is to help therapy be safe and effective. This function is carried out both by the content of the final contract and by the process. The process is good for both staff and patient. It has a quasi-legal aura to it that combines rights and enforcement. The process tells the patient that she is taken seriously, that staff have thought carefully about her, that every effort will be made to keep her safe, and that acting out is unacceptable. In addition, it instills an expectation for settled behavior and nonspecial treatment compared with other patients.

The more violent the past behavior of the patient, the tougher the contract must be. Some items are specific to an individual patient and are included at her request. For example, one patient said she had been injected with medications prior to participation in child pornography films: Her victim alter was terrified of needles, so a "no-IM" meds clause was included in her contract. For another patient items about confidentiality or some other issue might be helpful. A contract should fit on one page.

There will be minicontracts at a verbal level throughout therapy. These may include agreements to put an alter to sleep for a while, changes in frequency of sessions, rules about phone calls, or countless other matters. One of the most difficult aspects of the therapy is the suicidal drive of the patient (Ross & Norton, 1989b). No-suicide contracts can be drawn up with specific alters much as they would be for a non-DID patient.

I have found no-suicide contracts to be somewhat helpful, but not a panacea. When they are effective, it often seems to be because of the scrupulous honesty of the patient. Many DID patients have a strict code of honor and truthfulness, and will not break a promise. The problem is getting the persecutory alter to agree not to harm anyone. Once the promise is truly made, though, it is often kept. Alters may discuss openly the difficulty they are having sticking to the agreement and may only be able to contract for short periods. When suicide is viewed as euthanasia, the alter responsible for the self-destructive behavior may be unwilling to relinquish that option on a long-term basis. Sometimes the system is just out of control, and contracting is meaningless. As a general rule, a short-term contract is better than no contract.

Therapy can also go wrong when the contract between the therapist and the institution is faulty. This usually doesn't involve the therapist's job description or job contract, although it may when too many hours are being devoted to one patient. More often, subtle, unspoken agreements in the institution are violated by the therapy. These may be ideological, or may involve treatment modalities. Renegotiating with the institution can be a far more formidable task than settling differences with individual patients.

ESTABLISHING INTERPERSONALITY COMMUNICATION

Interpersonality communication is an essential interim goal of therapy and a step toward integration. Patients enter therapy with a wide range of types and degrees of interpersonality communication in place. There is also great variability from phase to phase of therapy, and from one region of the personality system to another. In the broadest sense, communication between personalities includes somatic memories, Schneiderian symptoms, dream intrusions by alters, and other DID phenomena that are symptoms as well as communications.

In our series of 236 cases (Ross, Norton, & Wozney, 1989), 71.7% heard voices arguing and 66.1% heard voices commenting, while in the series of 102 cases (Ross, Miller, Reagor, et al., 1990) 78.4% heard voices arguing, and 81.4% heard voices commenting. Voices are a form of interpersonality communication that is encouraged and cultivated during therapy. DID therapy is the only form of psychiatric treatment in which auditory hallucinations are deliberately amplified. As described in Chapter Eight, voices can take many forms.

The host personality often experiences voices as frightening signs of insanity at the beginning of treatment. Personalities in the background will simultaneously view them as conversations in a matter-of-fact way. This illustrates the necessity of understanding the meaning of any given communication for all personalities who are party to it. Once a treatment alliance has been formed with the host and another alter, the next step is to begin working toward open communication between them. Since the alter in the background may have traumatic memories to give back, this must be done carefully.

If the host is completely unaware of the other personality, the therapist can begin breaking down the amnesia barrier using neutral, nonthreatening material such as writing exercises, whispering, or transmission of visual images to the host. The idea is to desensitize the host personality to the process of communication, in order that she can eventually receive the difficult content. This can be conceptualized in behavioral terms as the construction of a hierarchy for systematic desensitization.

We might get an agreement from the host that the alter will try to send her messages. We then ask the alter, who is coconscious behind a one-way amnesia barrier, and with whom we have previously discussed the exercise, to say a number or to say "Hello." The host listens and writes down the message. We then switch to the alter and check as to whether the message has been received correctly. Step by step, we then have the alter transmit more complex neutral messages, until a conversation is established. Since the background alter is coconscious and can hear the host easily, the desensitization is unidirectional, except where there is two-way amnesia, in which case the desensitization must be done in both directions at once.

If the patient has trouble opening up the communication channel, formal hypnotic suggestions can be given to help. It is important to suggest that amnesia barriers will dissolve away at a safe pace, and that only as much communication as can be tolerated will occur. I can't see experimenting with flooding techniques in DID treatment, because patients can barely handle the degree of flooding they experience spontaneously. Such techniques might work with Vietnam veterans, but their trauma occurred in adulthood in a foreign country. Flooding someone with war memories is not the same as flooding them with incest memories.

Once the host can hear the alter's voice, I might ask the alter, with the host in executive control, if there is anything she wants to say to the host. The therapist can prompt therapeutic conversation, knowing the fears and concerns of the alters. For example, the alters are often afraid that the host won't like them, will be mad at them, will blame them, or will not be satisfied with their performance. A direct simple statement by the host that she likes the hidden child, and wants to talk with her, can ease the child's fears. It also makes the host feel better.

If there seems to be excessive trouble establishing communication between two personalities, there is a good chance that someone else is blocking it. In this situation, you have to explore further and try to deal directly with the blocking alter, who will have a rationale for what she is doing. I might say:

> I have a feeling that there's someone else there who's blocking the conversation between Susan and Susie. If there is, there's probably a good reason for the blocking. I'd like to find out what it is so I'd know what to do. Is there anybody there who knows about that who could talk to me?

If an alter comes forward, I ask for as much information as possible, then work to solve whatever problem is motivating the blocking. This could be a fear that Susan will go crazy if she learns too much. I deal with this by contracting for gradual establishment of coconsciousness, and ongoing consultation with the blocking alter as to how it's going. If a more unreasonable, hostile motive is at work, I might postpone further communication between Susan and Susie until the hostile alter is onside.

Once two personalities are able to talk freely, communication will continue outside therapy. If Susie holds abuse memories, the next step would be to begin working on coconsciousness for Susan. Work with Susie will already be ongoing behind the amnesia barrier, so that Susie is somewhat desensitized to the memories before they are transmitted to Susan. As in the procedure for voices, coconsciousness begins as an in-session phenomenon, with neutral content.

I get permission from both alters for a trial of coconsciousness, then switch to Susie. Prior to the switch I may do a formal hypnotic induction with suggestions for removal of the amnesia barrier. A typical instruction would be:

> In a moment, Susie will open her eyes and be here. This time, though, Susan will be awake and listening. Susan will be in the background but she will be awake and listening and watching. Susan will be able to hear and understand everything that's said. Then after I'm finished talking with Susie, Susan will come back and

she will keep the memory of the conversation with Susie. The memory will not be lost. Susie can you be here now?

I keep the discussion on a safe topic, then switch back to Susan. Before going back to Susan I will give an instruction for selective amnesia for any material touched on in the conversation with Susie that would be too difficult. This usually works very well. Once Susan is desensitized to coconsciousness, we then move toward more difficult content, and eventually Susan is fully coconscious for Susie's abuse. Susan will have a partial, vicarious experience of the trauma herself while watching Susie's recollection of it, then may have a more direct experience of it herself when she returns to executive control. Sometimes Susan does not complete her final assimilation of Susie's memories until after Susie has been integrated with her.

During the early phases of establishing coconsciousness, it is helpful to ask Susie to talk to Susan while Susie is out. Susie can then report to the therapist on Susan's responses. This gives Susan experience at being a background alter, and seems to help free up the communication channel. The same procedures can be used for all forms of communication between all combinations of personalities.

One can contract for increasing coconsciousness through internal images, diaries, dreams, or any other technique the therapist can invent. The metaphor of the family living in a DID house provides the frame for this work. The therapist has to move back and forth from room to room, and deal with everyone's anxieties and fears about talking with everyone else. Prior to direct communication between personalities, the therapist acts as a messenger and interpreter. Before exercises with Susie and Susan can begin, Susan will have been filled in on Susie's name, age, function, character, and concerns. This is the first step in desensitization.

As personalities begin to communicate more and more, a process of generalization sets in. The amount of information leakage across the amnesia barrier begins to increase in many ways. Feelings that have never been directly addressed in therapy leak from Susie to Susan, making Susan feel small and frightened. At the same time, Susie may start to feel a bit bigger, stronger, and braver. The therapist may notice "slips" at this stage of therapy that raise a suspicion of malingering. Alters may know things they are "supposed" to be amnesic for, and may try to claim amnesia for information they have disclosed. I view this more as trouble adjusting to coconsciousness than malingering, and usually let it slide by without much comment. Such slips are a phase-specific phenomenon in therapy that remit prior to integration.

As the alters move closer to integration, they come to a point where everybody knows and feels everything, and decisions are made democratically. The entire system does not arrive at this point en masse, however. In complex layered cases, it is common to successfully integrate some personalities before others are even suspected. Establishing coconsciousness is usually done simultaneously with establishing interpersonality communication, since the two reinforce each other reciprocally. The purpose of coconsciousness is communication, and the purpose of communication is coconsciousness.

Interpersonality communication is reinforced by the therapist in a number of ways. One is by modeling communication for the patient, which occurs when the therapist requests switches, and debriefs alters on conversations held behind amnesia barriers. I give lots of "strokes" for progress in therapy, and lots of reassurance. Also, I'm explicit about the goals of therapy, and my investment in them as a therapist. At some point in therapy, many patients berate me for being narcissistically invested in curing them. They may say that I am only interested in them as research guinea pigs or as case studies.

I deal with this by acknowledging that indeed I did go into medicine to heal people, and that I get much more personal and professional satisfaction from successes than from failures. I then ask the patient if they would prefer to have a doctor who was committed to curing them, and willing to work hard toward that goal, or one who didn't care one way or the other, and saw them for 15 minutes once a month. I point out to the patient that my narcissistic investment in her outcome is an asset for her, not a liability.

There is no need to be apologetic for commitment to the goal of integration, and the specific techniques that help the patient get there. The patient will stall and resist the work toward interpersonality integration in countless ways. This is as it should be for someone who has survived extreme trauma thanks to dissociation.

CONCLUSION

The preceding sections describe the principal techniques used in the initial phase of therapy. If a new layer of alter personalities is discovered late in therapy, these techniques may be used again at that stage. Similarly, many of the techniques described in the next two chapters can be used in the initial phase of therapy. The dividing of techniques into phases of therapy is a rough guideline only.

CHAPTER FIFTEEN

Specific Techniques of Treatment: The Middle and Late Phases of Therapy

The middle and late phases of therapy for dissociative identity disorder (DID) are long and involve most of the work. During this part of the treatment, many patients will feel, at times, that the effort is not worth it. Within a short-term perspective, this may be an accurate assessment. The patient may experience more distress as her dissociative defenses are being dismantled. Numerous posttraumatic symptoms may occur and the ability to cope on a day-to-day basis may deteriorate. This is not inevitable, necessary, or desirable, but may occur. Fortunately, this does not last forever, and eventually the patient moves into the less volatile, later stages of treatment.

The techniques in this chapter, like those in Chapter Fourteen, can be used throughout therapy but are characteristic of the middle and late phases.

ABREACTING ABUSE MEMORIES

The amount of formal abreactive work I do has dwindled to almost zero since the first edition of this book: I treated a private patient to initial integration starting in 1992, and arriving at integration in 1995, without any abreactive work being done in session. I have reconceptualized abreaction as being by definition *acting out*. Before, following Janet, I thought of abreaction as both a spontaneous symptom and part of the therapeutic method. Now I think of it as turning feelings and memories into behavior, rather than processing them cognitively and verbally. I am now more aligned with Freud on this point than with Janet.

When I say *abreaction,* I am referring to full-tilt behavioral reenactments of trauma with dramatic behavior, regression, clutching at the genitalia, expressions of horror, and loss of orientation to the present. My patients no longer abreact as part of their treatment plan. Their experiences are now better described as intense recollection, rather than acting out. Abreaction never was an end in itself and was always extremely painful for the patient. It is also stressful for the therapist, and in fact some therapists develop full *DSM-IV* posttraumatic stress disorder from working with severely abused multiples.

The rationale for therapeutic abreactions is a surgical analogy: The abuse memories are like foreign bodies; unless they are removed, the abscess cannot be definitively treated. This does not mean that every single abuse incident requires full abreaction, according to the abreactive model. Such work would take far too long. Generalization occurs in abreactive work, as in other aspects of the therapy, as a result of which reliving of key representative traumas cleanses the entire system.

Observing and guiding the abreactions is emotionally intense, technically delicate work for the therapist. The therapist must "be on his toes." To do the work, it is essential not to be too involved and not to take the abreactions too literally. The patient will experience an abreaction as an exact copy of the original experience, which it isn't. An abreaction is a highly stylized enactment of a reconstructed memory of a possibly real trauma. It is not a video playback of reality. The therapist is not really watching a rape, and the abreacting patient is not really a child.

Abreactions, though, are sincere, genuine experiences for patients. They are very dramatic, and can be exploited and embellished for secondary gain, but they can also be important healing rituals. To be healing, the ritual must have a frame and a meaning, and must be debriefed.

Abreactions can be countertherapeutic and destructive if not handled properly. Especially during inpatient work, when multiples may regress behaviorally, the reliving of childhood trauma can take the form of malignant abreaction. Malignant abreaction consists of chaotic uncontrolled runs of screaming, self-abusive, or regressed behavior during which the patient may switch repeatedly. There is no learning or transfer of meaningful information to other personalities. Malignant abreaction exhausts the patient, staff, and therapists, and triggers other patients to abreact.

Malignant abreaction must be suppressed with behavioral techniques, medication, and/or hypnosis. Left uncontrolled, it may destroy the therapy. Between such extreme chaos and the staged, contracted abreactions of outpatient psychotherapy, there is a spectrum of abreaction. Often, within the abreactive model, it will be difficult to tell when an abreaction should be limited and when the therapist should allow it to run its course.

There is a spectrum from a purely informational recall of trauma to full abreactive reliving in the present. As in other aspects of work with dissociative identity disorder, a desensitization model is required. This can sometimes be contracted for directly with the alter who holds the memories. The phobic stimulus is the traumatic memory and its associated feelings: The therapist must set up a systematic desensitization hierarchy for the patient and prevent flooding. The problem with many therapies containing strong iatrogenic pressures to false memories and false-positive DID is that there is no desensitization hierarchy. The therapy consists of massive flooding with decompensation, regression, and dysfunction setting in. These symptoms are then treated with more flooding.

The first step in systematic desensitization is to orient the child alter holding the traumatic memory to being in the same body in the present, and educating the alter about the safety of the present. The second step is to ask the host or a key protector personality to create an internal safe place for the alter and to assign an alter the job of being an internal good parent. Following this, I work on establishing neutral system communication with the child alter as described previously. The host has already been told by someone else in the system and/or by the therapist that the child alter was created at age six to be the victim of sexual assault by the father. A contract is then made for the child to describe the assault with the host coconscious in the background, then the child alter is called out. The child is then asked to begin describing the scene just prior to the assault, and then walks through the event itself.

While this planned recollection and retelling of the trauma is going on, all available internal soothing strategies are in use, and the therapist is grounding the system in the present by pointing out the present year, the location, the safety of the present, and the ongoing support and help provided by other alters. When this procedure is followed, full abreaction seldom occurs.

It is usually not hard to tell that an abreaction is taking place. The alter speaks as if the abuse is happening in the present, and there is a vivid recreation of the event. Facial expression, body posture, tone of voice, and autonomic state leave no doubt that an intense experience is occurring. A therapeutic abreaction has a curve with which the therapist becomes familiar, and usually lasts 5 or 10 minutes at peak intensity. The abreaction begins with a preamble about the setting, who is present, and where the father is at the moment. This progresses through an approach phase, during which fear mounts, then the overt sexual assault begins.

During this phase, the child may cry out, plead with the father to stop, clutch her pubic area, try to push father off, attempt to spit out semen, or curl up in the corner. After the peak intensity, there is a denouement during which the child may whimper, or express sadness. This is accompanied by a transition back to the present, as the alter reorients and realizes that the abuse happened long ago. The abreaction has an outline that parallels the arousal curve of the father. Following the abreaction there is a debriefing with the child and the host. "Debriefing" is not a dry, technical intervention, and may involve touch, holding, reassurance, and hypnotic suggestions for sleep, calm, or safety.

What I have learned through my personal experience and the collective experience of the field, is that full abreaction is not necessary for healing. In fact it is retraumatizing and regressive. Especially on an inpatient unit, abreaction has a domino effect: Uncontrolled, spontaneous abreactions can reduce a stable, rational adult treatment milieu to destructive chaos very quickly.

Many patients still view abreaction and misery as evidence that serious work is being done and proof of their pain and suffering. This is a cognitive error, and needs to be corrected. Once or twice a year, we do a temporary unit shutdown, bring all the patients together in the day room, and discuss the problem of spontaneous abreactions, acting out, and unit instability for one to two hours. This is always successful in shutting down the malignant abreactions that have been occurring. The explanation I give the patients for not tolerating excessive abreacting has several elements to it.

The first point is that there is no such thing as "spontaneous" abreaction on an inpatient unit, and probably not anywhere. If abreactions truly were spontaneous, they would be randomly distributed in time: They would occur at the supermarket as often as in therapy or in the hospital. In fact, abreactions are highly cued and context-dependent. They serve strategic interpersonal and intrapsychic functions, and are always acting out. They are highly responsive to the rules and limits of the treatment team.

Patients come from across the country to our unit, I remind them, because it provides a high-level, intensive subspecialty psychotherapy program. The purpose of the program is to work hard in a focused fashion for a short period. Abreactions destabilize the unit, increase other acting out, embroil the patients in conflicts and power struggles with each other and the staff, and prevent them from doing the work they need to do. Abreactions are therefore unhealthy and countertherapeutic and need to stop. Those who are too triggered by the milieu to stop abreacting will be transferred to the general adult unit for stabilization, for their own good and for the good of the milieu. This is done because staff are responsible for maintaining a therapeutic milieu and ensuring that those who are here to work are able to do so.

Defining abreactions in this way ensures that the only ground for objection by a patient is a declaration that she is not here to do serious work. This declaration, which is never made, would be responded to with transfer off the unit. With this approach, patients are trapped in a therapeutic loop because abreaction is now defined as acting out, hurtful to the other patients, evidence that the person is not serious about recovery, and grounds for negative countertransference.

If an abreaction seems to go on too long at peak intensity, this is a cue that the patient is stuck in it, and that there will be no therapeutic benefit, even within the abreactive model. Successful abreactions often involve cuing by the therapist, with inquiries such as, "What happened next?" or "And then what?" The therapist can use the past tense while the patient uses the present tense, without reducing the intensity or completeness of the abreaction: Patients seem to handle this incongruity easily with trance logic.

If the alter is stuck in the abreaction, the therapist must intervene. A hand on the shoulder, and firm commands that the child will go to sleep often work. The child is put to sleep, safety suggestions are given, and the host is called back. A suggestion for amnesia for the host may be inserted if necessary. Alternatively, a malignant abreaction may be converted to a therapeutic one that will then run its course. This is done in a fashion similar to termination of an abreaction, except that suggestions for progression through the memory are given. A short speech about the therapeutic purpose of the abreaction can be made, and this may be heard by an inner self helper or the system generally. Hypnotic suggestions can be given to the whole person at any time in therapy: During a malignant abreaction such suggestions help marshal rational, adult resources.

In an extreme case, an injection of 2–5 mg of lorazepam may be required. This is the best medication to use because it is a benzodiazepine, and is therefore much less toxic than antipsychotic medications. Other benzodiazepines are not as well absorbed intramuscularly. A private practice nonmedical therapist will not have this strategy available, so must try and try again with hypnotic suggestions and commands. Sometimes abreactions are very difficult to turn off. If there is too much uncontrolled switching and abreacting, consultation and/or admission may be required. The acting out should be explicitly defined for the patient as resistance to the work of therapy.

The recovery of abuse memories may occur in many ways besides abreaction. Memories may initially come back as flashbacks, dreams, hallucinations, vague premonitions of upcoming flashbacks, inner reveries, overheard conversations between alters, diary entries, or physical symptoms. Any such channel that seems to be becoming overactive, and crowded with transmissions, may be a clue that an alter is moving toward abreaction. Alters that have not entered therapy often make themselves known in this way.

For example, hallucinations of blood, accompanied by fear and feeling small, may occur. There may be an alter in the background who is deliberately causing the hallucinations. The therapist then asks to talk to "Someone I haven't met before who knows about the blood Susan has been seeing." If an alter comes out, she can usually explain why she is causing the hallucination, and describe the original bloody trauma, which may be a false memory. The therapist can then attempt to contract with the alter to stop the hallucinations, and concurrently work toward understanding the systemic purpose of pushing the memory into the host. Often an alter will give a casual rationale for the hallucinations along the lines, "I thought she should know about it." Another motivation might be to make the host so disturbed that she must be admitted: The motive here might be hospital dependency. Often the hallucinations are caused by a persecutor alter who reasons that the host is bad and should be punished.

Sometimes the therapist can contract for a more controlled recovery of memory without directly contacting the responsible alter. Some abuse memories seem to be held in a general unconscious and are not linked to any one alter. Another variation is a trance memory held by a specific personality. This can be recovered by hypnotizing the alter, who then describes the abuse she originally experienced in a trance state. This description may also occur in trance, so the alter must be brought out of trance in the session, prior to switching to anyone else. Memories recovered in this fashion have an increased risk of being false or distorted, which is one reason I don't do this kind of work.

When an alter has gone into trance during a trauma, she may be amnesic for it after an abreaction of the original event. In this situation, gradual or sudden recovery of the trauma can be contracted for in the same way as is done for the host. One alter I worked with had repeatedly gone into her parents' bedroom in the middle of the night during childhood, in a trance state, but had never used the knife she carried in a raised hand. All known personalities were amnesic for these episodes, but the alter remembered feeling like she was going into trance prior to the onset of the blank spells. There were many reasons for thinking that this patient was producing false memories, and members of her treatment team were convinced in 1986 and 1987 that the rapes she was reporting were factitious. This kind of abreactive/hypnotic/trance work introduces too much noise into the already complex memory equation.

Following any full or muted abreaction, much of the debriefing involves working on associated cognitive errors. Often the historical origin of the cognitive error can be identified during the abreaction: This seems to help the cognitive therapy be more focused and effective. During debriefing, I review the purpose of memory processing, congratulate the alters for their courage, repeat that it is safe now, and discuss the need for less intense abreaction in the future. A balance must be struck between comforting a child who has just been assaulted and working with a rational adult. Just as patients can get stuck in abreactions, so can therapists.

One must not treat the patient exclusively or predominantly like a child, or spend years repeating abreactions and simply comforting the child alter afterward.

Because planned abreaction is hard work and very stressful, it is an aspect of therapy that requires particular care and structure. It is that—an aspect of therapy—and should be considered as such, despite its drama. Clinical experience to date is that severely abused multiples must recall their trauma in a meaningful way in therapy to get better, but do not need to abreact.

I have discussed abreactions at some length, even though I don't myself do abreactive work in therapy, for two reasons: (a) to emphasize the necessary cautions, and (b) to provide a framework for therapists who will continue to do planned abreactive work.

AGE-APPROPRIATE ACTIVITIES WITH CHILD ALTERS

Working with child alters can be fun. That is why it can be difficult. The therapist could spend hundreds of hours playing with child personalities in a countertherapeutic fashion: Play can seem more pleasant than dealing with ambivalent attachment to the perpetrator and helping the patient take responsibility for herself as an adult. Throughout therapy, child alters should be worked with but not indulged. Despite childish handwriting, facial expressions, and body posture, they often function at a cognitive level far beyond their years, and often have a more complete and mature understanding of the personality system than the host does at the beginning of therapy.

Child alters can be more seductive than the overtly seductive, sexually acting out adolescent and adult personalities. They can be lonely, sad, or frightened, and can evoke parental and protective instincts in the therapist. They can be delightfully spontaneous, childlike, and trusting, giving the therapist powerful positive feedback for playing games with them. One of the functions of the child may have been to divert the father from incest, and she may divert the therapist from the painful work of therapy, in a parallel process.

No matter how frightening the memories, or confrontations with persecutors are for the children, the purpose of therapy is recovery, not play. The therapist needs to push gently at different times throughout therapy, while listening carefully to advice to slow down. Within the necessary framework, age-appropriate activities with child alters can be therapeutic. They have a number of different purposes, which are served by both process and content.

It is impossible to work at peak intensity all of every session. Like a play, novel, or movie, there is a rise and fall in the action of therapy, and interludes of different intensity are required. Both patient and therapist can benefit from a break. The break, which may be a walk, playing cards, or any other mutually enjoyable activity, is still part of therapy. Irrespective of what is said during a break, it provides the patient an experience of normal child-adult interaction. This will have value as corrective emotional experience, and as modeling of parental behavior for the patient, who may have children. Such interludes help build trust and safety both with the child and with hostile alters in the background.

If a trip out of the therapist's building is made, it may have an important desensitization component. The outside world often seems very big and frightening to child personalities. As well, the therapist has an opportunity to make in vivo observations, which may be useful later in therapy. Just being together in a happy way can help both parties to the social contact prepare for more difficult work. The interlude shows that the therapist values the child, and acknowledges his or her subjective experience of self and the world. This in turn indirectly validates the child's perception of the abuse as wrong and traumatic.

Often a child personality does not believe that many years have passed, and that she is now in a different city. One child was convinced that this must be true by looking at her hands and looking out the window at the snow: The patient grew up in a city that never had snow. Such educational interventions may progress to a walk in the snow, which consolidates the new cognition through touch, sound, smell, and even taste if the child eats a handful of snow.

One adolescent alter was extremely shy and nervous, and could only stay out for brief periods. She held a key position in the personality system and could communicate with many personalities at different levels in the system, so I wanted to be able to talk with her at greater length. Playing cards seemed to help her to relax and increase the length of time she could stay in executive control. Reading stories to children is another way of drawing them out into the therapy, especially when they have been severely abused.

Formal play therapy is a modality we use sparingly in our Dissociative Disorders Program. However, therapists at other centers have extensive experience with the use of dolls, sand trays, dollhouses, and other toys. These props are used in much the same way as they would be in work with an actual child, for establishing trust, disclosing abuse memories, resolving conflicts, and defining issues for verbal therapy. My feeling is that the work can be done without the props, but I am ready to believe that I underutilize toys.

Patients may bring shawls, bears, blankets, or other transitional objects into therapy, and these should be talked about explicitly by the therapist. If the therapist doesn't comment, the child may conclude that the therapist doesn't like her or her bear. Sometimes the bear becomes a copatient in the therapy. This occurs when the child alter projects onto the bear so intensely that the bear is alive. When this happens, the transference to the bear is extremely charged and plastic, and important work can be done. The child may divulge abuse secrets that only she and the bear knew about, or may enter a long monologue addressed to the bear in which she defines key issues in therapy.

The therapist may comment on how brave the bear is, how lucky the bear is to have the child with him, and how glad the therapist is that the bear was willing to share these memories. A promise may be made to have the bear back for future sessions. By working with the bear, the therapist can deal with displaced and projected material that would be too painful for the child to discuss directly. Talking with bears can be very useful and shouldn't be omitted because it isn't "proper" technique. The negative aspects of the transference will also come out in this work, and the bear will be at risk of being stabbed, burned, drowned, lost, or otherwise abused between sessions. If possible, abuse of the bear should not be allowed during sessions because the therapist who allows the bear to be hurt will be perceived as condoning child abuse.

There is no need to be concerned that talking with teddy bears will inevitably reinforce regression, promote psychosis, reward maladaptive behavior, or have similar harmful effects. Most DID patients understand the conventions of therapy well, and can make good use of this technique. If work with transitional objects does become counterproductive, then that is a problem in therapy to be discussed, understood, and resolved like any other. For example, one patient externalized her alters into a set of bears as a resistance to accepting them as human and part of herself.

One of the devices we use most often in working with child alters is drawing. The children can talk about the abuse through drawings in a deep, intense way (Cohen & Cox, 1995). They can often say more with crayons than they can with words. Most of the time no fancy skills are required to interpret the drawings. They will contain anatomical portrayals of particular abuse incidents, often with red blood. Knives appear frequently, as do confining rooms, views of houses from outside, and simultaneous views of various rooms in houses with abuse occurring in some. The drawings may be obviously disturbed at a glance, with furious circles of black and a chaotic welter of angry lines. I make a point of striving for common sense in commenting on drawings, in therapy and in discussion with colleagues.

The drawings can be done in session, between sessions, or in the art therapy room. A problem arises when a patient asks the therapist to display her artwork on an office wall. This is a no-win situation for the therapist. The least harmful option is probably to decline most of the time in most cases. For one thing, most of the artwork is not skillful or attractive, and will soon become a sore point for the therapist, who has to look at it every day. DID patients want and need to be "special," and will get into a competition with other patients for number one status, via displayed artwork. This needs to be nipped in the bud. I keep a file in my office, separate from the outpatient chart, for each DID patient, in which I save drawings, cards, notes by me, and other artifacts of therapy.

There is nothing intrinsically wrong with displaying patient artwork in the office, as long as the therapist is aware of the implications and complications of doing so, and is prepared to deal with them. Most of the time, putting artwork on the wall will be a "big deal" for the patient, and depending on the degree of conflict in the system it may make some alters very angry. I prefer not to create more problems in therapy when there are already many to deal with. There are only a few absolute rules in therapy, and *display no artwork* is not one of them.

Age-appropriate activities with child alters are a useful component of therapy that can easily get out of control. It is probably better for a beginning therapist to err on the side of too few of such interventions rather than too many. I have heard tales of incredibly bad therapies perpetrated in the name of "reparenting," which I would describe as gross malpractice if called to testify. The therapist is a therapist not a parent, and the patient is a patient not a child. Age-appropriate activities with child alters are an aspect of therapy that can easily bring the treatment of DID into disrepute.

The amount of age-appropriate activities I do with child alters has dwindled down to almost zero, in parallel with my deemphasis of abreaction. The particular props or techniques used in such activities are probably less important than the process of interaction at a childlike level. The techniques do not need to be described in detail the way calling out alters or dismantling amnesia barriers do, and are mostly nonspecialist in nature. The therapist needs to view his play as serious work, the way children do, then his work can become serious play.

WORKING WITH AGGRESSIVE AND PERSECUTORY PERSONALITIES

Working with persecutors, who are present in 84.0% of our series of 236 cases, is one of the most difficult aspects of therapy. Dealing with these personalities is technically demanding, emotionally stressful, and potentially dangerous. Some DID patients who have committed violent crimes and been in prison might be untreatable because of their aggressive personalities. For example, one alter personality described on videotape having raped a 76-year-old virgin nun on Halloween night, a crime for which the patient was executed in 1992. The alter claimed that although he had raped the woman on behalf of the host personality, the nun was alive when he left, and must have died subsequently of a heart attack. The alter's account could not have been consciously malingered, because in fact the victim died of multiple stab wounds. Another alter, perhaps too violent to be approached in therapy, must have come out and done the stabbings behind an amnesia barrier. In regular clinical work, however, the angry personalities can usually form a treatment alliance and achieve stable integration.

I have discussed techniques for establishing trust and safety earlier, and these are often used with the aggressive internal states. It is a general principle of DID work that the therapist should always gather as much information as possible before contacting a new alter, and in fact at all times throughout therapy. If the therapy of DID is viewed as a form of intrapsychic strategic family therapy, then reconnaissance is essential for effective planning.

The first hint that an aggressive alter is present is often a disclosure of internal intimidation by a frightened personality. The identified personality will give out information in small parcels, and repeatedly emphasize that "there's going to be trouble." The trouble can take the form of wrist slashing, headaches, internal bullying, increased blank spells, interference with function, or imposition of unpleasant states on the host personality. The strategies for dealing with such problems vary a great deal from situation to situation, and case to case.

Hostile personalities tend to belong to one of a few different subgroups. How the therapist deals with them is determined partly by the subgroup. Some uncooperative personalities are not violent or frightening for the therapist, and represent a more benign resistance to therapy. For example, one adolescent personality began making the patient miss sessions by taking executive control before the patient could leave home, and not relinquishing it till after the scheduled time was over. I dealt with this situation by using a paradoxical intervention.

The adolescent alter came out in a session at my request, and made it clear that there was nothing I could do to ensure that the patient made her appointments. I therefore stopped making appointments with the host personality altogether, and said I would only make appointments with the adolescent at her request, which I did. This made it impossible for the alter to exert power through dissociation, and gave complete control to her. I already knew that this alter wanted to be in therapy herself, so I made her the patient. The host personality thought this was very unfair, and said, "Why should *she* have appointments and not me? *I'm* the one who's in therapy." I replied that that was too bad, but that was how I was going to handle it. The adolescent alter didn't miss appointments anymore, quickly became a helper in the therapy, and was subsequently integrated.

The therapist should always try to avoid power struggles because they are usually impossible to win. I always give power to the patient, including persecutors, in such situations, within clear limits, while making it clear that self-abusive or destructive behavior is not acceptable. The main point is this: The patient has to be more invested in recovery than the therapist. If the opposite is true, the therapist, being desperate to cure someone, will be outmaneuvered and outpowered over and over. The therapist must relinquish all power and investment in outcome at the direct transactional level, in order to secure it at a metalevel.

Another type of aggressor is usually adolescent, feels mostly or exclusively anger and rage, and verbally assaults the host personality and the therapist. Such personalities usually feel bad about themselves, and are misguided helpers. Working with them involves firm behavioral limits and a focus on cognitive errors, including the delusion of having separate bodies. One of the key early interventions is to get such persecutors to acknowledge that they experience a broad range of feelings, because they often view themselves as exclusively angry. Telling jokes is a good way to do this, as the alters usually have a good sense of humor. Once you get the alter kibitzing, you can point this out.

Simply telling the persecutor that you view her as part of the whole person, that you assume she is there for a good reason, and thanking her on behalf of the whole patient for carrying the anger, is helpful. The persecutors usually feel rejected, unloved, and feared internally because of their anger. It is a novel experience for them to listen while the therapist explains to the host personality the invaluable work a persecutor has done on her behalf by holding the anger: A revolution in self-concept can occur for the persecutor when the host agrees and expresses thanks. Most persecutors are sad. It is a relief for them when someone understands the burden of carrying all that anger, and it is a further relief when the anger is normalized and legitimized. I always tell the patient that it is normal and inevitable to be extremely angry about the abuse, and that it would be abnormal not to be angry. Persecutors often think they are bad for being angry.

Standard techniques for dealing with anger such as devising alternate strategies for handling it, controlled ventilation, interrupting transactional sequences with an endpoint of anger as early as possible, and reinforcing control are as useful for the DID patient as for anyone, though their implementation can be complicated. A desensitization model is useful for anger, as it is for traumatic memories. The purpose of structured anger management groups, or similar work done in individual therapy, is threefold: to move through a desensitization hierarchy; to correct cognitive errors about anger; and to practice healthy anger management strategies.

If persecutor personalities attempt to attack the therapist, they must be physically restrained. Earlier on in my work—because of my inexperience—I had to do this more than I do now. One of the errors I made in an early case was to certify a patient and admit her on an involuntary basis after a hostile alter abruptly left the session. This error on my part fed into a self-perception as dangerous and volatile on the part of the alter, and put me in a position of coming on as "the law," which stimulated further aggression. In a similar situation, I would now simply wait for the patient to phone or for the next appointment time.

A good way for the therapist to stay out of trouble with hostile alters is not to do anything. This is a technique I learned in general adult inpatient work and on call. If there is a crisis, the best intervention is often not to do anything for a while. Then when you finally call the patient or come down to the ward, the whole thing has blown over. This takes judgment, because there can be real emergencies, or minor problems that are best dealt with quickly and simply. Overall, I think it is more therapeutic to be underavailable for the patient than overavailable. The hostile alters won't have to test and push as much if the therapist is less reactive. This is different from being "neutral" as a general stance, because it is a specific strategy not an overall principle of therapy.

Another type of persecutor is the internal demon, the alter identified as the incestuous father, and other paranormal alters. These are often difficult to engage in therapy. They sometimes require containment and outmaneuvering. One way to do this is to work with the other alters in the system, who are often severely intimidated. The therapist works with the host and the frightened children to develop magical shields, safe places, and protective formulas to ward off the persecutor. Usually one is dealing with a school playground bully who really wants to be contained and loved.

The therapist explains to the children that the alter is not really the devil or the father but is just pretending in order to scare them. The persecutor listens to all this intently, and fumes and rants in the background. Stating a paradox can be effective: "The more he tries to scare you, the more frightened he is to talk with me. You'll know if he says lots of mean things, and tries to scare you, that he really wants someone to pay attention to him, and love him. He was hurt too." This puts the persecutor in a paradoxical position of demonstrating his vulnerability by acting tough. "Maybe if he was really tough, he would be brave enough to talk to me, instead of just acting tough and scaring the children." It is tougher to be vulnerable than to be tough, as the patient learned from the abuse. These strategies are a way of taking the wind out of the persecutor's sails by creating a more benign perception of him in the rest of the system.

The persecutor may come out in a session and heap scorn on the therapist's paradoxical strategies, claiming to see through them. That is a sign that they are working, because the alter has slipped to a backup level of resistance, and is debating with the therapist rather than refusing to talk. I reply that no trick is involved and that my statements are simply the truth, which they are. It is the context that contains the paradox, and I don't comment on that. It is important not to get too elaborate and tricky and to "play it straight" most of the time. Sometimes it just takes a long time and a lot of repetition to stop the persecutory behavior: The therapist has to be able to tolerate superficial wrist slashes, minor overdoses, and other self-abuse in order to preserve the long-term goals. This behavior should be tolerated but not condoned, even implicitly. Sometimes I acknowledge that I would like the self-abuse to stop, but that I can't make it stop.

A comment similar to a transference interpretation can be made. The patient didn't deserve the abuse as a child, she doesn't deserve the abuse now, and the therapist doesn't deserve abuse from the patient. As a child, the patient could not stop the abuse, but the therapist is an adult, won't tolerate abuse, and will stop the therapy if the assaultive behavior can't be contained. The therapist has to be prepared to lose the patient in order to treat her.

The furthest I have been pushed by a persecutor is to part ways in front of the hospital late in the evening: I went to my car and the patient went running off barefoot to jump in the river and drown herself. The next day there were headlines on the front page of a local newspaper, describing an incident in which a woman claiming to have 33 personalities was pulled off the bridge at the last moment by a passerby. Only the passerby was interviewed by the reporter. The police had brought the patient back to the hospital from the bridge twice that evening before we parted in the parking lot. Some might say that that was an unacceptable gamble to take, under any circumstances. I say that there was no possibility of productive therapy if I was not prepared to take that risk.

At a fundamental level, you have to be prepared to let the patient die, otherwise you can't help her. An incessantly worried and frightened therapist, who is desperate to "save" the patient, won't be able to tolerate the work and will be entrenched in the rescuer position. His patients will either drop out, become chronically infantalized, or act out destructively. DID can be a malignant and untreatable illness because of the unrelenting destructiveness of the persecutors. It is not kind to engage such patients in an ineffective "therapy" that adds to their conflicts and suffering. All you get is an unhappy patient who has to overdose more often than she would without therapy, because of her therapist's vacations. Having said that, I have to emphasize that it is difficult, if not impossible, to predict which patients should not be treated, other than in extreme and obvious cases.

Dealing with persecutors may require hospitalization, which I will discuss in Chapter Sixteen. The overriding concern in work with persecutors of all kinds is to establish a treatment alliance with them. I usually do this by hiring them as consultants to the therapy. I tell the persecutor that I assume she has a good reason for what she is doing, and that her behavior makes sense from her point of view. I ask her to explain why she is abusing the other personalities emotionally and physically, so that I can understand. In conjunction with that, I ask the persecutor to tell me right away if I am doing anything she doesn't like. I don't promise to immediately stop whatever it is, but I agree to discuss, negotiate, and seriously consider changing my approach. I tell the alter that I don't claim to be perfect and that in fact I am guaranteed to misunderstand and do the wrong thing once in a while.

By treating the persecutor as a valued colleague, the therapist gives her a revolutionary experience: being respected as an adult. This is similar to work done with acting-out adolescents who have been branded as bad actors, and are fulfilling the prophecy. I establish a collaborative empirical contract with the persecutor to consider alternate strategies for reaching her goals. Discussion thereby replaces confrontation.

Many persecutory alters are hostile to therapy because they think it will increase the host personality's suffering, which in fact it will transiently. As soon as this motive is identified, I acknowledge that the hostile behavior is actually protective, and that it has been very helpful over the years. I remind the persecutor that it is smart not to trust me too much, because others who seemed trustworthy in the past have been abusive. This reminder is essential with patients who have been sexually abused by previous therapists. I go on to acknowledge that if the whole person really couldn't get better, recovering abuse memories would not be worth it. I agree with the persecutor's negative short-term cost benefit analysis, but predict a positive long-term outcome.

Once the persecutor has agreed to monitor the therapist and collaborate on protecting the host, most of the behavioral problems will have been solved. Persecutors, like helpers who present as cooperative and benign, often resent the therapist's intrusion in the system. They feel that it implies that they did a lousy job taking care of the patient. The persecutor must be reassured that this is not the case. I usually emphasize that I am only available for brief periods every week, and that the alters have full-time responsibility 24 hours a day. It is logistically impossible for me to usurp their role, and in fact I want to help them help the host more effectively.

Persecutors often present as tough and uncaring, but this is nearly always a facade. Pointing out that their apparently destructive actions are actually meant to be protective softens the tough stance. It also helps to reduce the level of fear and alarm in the rest of the system. One way to demonstrate the advantage to the persecutor of bargaining with the therapist is to negotiate a deal with other alters that is directly beneficial for the persecutor. For example, an alter who controls switching might agree to let the persecutor go to a bar if the persecutor agrees to stop fooling around with razor blades and scaring the children. David Caul referred to this kind of work as "horse trading," a good term.

Most persecutors can be brought into the therapy without extreme difficulty. They have a number of positive qualities including energy, commitment, staying power, assertiveness, and toughness that may be deficient in the host personality. They often have a frank, honest, no-bullshit approach to life. Integrated, the persecutors donate these valuable qualities to the host personality. I tell the host personality that the persecutor's anger is the best antidepressant on the market, and point out that it is impossible to be depleted and depressed and enraged at the same time: This is a sales pitch for system communication and cooperation, and eventual integration. In forensic cases, persecutors may be sadistic sex murderers who have committed numerous crimes, and be beyond rehabilitation. The therapist should always enter negotiations with persecutors cautiously, and with eyes and ears open.

COGNITIVE RESTRUCTURING TECHNIQUES

The purpose of this book is to help trained mental health professionals learn how to diagnose, understand, and treat DID. It is not to create therapists out of laypeople. Similarly, the purpose of this section is not to create cognitive therapists de novo in a few pages. Cognitive interventions in DID work should be grounded in an understanding of the cognitive therapy of anxiety (Beck & Emery, 1985) and depression (Beck, 1976; Beck, Rush, Shaw, & Emery, 1985). Because the cognitive therapy of DID is innovative and systems-oriented, additional reading is recommended, specifically *New Directions in Cognitive Therapy* (Emery, Hollon, & Bedrosian, 1981) and *Cognitive Therapy with Couples and Groups* (Freeman, 1983). Courses and workshops in cognitive therapy are available at a variety of professional meetings.

There is an unresolvable controversy in the field as to whether cognitions cause affects, or affects cause cognitions. Psychoanalytical therapists tend to feel that drives and feelings are primary, and that dealing with cognitions is too superficial and "intellectual" to result in real insight. The opposite dogma is that affects are epiphenomena of cognitions. My view is that the therapist intervenes in a *field,* in which cognitions and affects are interconnected by a complex variety of causal chains, feedback loops, and other regulatory mechanisms. Cognitions are one potential point of therapeutic entry into the field. I don't think that the debate over the relative primacy of affect and cognition will ever be fruitful, therefore I don't concern myself with it much.

In doing cognitive work, it is necessary to provide a rationale for the patient that makes sense, however. This is different from a theory or model. If I feel that an explicit rationale is necessary, I tell patients the following story:

> Sometimes what you feel is determined by what you think. When this is true, the best way to change how you feel is to change how you think.
>
> Let me give an example. Imagine you are upstairs in your bedroom at bedtime, alone. You hear a noise downstairs. You think to yourself, "A burglar has broken in and he's going to come upstairs and rape me." You will react with feelings of fear, panic, and alarm, and your behavior may be to hide, call the police, or get a baseball bat. On the other hand if you hear exactly the same sound, and think to yourself, "The dog knocked over his water dish," your reaction will be very different. You may feel annoyed, or not feel anything in particular at all. Your behavior may be to get up and check on the water dish, or if you're tired you might decide to leave it till morning and go to sleep.
>
> This illustrates how different thoughts can result in very different feelings and behaviors in exactly the same situation. Part of the work we're going to do together is going to involve looking at your thought patterns in detail to see if they are causing you to feel upset, anxious, or depressed, and to see if you can learn to feel better by changing your thought patterns. Let me tell one other story to explain how this will work.
>
> Think about what happened when you learned to ride a bike as a kid. At first you had to think to yourself, "I have to put my left foot here, then I swing my other leg up, then I do this, then I do that." You had to think very laboriously about each little step in what you were doing. Soon, though, bicycle riding became automatic and you didn't have to think about it at all. The same is true with the thought patterns we're going to be looking at in therapy. You've repeated the patterns so many times that they've become second nature, almost like they're automatic.
>
> Because of this, we're going to try to reverse the process of learning to ride a bike. We're going to take the automatic thoughts, make them fully conscious again, examine them in detail, like I said, change some, and then see if that helps you feel and live better. In your case, most of the thoughts were ingrained in you by the abuse, as we've been talking about.

Most of the time I don't provide a rationale for the cognitive interventions, I just blend them into the therapy. The patients have no trouble understanding what is being done. I rarely use the technical terminology of cognitive therapy in the sessions, except perhaps to refer to automatic thoughts, cognitive errors, or errors in thinking. With DID patients, pointing out cognitive errors can be experienced by the patient as blaming or belittling, so one has to continuously check for the effects of cognitive interventions. This is true with all techniques used throughout therapy.

The classical cognitive errors such as catastrophizing, and selective generalization are common in DID. They can be dealt with using standard strategies. The cognitive therapy of DID is different from that of depression or anxiety primarily because incompatible and contradictory cognitions are held and endorsed by separate personalities. Mapping the cognitions involves calling out the different alters and dealing with them psychotherapeutically at the same time. Because of the dissociation, pure, classical cognitive therapy is impossible in DID, and the work must involve noncognitive techniques never discussed by Beck and his colleagues. I don't think it makes sense to speak of the "cognitive therapy" of DID as an entirely distinct method from systems or psychodynamic work.

An exhaustive explication of the use of cognitive techniques in the treatment of DID would require a separate monograph. Therefore I am going to be illustrative. In our paper (Ross & Gahan, 1988a) on the cognitive analysis of DID, the first assumption we list is *Different parts of the self are separate selves* (see Chapter Six). One of the cognitions this leads to is the erroneous belief that different alters have different bodies. This is a crucial error to address in therapy because it helps maintain the self-destructive behavior of alters, who in effect attempt to murder the self.

I might challenge this belief in a number of ways. The first step is to take a full life history of the alter who is claiming to have a separate body. Often she will endorse several other subcognitions including the belief that the abuse never happened to her, and that the host's parents are not her parents. The belief in a separate body is usually part of a more massive denial and dissociation of the reality of the abuse. Having taken the cognitively oriented history, I might then go on to focus on the time and mechanism of origin of the alter.

Different alters claim to have different origins. Persecutors sometimes state that they were discarnate entities floating in the ether prior to entering the patient's body. In such cases, the persecutor will usually acknowledge that the body is the host's body, and she will claim to have an unaffected astral body, which is not harmed by the cigarette burns or wrist slashes. In this instance, I would then explore the cognitions in the second set derived from the belief that the victim is responsible for the abuse.

When an alter claims to have a separate physical body, I might ask about where she lives, what she eats, where she buys her clothes, and how all of this is distinct from the host personality's activities. The alter can rarely give a satisfactory account of these day-to-day matters, so the questioning plants the first seeds of doubt. I then restate the alter's perception as a logical proposition and get her to make an experimental prediction, which I know will be refuted by the facts.

The classical example of this strategy involves recent wrist slashing. Through Socratic questioning, I get the alter to endorse a chain of cognitions that maintain the locus of control shift: I have a separate physical body—I forced the host to slash her wrists—I did this because the host is bad—the host is bad because she caused the abuse to happen—she deserves to be punished—I was never abused—I'm not bad—I don't deserve to be punished—the slashing doesn't affect me—there are no slash marks on my arm. I then ask the alter to roll up her sleeve. When she sees the same slash marks the host inflicted on herself on her own arm, the entire chain of cognitions is shaken.

It is important to link together as complex and central a group of cognitions as possible, to maximize the impact of the intervention. I then review the empirical findings. The alter acknowledges that there are slash marks on her arm, that they look just like the ones on the host's arm, and that she doesn't know how they got there. Next, I propose an alternate hypothesis to account for the findings—that the two personalities are dissociated aspects of the same mind. This hypothesis is then discussed, the alter provides arguments in favor of the old theory of separate bodies, and these are analyzed, weighed, and refuted as persuasively as possible.

Alters usually abandon their cognitions in a stepwise fashion. The demonstration involving slash marks may rapidly result in an acknowledgment of a shared body, but the alter will still insist that the abuse never happened to her. "It happened to this body, but it didn't happen to me," is a common statement. I may not challenge that belief. Instead I might acknowledge it, and say that the belief in separateness was an effective and necessary survival strategy during childhood. I emphasize that I appreciate that the psychological reality for the alter is that the abuse did not happen to her. I say that this is as it should be.

I then divert attention to the fact that the persecutor has a stake in the welfare and survival of the body she inhabits. If the body dies, she dies. If the alter acknowledges this, a contract for no self-harm may be possible. Other persecutors will restate their conviction that they are discarnate entities with no stake in the survival of the physical body. In that instance, I then proceed to an examination of the alter's motives for self-abuse. My intention is to try to redefine the slashing or overdosing as helping strategies that could be improved. If this can be done, then a contract for a moratorium on self-harm while alternate strategies are being considered may be possible.

Often one has to nibble away at the cognitive fortress like a mouse trying to break into a castle made of cheese. The personality system will have an elaborate rationale in place for its self-destructive behavior, but there are always flaws in the logic somewhere. Once these are located, they can be chewed away at until a sizable breach has been established.

The cognitive work also has a computer-game feel to it, as the therapist analyzes the system and tries to figure out the entry codes. The cognitive interventions are like viruses inserted into the system, which then replicate and dismantle it from within. Much of the dysphoria and self-abuse is driven by the core assumption: *The victim is responsible for the abuse.* This error in reasoning originated in early Piagetian stages of development, but the patient now has a mind capable of formal operations, which can unlearn the earlier modes of thought.

I use a number of strategies for this problem, the main one being an explanation of the locus of control shift. The belief that "I must be bad" has a narcissistic quality to it that can be challenged. Using a Socratic approach, I get the target alter to review her beliefs about children in general. Usually she will agree that children in general are not capable of adult responsibility for what happens in their lives.

If a child gets sick, that is not her fault. If a child's father dies in a car accident, that is not the child's fault. But one can understand how a child might reason incorrectly and conclude that Daddy died and went away because he didn't like her, and it was her fault. As adults, we can understand the child's reasoning, and know that it is mistaken. I then ask the patient how she feels about the little girls in our city who are currently being sexually abused by their fathers. Is it their fault? The patient will usually insist that there is no way it could be the girls' fault, and say she would like to rescue them. In a group therapy, I punctuate my explanation of the locus of control shift with the observation that all group members view all other group members as victims, not causes, of their abuse: All members make the locus of control shift only for themselves. This proves that the proposition *the abuse happened because I am bad* is an intrapsychic strategy, not a general truth.

I clarify that in general children are not responsible for traumatic things that happen to them. In particular, little girls who are being abused today are not responsible. The adult is fully responsible, and the behavior is criminal. If these things are true for all children in the world, why aren't they true for the patient? Is she so special and different that she's the one child in the world who is responsible for her abuse? This line of questioning puts the patient in a position of being grandiose if she claims responsibility for the abuse. Since she feels worthless, the logical structure has to break down. Its internal inconsistencies have been revealed.

Such interventions do not work instantaneously. It takes a great deal of repetition, negotiation, and other work to cure the cognitive errors. Additionally, one can ask the patient as an adult to review all the strategies available to her as a child to deal with the abuse. She could tell, but nobody would believe her, and she would be abused even worse. She could fight, but that would be ineffective and would escalate the abuse. She couldn't run away at four years old. She didn't know how to kill herself. She could try to be perfect, but that didn't work. So she shifted the locus of control, the best and most brilliant strategy.

In conjunction with a review of strategies, I examine motive. Did she enjoy the abuse, did she ask for it, did she want it? Does she think that girls who are being abused today like it and want it? So how could it be her fault? She may restate her arguments that it would have stopped if she had been perfect. I then ask if it is reasonable to bring children up in an environment where they will be raped if they don't vacuum well enough. At some point, tears will break through, then anger, then a declaration that the father is a bastard and the patient wants to kill him. I respond to this by evoking memories of the positive aspects of father, and the feelings of alters who were treated well by him. The patient must learn to tolerate ambivalent attachment to the perpetrator without dissociating, and in any case I want to discourage murder.

This set of interventions can be complicated if the alter enticed the father into bed in order to divert him from a sister in another bed, when he crept into the bedroom at night. This was honorable and courageous behavior, and didn't prove that the patient wanted or deserved the abuse. Often the patient will have experienced sexual arousal during the abuse and will cite this as proof that she is bad, dirty, to blame, and really wanted it. I deal with this by asking the patient how her fingertip would react if she placed it on a hot stove. It would blister if she didn't pull it away quick enough. Blistering and reflex withdrawal occur independently of our thoughts and motives, and are natural bodily responses to stimuli.

Similarly, the human body is designed to be sexually aroused by certain stimuli. This has been very useful in evolution to ensure the propagation of the species. It's why vibrators work. That your body found the abuse pleasurable doesn't in the least prove you wanted it or enjoyed it emotionally, anymore than blistering proves you like getting burned. Much of the cognitive work is educational in nature, and only some is more formally argumentative.

A difficulty can occur in patients with highly structured, layered personality systems. One can deal with and disarm hostile, abusive alters with cognitive and other techniques in one layer, then encounter similar alters in another layer who have observed the "mind games" and declare they aren't going to be taken in by them. My cognitive interventions have also been called "hocus pocus" by alters in such systems. So far, I have found that the same strategies seem to work layer by layer, although the bag of tricks has been used already.

The third set of cognitions based on *It is wrong to show anger* are susceptible to cognitive restructuring. Part of this involves a short lecture on the utility and natural beauty of anger, the righteousness of anger, the energy value of anger, anger as a motivator, and so on. The patient's anger must be redefined as biologically normal, legitimate, and healthy, but in need of containment and channeling. Anger is not desirable in itself, and it occurs in a transactional context. Neither is it intrinsically undesirable. It just is. Anger gets bad press in our culture, and many patients have been subjected to severe ideological suppression of their anger by "religious," sexually abusive parents.

I borrow a page from the feminist handbook and point out that much of the social change brought about by the women's movement was motivated by healthy anger. I also work hard to get the patient to see that the abusers controlled and abused the patient by coercive persuasion, mind control, or brainwashing, in which the patient was told she was bad for having normal angry responses to abuse. Because several alters contain all the anger, whereas others have never been angry, I review the utility of dissociation once again. The goal of the therapy is to remove the boundaries that keep thoughts, feelings, memories, behaviors, and skills compartmentalized in separate personality states. In part, the cognitive errors are the intrapsychic machinery that maintains the dissociation: When the errors are corrected, the leakage of anger and other feelings from alter to alter increases.

I might ask, "Who says anger is bad? How do you know that?" knowing full well that the parents said it. A common reply is, "I just know it's bad." I counter, "How do you know that? Did you find some stone tablets with *Never Get Angry* written on them? Is *Never Get Angry* a scientific law that you studied in physics?" *Reductio ad absurdum,* playful parody, and exaggeration, even sarcasm, can be useful techniques. The patient then might say, "I know it's bad to get angry because I always got beaten up if I got angry at home." I go on, "Oh, I see. You're saying that your parents are healthy, well-adjusted people, and that you value their opinions on how to raise children. If they said anger is bad, they must be right. They were right that it was okay to abuse you, they were right that it was okay to kill your cat, so they must be right about this too. Is that it?"

The next comment by the patient might contain several four-letter words. This is good because it mobilizes the patient's anger, and I point this out, and approve of the anger. There has just been a revolutionary transactional sequence for the patient. I push patients hard on their cognitive errors.

Another way to work with cognitions is to get alters who endorse incompatible cognitions to state them out loud while the others are listening. The alters then have a disagreement among themselves that they have to resolve. This provides practice in internal democracy. The conversation generates irrefutable evidence that the patient as a whole does not endorse any of the cognitive errors, that the whole is greater than the sum of its parts, and that the alters exist to ensure that ambivalence is dissociated and experienced as certainty by parts that hold only one pole of the ambivalence. Life is both simpler and more complicated after integration. With coconsciousness, the alters can begin to understand directly how they function as a dissociative system with complex linkages between subregions, rather than as separate, independent people.

Because cognitive therapy is always cognitive-behavioral, graded exercises are useful. These can be applied to the fifth core assumption: *The primary personality can't handle the memories.* Through graded return of memories and gradual attainment of coconsciousness, this assumption and its cognitions are experimentally refuted. This assumption is an example of dichotomization: the options at first appear to be complete amnesia, or complete recovery of memories with insanity. Fears that one alter won't like another can be disconfirmed by having the fearful alter listen in while the issue is discussed with the other personality.

In parallel to what occurs in the therapy, many of the cognitive techniques are scattered throughout other sections of this chapter. Cognitive interventions interact and synergize with other techniques.

It isn't only patients who make cognitive errors. The resistance to DID among mental health professionals can be analyzed in terms of cognitive errors, as I did in Chapter Ten. For example, Fahy (1988) in a review that is dismissive of DID as a legitimate nosological entity, says that the failure to define a personality is a major weakness of the *DSM-III* criteria. He then characterizes DID as "hysterical" without defining that term. This is an error of reasoning and analysis. Something approaching closer to a classical cognitive error is the incorrect belief that a diagnosis of DID provides the patient a license for irresponsibility.

Once this assumption is made, a set of attitudes and behaviors hostile to DID follows logically. If the assumption is dismissed, the attitudes and behaviors simply melt away. Cognitive therapy has a Zen flavor to it in that the therapist doesn't so much teach patients what to do, as teach them what not to do. Once they stop doing what they shouldn't be doing, everything works well and naturally. This is only a part truth about the therapy of DID. The main point I want the reader to carry away from this section is that cognitive interventions are only one "personality" within the entire therapeutic system, not a freestanding entity.

NEGOTIATING WITH ALTER PERSONALITIES

Some of the principles and techniques of negotiation with alters have been referred to previously. The therapy of DID can be thought of globally as analogous to labor-management negotiations. The therapist alternates between roles of mediator and arbitrator. Enforced arbitration occurs with involuntary hospitalization, violation of absolute rules of therapy, putting alters to sleep hypnotically, hiring alters as internal enforcers to keep other personalities in line, and similar unilaterally enforced actions. These are temporary measures in an ongoing process of therapy, unless termination occurs. Even unilateral actions by the therapist have been negotiated with some other part of the system.

A goal of treatment is to convert the patient from a dysfunctional, war-stricken state to a more functional political organization. The patient enters therapy with hostile, uncooperative, frightened, abusive, and hidden personality states that have limited coordination with each other. The role of the therapist is to analyze the system, identify the specific conflicts and problems, and negotiate solutions with the involved parties. This is similar to the role of a consultant to a large corporation who generates a plan for improved corporate function. As a system, the DID personality system is as complex as a large company.

Businesses have similar problems to the DID patient: Marketing does not communicate with finance; payroll is having trouble converting to a new system; the lines of communication are unclear; one vice-president has an alcohol problem; another is pursuing his career goals at the expense of the corporation; the company is reacting in a self-destructive way to certain market forces; the original structure of the company cannot adapt to a changed business environment; a hostile takeover by a corporate raider is feared; the secretaries are unhappy with office noise levels; cash flow is down; and so on. The systems analyst has to take numerous types of problems into account.

Anyone who can analyze and treat complex DID could learn to improve the function of large corporations: The logic of the analysis is the same. The DID therapist would have an advantage over most consultants because of his awareness of the emotional determinants of system dysfunction. For example, if I were asked to consult to a corporation, I would make a point of interviewing the secretaries personally. In my experience, they often have a unique and profound insight into the function of systems in which they are employed that you cannot get from management. This is analogous to interviewing everybody in the DID personality system.

DID treatment is the same. You have to talk to everybody, find out what the problems are, and then work out solutions. For example, a woman was admitted for intensive inpatient work. She complained that a record of "Old McDonald Had a Farm" was playing over and over in her head. She found this very distressing and feared she was going insane. Brief inquiry easily established that an older male alter was playing the records for a frightened child, who liked them. The male agreed to try to learn how to play the records without the host hearing them, with hypnotic help from us. Our next strategy was to have the male find out what tapes the child would like to listen to that the host would also enjoy. The patient could buy these and play them on her Walkman, and the child could listen to them.

This negotiated solution would remove the symptom, demonstrate to the child that it was safe to enter therapy, reinforce the protective role of the male, establish coconsciousness for nonthreatening, pleasurable experience, demonstrate to the host that she was not insane and that her symptoms were treatable, and provide a concrete example of the benefits of negotiation. Yet it is simple and practical. The involved alters could consent to the intervention as is, or propose and negotiate modifications.

Negotiation is a pervasive aspect of therapy that, once grasped in principle, is used in a pragmatic fashion. The method of therapy, I can't repeat too often, is to ask and find out, then problem-solve. Sometimes the therapist will feel as if he is dashing around chaotically putting out fires, without an overall direction. This is a sign of inadequate analysis and problem prioritization. Most of the work goes on at a microlevel and involves solving countless little problems such as the auditory hallucination of "Old McDonald Had a Farm."

USING METAPHOR, RITUALS, IMAGERY, AND DREAMS

This is a rich and imaginative set of interventions. It has been taking a lot of heat from the false memory camp. There must be some sort of neuropsychological link between abuse, dissociation, and visual imagination. DID patients often have very intense visual modes of thought. They are good at thinking in metaphors and using guided imagery techniques. These interventions can be so creative and interesting for the therapist that they become countertherapeutic: It is important to keep a clear focus on current function in the real world.

Some patients have highly structured internal environments in which the alters can move around. Bringing a frightened child into therapy may involve a hypnotic expedition to a distant room in an internal house by a helper personality, with guidance from the therapist. One patient had a child alter who was locked in a room. The other personalities were terrified to open the door of the room and let the child out because they knew something bad was going on in there. A great deal of work was done fusing some of the alters, putting some to sleep, negotiating with adult alters to protect other child personalities, and preparing for the therapist to open the door.

The other personalities could detect a pinelike odor coming out of the room that smelled like a cleaning agent called Pinesol. With hypnotic preparation, I went into the building, opened the door, and called the alter over. She was in a room in which pornographic movies were being made. She and other children, many drugged or drunk, were taking part in hardcore sex while being filmed. I was able to accompany the child out of the room because nobody but her could see or hear me. In the hall, there was a struggle as she tried to get away, and we were able to escape from the building. I brought her to the hospital and she found a safe place to be in her inner world. The door to the room was reported to be permanently closed, but the memories were not lost. They were now memories of the past rather than ongoing abreactive experience. The odor was from Pinesol used as a cleaner by the pornographers. With this intervention, a range of frightened, agitated, and highly anxious behavioral states went into remission. The intervention was effective whether or not the memory was confabulated.

My office contains a number of amulets, medicine bundles, and shamanic power objects that testify to my authority and healing power, and that reveal to the patients that therapy is a prolonged spiritual ritual. I have magically transformed these possessions into objects consistent with the cultural expectations of my patients. Nonshamanic people who enter my office see only degrees on the wall, professional books, and other artifacts of the late twentieth century. I, however, know that all therapy is a mysterious ritual.

Therapy can be guided by both global metaphors and micrometaphors. The patient's personal metaphor of integration provides organization and direction for all the work. An example of a micrometaphor occurred in therapy with a patient who could not understand why there was so much commotion in her personality system, with alters constantly changing alliances and positions. Since a number of child and adolescent alters were involved, I pointed out to the patient that there was trouble on the school playground. She grasped this immediately.

The metaphor seems simple but it is complex. It brings to bear on the therapy a wealth of assumptions, tacit knowledge, cultural expectations, and direct experience about the social structure and function of school playgrounds. There are bullies, shy kids, outcasts, older kids, younger kids, and a few protective teachers who also know how to spoil the fun. Commotion on the playground, rather than being a sign of mental illness, is evidence of exuberant life. Changing alliances and positions is part of the natural order of playground life, and not necessarily cause for anguish or alarm.

The patient immediately set about the task of organizing the playground a little, getting someone to look out for the young children, finding a friend for the lonely adolescent, and putting limits on bullying. We sometimes put alters to sleep, frequently call out alters, and talk about eventually terminating therapy: All of these are metaphors, the last communicating sinister but unacknowledged feelings about patients. Is therapy really something to be "terminated"? Why don't we talk about metamorphosing patients out of therapy, or transmigrating them? Why have we chosen an official term that evokes extinction?

Particular metaphors or imaginative rituals should not be reified, or blown up into a method or school of therapy. They may make an interesting case presentation or clinical tip, and can be the subject of a 15-minute conference presentation. Usually, they should not be more. Rituals can be borrowed from whatever mythology the therapist and patient find congruent. I might tell an alter that I am going to get tough with her, or set limits: more metaphor. This paragraph contains metaphors involving the following words: reified, blown up, school, tip, borrowed, congruent, get tough, set limits, and contains.

Therapy is no more metaphorical than molecular biology, however. I remember noticing in premedical studies that the scientific study of DNA is almost all metaphorical. In a single paragraph one finds metaphors about genetic blueprints, mapping DNA, transcribing DNA, messenger RNA, the genetic code, cellular architecture, bonding, reading DNA, information encoded on chromosomes, and the gene pool, to give a sample of the basic vocabulary of genetics. Science is as fundamentally metaphorical as poetry, but the metaphors of science are connected to physical reality in a special way that yields modern technology. The metaphors of DID therapy are connected to reality in ways that dramatically modify observable behavior, as demonstrated by our treatment outcome data. DID therapy deals with "facts" just as much as molecular biology, but the facts are psychological in nature.

I make these remarks to indicate that the use of metaphor in DID therapy is not soft, hazy, romantic, or poetical, in the usual current senses of those terms. These techniques are used for specific purposes, the effects of which need to be monitored.

Although other therapists do dream work with DID patients (Barrett, 1994, 1995; Franklin, 1990; Gabel, 1990; Marmer, 1980; Paley, 1992), I do none. This is probably a limitation of mine, and I should probably do some form of dream work. I am more interested in the paranormal properties of dreams than in their personal psychological meaning, so will probably never investigate dreams within the context of psychotherapy.

For DID patients, dreams are like hallucinations. In dissociative patients with childhood trauma histories, dreams and hallucinations can be intrusions of trauma memories. On the other hand, they can just be dreams and hallucinations. Dream material is at best a highly unreliable source of accurate recall. Staged recovery of memories can occur through dreams, hallucinations, internal movies, abreactions, and flashbacks, but all these methods increase the likelihood of memory distortion and confabulation. New dreams can precede the uncovering of a new layer of personalities in highly structured patients.

To do DID dream work, the therapist should proceed on the hypothesis that the images and events make sense psychologically, but are not necessarily memory traces of historical events. This will set the correct tone for clinical inquiry. If dreams are coming too fast or are too disturbing, and direct contact with the alters in the background has not been established, several techniques might be helpful. Hypnotic suggestion might help, or the therapist can talk to "whoever is controlling the dreams" by talking through the host, or whichever alter is in executive control at the time.

I might say:

> I'm talking to whoever is controlling the dreams about blood that Susan has been describing. I don't know for sure, but going on how it has worked in the past, this probably has to do with something bad that happened. If that's true, it's good that the memories are coming back. The problem is they're coming back a bit too fast, and causing Susan a lot of distress. So I'm asking whoever is giving the memories back to slow things down a bit. Actually, I'd like to talk directly with whoever it is, if that's possible.

I might then use indirect techniques for contacting the dream controller. I might also make reassuring or other statements to the presumed alter in the background.

Hypnotic interventions, audiotapes, trazodone, and benzodiazepine medications may all help to control traumatic dreaming, but often the patient just has to tough it out to some degree. Guided imagery interventions can be thought of as journeys into a waking dream world, and may be helpful for control of both daytime symptoms and traumatic nightmares.

For example, a child personality may run away into a dark place and not know how to get back. If a marker has been placed on her beforehand, the therapist can give a hypnotic suggestion that because of the marker his voice is bringing the child back to the therapy room. I would give relaxation instructions and say:

> I'm calling for Susie now. Susie is far away and nobody knows where she has gone, but it's safe now for her to come back. I'm calling now for Susie, and because of the marker I gave her, my voice can reach her and bring her back. My voice is traveling out into the darkness, guided by the marker, and is bringing Susie back to talk. Susie, you feel yourself coming back now, everything is safe, it's Dr. Ross calling you and bringing you back to talk. My voice is traveling out into the darkness to find Susie and bring her back.

This is a cultural equivalent of the circumpolar shaman sending spirit guides out over the arctic landscape to locate game. Patients can be given any of an infinite variety of objects to carry with them, for numerous purposes. One of my cotherapists gave a patient an ornamental rock that she held in order to guide her back to the office, after her child personality had been out. She was a patient who had a prolonged, foggy state during switches back to her host personality. Another therapist gave a patient a pen of his to carry for strength, a gift that crystallized erotic and other transferences. The fact that it was a standard issue hospital pen taken from a supply cupboard did not detract from its therapeutic power.

One alter personality said to me, "I can't talk to you because I'm dead." My response was to say that I was sorry the alter was dead, and to ask what it was like being dead. I learned from this alter that being dead meant being hidden in a safe place far away where no one would ever look for her. In another patient, such an alter might first be contacted in a nocturnal dream, in which the host was journeying to a distant world.

One of the most important rituals is the actual integration ritual, which I will describe in Chapter Sixteen. There is no need to list countless examples of metaphors, rituals, and imagery because they all conform to general principles. The information transmitted through dreams is often fragmentary at first. To clarify it, the therapist uses other techniques, focused on contacting the alters who hold the memories consciously. I will conclude by describing a technique used by George Fraser (1991).

A good way to map the system, resolve issues, and recover memories is to hold inner board meetings. The patient relaxes with a brief hypnotic induction, and the host personality walks into the boardroom. The patient is instructed that there will be one chair for every personality in the system.

Then a general suggestion is given for all members of the system to enter the boardroom and take a seat. Once this is done, the therapist chairs the meeting, takes roll call, and coordinates negotiations between board members. Often there are empty chairs because some alters aren't ready to enter therapy. The empty chairs provide useful information, and those present can be asked what they know about the missing people. There should be a number of doors in and out of the boardroom because some alters might not feel safe using the same entrance as others.

The boardroom contains a projector and screen on which abuse memories can be replayed. Alternatively, selected alters can adjourn to a separate screening room. Watching the abuse on a screen is done with specific hypnotic suggestions that the host will see the movie but not feel the feelings. This allows for safe, staged recovery of memories without full abreaction. Such internal meetings can be held in a variety of settings. They are a way of rapidly establishing coconsciousness and cooperation for selected issues and material.

Another common use of guided imagery is to find safe locations for the children in the inner landscape. This can include safety from memories, external abusers, and persecutory alters. Children can be asked to go away and play while particularly difficult adult work is being done. This set of interventions is high on the list of targets for ridicule by skeptics. Rituals, dreams, metaphors, and imagery directly tap the hypnotic/dissociative virtuosity of the patients, and teach them that their gift can be used for recovery and improved function. As I said at the beginning of this section, though, these techniques can get out of control if the therapist becomes more interested in his own creativity than in the patient, and therapist and client can both get lost in the inner virtual reality.

HYPNOSIS AND RELAXATION TECHNIQUES

Richard Kluft (1982, 1985c) has written specifically on hypnotic techniques in the treatment of adult and childhood DID. He has also published a very interesting paper on the use of hypnosis to recover lost objects (1987c). It is a bit difficult to provide a catalog of the uses of hypnosis in DID work because it can be used to augment virtually any intervention (Gruenewald, 1971; Howland, 1975; Schafer, 1986). In one sense, everything done prior to integration is a hypnotic intervention, because some part of the patient has been continuously in trance since early childhood.

The main caution concerning hypnosis is not to use it for recovering memories. There is abundant evidence that hypnosis can stimulate confabulation, although it can also augment accurate recall. Hypnotic techniques result in a greater quantity of recalled material overall, which includes a greater amount of confabulated material than was present at baseline. It is impossible to tell purely on clinical grounds which elements are real and which are not. Therefore hypnosis inevitably introduces more noise into the memories if used for memory recovery.

When people ask me if you have to use hypnosis to treat DID, I say "No." I point out that the aim of therapy is to bring the patient out of trance, not to put her in it. All this is a bit semantic, but I think that anyone who is making massive ongoing use of dissociation is in some sense continuously hypnotized. The idea that DID is a disorder of autohypnosis is questionable, because the original induction was probably done unintentionally by the abuser. It is arbitrary whether one calls this autohypnosis or heterohypnosis.

One adult patient was not showing as much improvement as she should have been, despite the integration of 50 alters, and her apparent substantial strengths. I then discovered that, according to her, her father was still having intercourse with her at least twice a week, and had been doing so continuously since childhood. The final layer of alters contained a mute victim alter, and was divided into a good and a bad side. The father would knock on the door, and the host would switch to one of three enabling alters under the control of the leader of the bad side, who would open the door. Once the father entered, the bad leader would switch the patient to the victim. When the father (actually the father's alter, since the father's host personality was amnesic for the abuse) interrogated the patient for information about whether the ongoing abuse had been disclosed in therapy, the bad leader had one of the enablers talk for the mute victim-alter, without a switch of executive control.

However the leader of the good side temporarily took all memories of disclosure in therapy out of the minds of the enablers at the moment they began to reply to the father. When the father left, the patient switched back to her host personality, who was amnesic for the entire episode. Setting aside the problem of false memories, attempting to decide which parts of this patient are in trance at which times is a scientifically impossible and therapeutically irrelevant task. One could say that the host personality is hypnotized by the father, while the enablers are hypnotized by the leader of the good side; that the entire personality system is in autohypnosis; or that only the host has gone into autohypnosis on the grounds that only she experiences amnesia. This doesn't resolve who is putting the father in trance.

I don't think it is true that the host is awake, while the alters are in a trance state when in executive control, as some people assume. Some people seem to think that when you are talking to any alter but the host, the patient is in trance. This is an arbitrary distinction with no empirical basis. Besides, different alters can be the host at different times. This means that it isn't necessary to do a hypnotic induction to contact an alter. In fact, the reverse can sometimes be true: You have to hypnotize an alter to get the host back.

Another problem in deciding what is and what isn't a hypnotic intervention, is the difficulty distinguishing between a relaxation exercise and a hypnotic induction with DID patients. I remember one patient with whom I wanted to call out an alter for the first time. I explained what I was going to do, then said, "Now I want you to close your eyes and be as relaxed and comfortable as possible." She closed her eyes and immediately exclaimed, "Boy! Do I feel relaxed!" I hadn't even started my relaxation procedure yet! Two more sentences from me and she would be in deep trance.

DID patients can go into trance states instantly in response to innumerable internal and external cues. In some sense, patients probably go into trance walking across the parking lot to get to the therapist's building: From this perspective, patients are never fully awake till after integration. Advocates of the theory that DID is an artifact of hypnosis have to be careful how they define an induction, and how they differentiate auto and heterohypnosis.

It is known that there are awake, alert hypnotic states, and that induction procedures need not involve relaxation, sleep, focus, or fatigue imagery. Thus, most interventions in DID may have a hypnotic component. A formal induction procedure is rarely required. I rarely if ever use formal inductions in therapy, even when getting into a new layer of personalities. The main use of formal inductions for calling out alters seems to be anxiolysis. The personality in executive control and the alter about to emerge are nervous about switching, and need calming and reassurance about it for a while.

Formal inductions serve only to mobilize the patient's dissociative skills for particular therapeutic purposes. I use a relaxation and warming up induction out of personal preference. I like it because it gives permission for hypnotic amnesia through sleep suggestions, is anxiolytic, can be generalized for relaxation training, is pleasant, and involves the entire body.

Hypnosis can be used for adjunctive pain relief, improved sleep, and general relaxation. Audiotapes can be made for DID patients with an induction and whatever suggestions are suitable. This may include increased confidence, reduced stomach pain, or any other instruction. I have reviewed the use of posthypnotic suggestions for safety in an earlier section. Formal inductions are most often used to facilitate contact with alters, increase interpersonality communication, and stop malignant or unproductive abreactions. Hypnosis should not be thought of as a technique in itself either to use or not to use. Although an induction can be done at a specific point in time to augment another intervention, hypnosis is never something the therapist does for its own sake.

There is therefore no need to list further examples of the use of hypnosis in DID work. It can facilitate many or all aspects of the work, but patients can be treated without a defined verbal induction ever being done.

AGE PROGRESSION AND AGE REGRESSION

Personalities can be grown up or made younger for many purposes. Both age progression and age regression can be augmented by a formal hypnotic ritual. In the 1980s, some therapists (Bornn, 1988) made specialized use of prolonged, massive age regression in selected inpatient cases. I have never done that, and I am not going to talk about such extraordinary interventions. I also do not do intrauterine or past life work, although DID patients report spontaneous past life intrusions among their other paranormal experiences.

I have watched a non-DID patient age regress to the intrauterine state and complain about an unsuccessful illegal abortion, but I did not believe that this was a real memory of an event that occurred at two months' gestation. Such memory is impossible. The patient experienced the memory as intense and real, however, and it clearly symbolized chronic feelings of being unloved and rejected. Another patient described listening to an argument between her parents while a fetus, understanding the words, and reacting to their meaning.

Age regression and progression are techniques that, like abreaction and formal hypnotic induction, have disappeared from my practice in the 1990s. I find them unnecessary. However, some therapists may find such interventions helpful in selected cases, so I will describe them briefly. If I were to do an age progression now, I would make sure to emphasize this is a reconfiguration of the patient's inner world that she is doing, not I; that she is in control; and that I am only consulting with her on what she might try doing. I want to empower the host to be in control of her system, which helps bump her out of the victim position. I don't want to be the controlling good father who opposes the bad father from the past.

Age regression can be used to take an alter back to before the time of a trauma that is causing an otherwise untreatable symptom. One child alter was constantly screaming inside about a murder witnessed many years earlier, which was probably confabulated. This screaming and an associated conversion symptom went into temporary complete remission when the alter was regressed to an age two years earlier than the murder. This was only a temporary technique until a more definitive solution could be worked out, the alter integrated, and the symptoms cured.

The host personality or the alter may say that she doesn't know how to do age progression. I reassure her that her mind created the inner world in the first place, and that she can restructure it simply by deciding to do so, which is true, given that the defensive functions of the virtual reality are taken into account. I then simply instruct the host personality to grow the alter up to the desired age, and wait while she does so. I point out that because the alter is older, she will understand that the trauma happened a long time ago. It is in the past now, the alter is safe, and she understands better and can talk about it.

Such age progression is useful for infant alters, frightened children who are stuck in the past, lonely alters without friends, and others who could benefit from the ability to function at the level of formal operations. Age progression demonstrates that alter personalities are not people, psychologically or legally. Age progression can be done rapidly—a decade in less than a minute in some cases. In other cases, it may be necessary to stop every year for a brief birthday party, or other alters may hold an internal birthday party every few days to help the child grow up quickly. Age progression can be spread out over minutes, hours, days, or weeks, and can occur spontaneously.

For one patient treated in the 1980s, I age-progressed a child alter because the host personality didn't feel it made sense to integrate that personality with her adolescent protector if they were different ages. Some therapists make a point of growing up alters to the chronological age of the patient prior to integration with the host, but this is not necessary. The vast majority of the work can be done with the alters at their presenting ages, but age progression can be helpful in some cases. Before undertaking age progression, there must be consultation with the necessary alters, which include the one to be aged, the host, and often a protector/observer.

WRITING EXERCISES

Some patients write volumes and volumes in their journals, diaries, and notebooks, and bring in a far greater amount of material than the therapist can possibly read. This requires limit setting. One patient liked to write in session, which seemed to work well for her. There is a wide variety of ways in which written materials can be used. Writing can be used for both diagnostic and therapeutic purposes, as illustrated by a case I consulted on.

A young woman was inflicting serious knife slashes on her face during the night, and was completely amnesic for the behavior. Nocturnal epilepsy with automatisms? No. In consultation I recommended that she leave a notepad and pencil by her bed on a night table, and that she write a request for anyone there to send her messages on the notepad. Such messages began to appear and resulted in entry into her personality system and eventual extinction of the slashing.

Similar requests can be made of alters who are known but who are reluctant to participate in therapy. These requests can be made by talking through the host in session and asking the alter to write at home. The host can either leave a set of specific questions for the alter to answer, or an open-ended request to talk may be sufficient. This may result in furious scratchings or rational conversation. In either case, important information is transmitted and the process of communication has begun. With hostile alters, it may be safer for the therapist to begin communication in this indirect way with the hostile personality taking executive control at home rather than in the office.

Daily journals can be a kind of internal internet forum for coconsciousness, with alters taking turns writing, and commenting on what others have had to say. The penmanship can vary dramatically from personality to personality (Yank, 1991). I described the use of writing exercises in the section on establishing interpersonality communication.

Another way in which writing can be of benefit in DID work is encouraging creative writing, such as poems, stories, and autobiographical sketches. I see such work as healthy, normative, and therapeutic. Although

the patients' poetry is not technically advanced, it is much more interesting than most of what I've seen in literary magazines. This is so because of
the seriousness of the DID subject matter and the integrity of the expressed
feelings.

The purpose of this section is to highlight writing exercises as a distinct
set of therapeutic techniques. There is no need to provide further detail or
examples, since the principles are readily grasped. I have already discussed
artwork in a previous section, so will not say more about it now, although it
is listed separately in the Therapist Dissociative Checklist.

USE OF AUDIOVISUAL MATERIALS

Everything that applies to using videotapes in therapy also applies to the
use of audiotapes, except that the impact of video is greater. The only exception to this is prescribing audiotapes for relaxation, better sleep, and
symptom relief.

I sometimes request permission to videotape for educational rather than
therapeutic purposes. So far I haven't had any trouble with this and patients have been happy to contribute to the education of other mental health
professionals. Patients are aware of the difficulties in modern society that
act as a barrier to the diagnosis and treatment of DID, and like contributing
to public education. Some patients would like to do so but can't for confidentiality reasons. In an indirect way making such educational videos is
healthy for the patient, but this is a minor side-benefit. Actually, patients
are happy to do us a favor, but since they are vulnerable to exploitation of
all kinds we have to be sensitive and careful about the matter. Written consent for videotaping for educational purposes is essential.

I have had mixed experiences allowing television film crews into our
Dissociative Disorders Program. In one instance the Program and I were
victims of a scam: The film producer said that the purpose of the filming
was to do an educational program supportive of DID, when actually it was
to select clinical vignettes out of context to make the treatment look stupid.
In a subsequent experience, the presence of the film crew resulted in an escalation of cute child alter behavior and spontaneous abreactions that was
contained with some difficulty. The film crew in this instance was generally respectful and considerate. My conclusion is that I am highly reluctant
to participate in any further filming of patients unless I am the producer.

The main use of video is to facilitate interpersonality communication,
and to give everyone in the system a chance to observe switching and different alters from the outside. We use video for such purposes in a regularly
scheduled weekly group, although I consider the medium to be inessential
and adjunctive. Like everything else in the therapy, video should be used in
a planned, negotiated way. When this is done, video can be a powerful prod
to increased communication and cooperation between alters.

Severe reactions of panic, fear, agitation, and distress can occur if material is observed for which the host wasn't ready or if the host thinks she looks crazy on tape. Such reactions may be dealt with by spontaneous amnesia for the watching of the videotape. Therapists need to understand clearly that they can't force premature coconsciousness through audiovisual materials because protective amnesia barriers will be created. Video, like any other technique, can be countertherapeutic, slow the pace down, damage trust, and create iatrogenic complications in a therapy that is not well designed.

Another use of videotape is having patients watch educational programs on DID. This can be helpful, and may act as a kind of vicarious group therapy if the patient gets to see someone else switching on TV. Anyone planning to do a workshop on DID must realize that there will likely be diagnosed and/or undiagnosed DID patients in the audience, among the lay or professional attenders. Provocative tapes may stimulate switching, panic, emergency trips to the washroom, or other reactions in audience members. That is why I use videotape sparingly in educational settings, and not to illustrate abreactions.

An application of audiovisual technology I used in Canada, and which I am now investigating in the United States, was live telelinkage to professionals outside Winnipeg for ongoing consultation. Live interactive video linkage will probably be a component of health care in the twenty-first century, in some form. When the alternative is no direct observation by the consultant at all, this may be the most effective way of proceeding with long-distance consultations, and even therapy sessions. Psychiatry needs to be in the space age just like cardiology: Cardiologists can instantaneously read electrocardiograms (EKGs) done hundreds of miles away.

In one antidepressant study I was involved in Canada, computerized EKG analyses were fed back to us from the United States within five minutes through the phone system. They had to be overread by a cardiologist in the United States. The computerized analyses were deliberately conservative and yielded false positives rather than false negatives. With similar provisos and precautions, there is no reason that expertise in DID cannot be tapped effectively with remote video technology.

MEDICATIONS

There are many problems about the use of medications in DID. The most common error is countertherapeutic polypharmacy in undiagnosed patients. Undiagnosed DID patients get a lot of meds. In one consult I did, the patient was on paroxetine, lithium, trazodone, buspirone, lorazepam, clonidine, and risperidone for rapid cycling bipolar mood disorder.

In our series of 236 cases, 63.3% had received a benzodiazepine, 59.5% a non-benzodiazepine sedative, 68.9% antidepressants, 54.5% antipsychotics,

21.9% lithium, and 12.1% electroconvulsive therapy (ECT). We don't know how many of these prescriptions were warranted or how many helped. There is no indication for ECT in the treatment of DID. Most courses of ECT are probably prescribed for DID patients who do have depressions, mixed with dissociative Schneiderian symptoms. An important study would be a retrospective analysis of the efficacy of courses of ECT given to DID patients prior to their diagnosis. I'll bet the efficacy is the same as it would be for sham ECT.

This is an important issue because ECT is a humane and effective treatment which I have prescribed to selected nondissociative patients with dramatic benefits. If a DID patient does actually have a psychotherapy and medication-nonresponsive psychotic depression, then ECT can be properly indicated for that depression. ECT is absolutely contraindicated as a treatment for the DID itself. In practical terms, we have not prescribed a single course of ECT in over 1,000 inpatient admissions to our Dissociative Disorders Program, so it does not appear to be a useful or necessary treatment.

Likewise, there is no indication for the use of lithium in DID. It could be prescribed properly only for concurrent bipolar mood disorder. In practice, that would be difficult because of compliance problems. I have prescribed lithium to one DID patient on a trial basis, during the active phase of her psychotherapy. It had no beneficial effect. This woman had a 10-year history of classical rapid-cycling manic-depressive illness, as well as DID. The manic-depressive illness had been in complete remission for 18 months since integration on no medication when the patient was lost to follow-up. As a single-subject study, this is an extremely powerful finding. I have to emphasize that the manic-depressive history in this case was a vividly clear textbook description of rapid cycling illness.

I have seen lithium work well in a few cases of truly concurrent DID and bipolar mood disorder, and I have seen a few DID patients experience stabilization of their switching on lithium, but I am not yet convinced that this is more than a placebo effect. In general, the risk of overdose and toxicity outweighs the benefits of a trial of lithium in DID. The use of anticonvulsants for mood stabilization in DID involves the same problems as lithium, except for less toxicity and danger in overdose.

There have been no systematic or controlled studies of the use of any medication in DID. This means that there is no rigorous scientific basis for any prescription written for a DID patient, and that every prescription is an empirical trial. This applies to both benefits and side effects. It is important not to make exaggerated claims for either the efficacy or the harmfulness of medications in DID in the absence of data. A report by Loewenstein, Hornstein, and Farber (1988) provides the only small-N open-label pilot study of the psychopharmacology of DID.

Most DID patients develop clinical depressions, so the question of antidepressant medication comes up frequently. I have seen many clear examples of beneficial response to antidepressants in DID. The majority of inpatients with DID are clinically depressed and warrant a trial of a serotonin reuptake blocker antidepressant. A general rule of thumb is that medications have a better chance of working if the symptoms are spread across the entire personality system. If only one or two alters are depressed, while others are euthymic, that is a relative contraindication to a trial of antidepressants.

The tricyclic antidepressants are extremely dangerous in overdose. Some people will die from ingestion of two weeks' supply of a therapeutic oral dosage of tricyclics. If such a medication is to be tried, the absolute maximum to be dispensed at one time is a week's supply. This will not guarantee that the patient is not stockpiling. Compliance with tricyclic prescriptions can be monitored with blood levels, but there are no data on possible differences in therapeutic blood levels for depressed DID patients, compared with people who have nondissociative depressions. Use of the tricyclic antidepressants in DID has disappeared in the 1990s because of the greater safety and lower toxicity of the new compounds. The only tricyclic prescriptions we see in DID anymore are from state-run programs that, as a cost-containment measure, refuse to prescribe the safer serotonergic drugs, that have not yet gone generic.

As with all medications, unusual, idiosyncratic responses to neuroleptics seem to be the norm in DID. I have almost entirely dropped the antipsychotic medications from my practice. I gave one patient a tardive dyskinesia from a prescription for 25 mg of thioridazine at bedtime. Her dyskinesia of the diaphragm and periocular muscles took a number of months to resolve. I think that antipsychotic medications can dampen down auditory hallucinations in some DID patients through nonspecific sedation, which produces an illusion of specific antipsychotic effect in the undiagnosed patient.

The conventional antipsychotics have numerous side effects to which DID patients are often highly sensitive. They do not appear to have any specific antidissociative action. On our inpatient unit, they have been replaced by benzodiazepines, which are safer, more effective, less toxic, and easier to administer. I rarely prescribe nonbenzodiazepine sedatives to any patients, so won't discuss them. DID is a strong relative if not an absolute contraindication to the prescription of barbiturates. In any case, the barbiturates have only a handful of proper indications in medicine. In some patients, we may use a sedating phenothiazine at bedtime or for behavioral containment if there is a problem with benzodiazepine abuse.

The one antipsychotic drug we use regularly in our Dissociative Disorders Program is risperidone, which seems to be very helpful for some patients, especially those I would give the non-*DSM-IV* diagnosis of schizodissociative disorder, as discussed in Chapter Eight. Risperidone is relatively free of side effects, is not addictive, does not produce a high, and does not cause physiological dependence. It seems to tighten up the DID patient who is more unfocused, vague, or idiosyncratic than usual in her thought processes. Whether this is an antidissociative or an antipsychotic effect, I cannot tell. The dosages used are the standard ones for psychosis.

Trazodone is a very useful medication in DID because of its low toxicity, safety in overdose, and lack of abuse potential. I commonly use it as a sedative-hypnotic in dosages up to 400 milligrams at bedtime. It helps with sleep, and reduces headache and traumatic nightmares. Although it is an effective antidepressant in its own right, I commonly give trazodone at bedtime and a serotonergic antidepressant during the day.

Another medication that can be used in DID is buspirone, also because of its safety and low toxicity. It can be used as an anxiolytic (Ross & Matas, 1987), probably as an antidepressant in doses above 40 milligrams per day, and to augment the effects of serotonergic antidepressants. One of its uses is to reduce the benzodiazepine requirements of the patient. DID patients usually require at least 30 milligrams per day, given in two or three divided doses, to obtain any benefit.

This leaves the benzodiazepines. Many but not all DID patients are at high risk of benzodiazepine dependency and abuse prior to integration, and this is a constant problem. Anyone who is going to prescribe these medications to DID patients must have a clear plan of action, in terms of dosage, rate of dosage increase, maximum dosage, and dosage reduction schedule. This need not be spelled out in obsessive detail in advance, but there should be a clear decision tree in place for each contingency.

DID patients can tolerate enormous doses of benzodiazepines. I am impressed by the efficacy of benzodiazepines in easing anxiety, posttraumatic stress symptoms, insomnia, nightmares, acting out, chaotic switching, and demanding behavior. It is striking how DID patients can tolerate rapid increases and decreases in dosage without sedation or withdrawal. It seems that the level of neurotransmitter hyperarousal in some DID inpatients is so high that they do not reach the threshold for sedation until doses above 20 milligrams per day of lorazepam are reached. Even at ultra-high doses, patients may complain of only partial efficacy, even though they do not appear to have prior tolerance or cross-tolerance.

We no longer require ultra-high benzodiazepine regimes on our inpatient unit because of the refinements in our psychotherapy and milieu and behavioral management. We rarely require intramuscular injections of lorazepam or neuropleptics for behavioral management.

When indicated, for inpatient work the benzodiazepines of choice are lorazepam and clonazepam. Lorazepam is the only benzodiazepine that is well absorbed orally, sublingually, and intramuscularly. It is also available in generic form and is inexpensive. If a patient is assessed as being unlikely ever to need an IM injection, then any of the medium- or long-acting benzodiazepines could be chosen. Clonazepam may have superior efficacy for posttraumatic and panic symptoms, and certainly is not less effective, and is therefore indicated for DID, given that most DID inpatients suffer from both PTSD and panic disorder.

A typical prn order for high-dose lorazepam for an inpatient is 2–5 mg po or IM prn up to a maximum of 20 mg/24 hours. This can be given as often as every 30 minutes until the desired effect is achieved. A base dosage of lorazepam can be added to this prn regime at admission or later on depending on requirements. For example, a patient who receives at least 10 mg of prn lorazepam a day for the first week of admission should then get 10 mg/day in divided doses as a non-prn prescription. Prn's are then added onto this as required, and the base dosage is worked upward from there. The goal is to have as few prn's as possible with the maximum benefit. Such regimes are more likely to be required on dissociative disorders units with less experience or for patients admitted to general units.

In prescribing ultra-high doses of benzodiazepines to inpatients, one has to calculate the fastest rate of withdrawal possible, and the maximum dose one is willing to prescribe postdischarge. If this dosage is exceeded during admission, withdrawal to the discharge dose has to begin far enough in advance of the projected discharge date to be physiologically acceptable. It may be difficult to predict either the discharge date, or the acceptable maximum outpatient dosage, but miscalculations may result in a prolonged admission just for dosage reduction.

In some cases, it may be advisable to deliberately oversedate the patient with benzodiazepines if acting out, self-abuse, verbal abuse of staff, and assaultive behavior get too far out of line. This can be done with complete safety, whereas the neuroleptics are fraught with complications and side effects. Ten milligrams of IV diazepam can save the hospital several shifts of constant care nursing, the patient a lot of bruises, and the patient-staff relationship a lot of damage. In some instances, the attending physician may put the patient to sleep until the next morning. This can be achieved with *IV* diazepam supplemented by oral or IM lorazepam should the patient wake up during the night.

I think that IV diazepam is underutilized on general inpatient units in favor of neuroleptics. It is extremely useful in anticholinergic delirium for instance, and for any behavioral disturbance that cannot be managed with more conservative techniques.

Although most DID patients experience panic attacks, it is often not a realistic goal to strive for complete blockade of panic with benzodiazepines, as one would in a nondissociative panic patient (Walker, Norton, & Ross, 1991). The goal is to reduce both general and panic anxiety to a level that allows psychotherapy to be productive.

Two types of clinical trials should be conducted in DID: One is comparison of a given drug in DID patients with the general literature. For example, the blockade of outpatient panic attacks with alprazolam or clonazepam in DID could be compared with the results in the panic disorder literature. The point of the trial would be twofold: to determine the phenomenology of panic in DID, and to compare the response to medication with that in the panic literature. The other trial, which could be combined with the first, is a comparison of active medication and placebo in treatment of DID comorbidity. Simply establishing that clonazepam has a certain efficacy in panic disorder accompanying DID would not be sufficient, because the placebo response rate may be higher in DID patients than in the panic literature.

In view of Loewenstein, Holstein, and Farber's (1988) report of the efficacy of clonazepam in the adjunctive treatment of posttraumatic stress symptoms in DID, and because of its apparent efficacy in a variety of psychiatric disorders, as well as its long half-life, clonazepam is probably the benzodiazepine of choice for a moderate-dose outpatient trial. As these authors point out, specific target symptoms must be identified and tracked, and a subgroup of responders must be identified within the entire DID population.

The other medication that can be useful in DID work is sodium amytal (Dysken, Chang, Casper, & Davis, 1979; Dysken, Kooser, Haraszti, & Davis, 1979; Hall, LeCann, & Schoolar, 1978; Marcol & Trujillo, 1978; Marcum, Wright, & Bissell, 1986; Naples & Hackett, 1978; Pellegrini & Putman, 1984; Perry & Jacobs, 1982; Ruedrich, Chu, & Wadle, 1985). Sodium amytal is a short-acting barbiturate that is administered intravenously. In Canada, I mixed 500 mg in 10 cc of sterile water and administered it at one cc per minute through a #23 butterfly needle. The medication is injected until the patient is drowsy, which may occur by 300 mg and almost always by 500 mg. I never went above 500 mg, although this can be done. Patients can usually walk well by one hour postinfusion, which means they can go for a cup of coffee then go home, although they shouldn't drive till the next day.

If the medication is administered at 50 mg/minute, the only complication that occurs is excessive sedation. When it is administered too fast, the patient will stop breathing and die if respiration is not assisted. I always did my sodium amytal interviews on the inpatient ward, where a crash cart and hospital paging system were immediately available. The excess sedation which sometimes occurred wore off quickly, and I then continued the interview. Patients concurrently taking monoamine oxidase inhibitors may require lower doses of sodium amytal, and may get profoundly sedated by usual doses.

I have not used sodium amytal or intramuscular or oral barbiturate interviews for about four years. This is partly because the rules of the health care system in the United States make IV sodium amytal too expensive, due to the requirement for an anesthesia consult and a physician or nurse anesthetist to administer the drug.

Sodium amytal is a chemical alternative to verbal hypnosis. It seems to overcome resistance by massive anxiolysis combined with anesthesia of cortical function. Sodium amytal is an anesthetic. One uses it to put resistance to sleep. I usually combined a verbal hypnotic induction with the administration of the sodium amytal. I timed suggestions for warmth, relaxation, and hypnosis to the expected onset of the narcosis, which usually starts after 2–3 cc, and is pronounced by 4–6.

Another metaphor for sodium amytal is that it is a battering ram. It gets you into the system. One can use sodium amytal interviews in DID for contacting difficult-to-call-out personalities, and to gain access to otherwise hidden regions of the personality system. The drug can only be used a few times for such purposes because serial administration may create a craving for barbiturates. The physician may create a feedback loop in which the system will reveal an alter only if rewarded with barbiturate.

Like other elements of the therapy described in the first edition of this book, sodium amytal, and all barbiturate and benzodiazepine-facilitated interviews have become unnecessary in the 1990s due to refinement of other treatment methods. In the current legal climate, the possible clinical benefits of IV sodium amytal are outweighed by the medical-legal risks. A sodium amytal interview will always be strongly criticized by the plaintiff's experts in an iatrogenic DID or false-memory lawsuit. Like hypnosis, sodium amytal should not be used for memory recovery.

Like IV diazepam, sodium amytal is underutilized in general psychiatry. It can be used to switch a patient out of catatonia, panic, delirium, and the state we call an alter personality. The effect on delirium is transient and really only switches the patient to a behaviorally quieter delirium. Sodium amytal can be thought of as a state switch facilitator. As interest in dissociation increases, there may be a resurgence of interest in sodium amytal in general psychiatry.

Let me give an example of the use of sodium amytal in inpatient DID work. A rapid-switching patient had been on the ward for months with no therapeutic progress. She had four identified personalities including the host, a helper, an abreacting child, and a self-abusive, grunting, spitting, biting state. She spontaneously switched to the child and abuser a number of times per day, but we were unable to effect any change in the behavior of either alter. Patient and staff were getting drained by the frequent physical restraint, and the repeated X-rays. On one occasion, she was transported to emergency in a neck collar with spinal immobilization.

Not expecting much benefit, and at a complete therapeutic impasse, we tried a sodium amytal interview. The interview readily opened the door into her polyfragmented personality system, and she reached integration within five months. Prior to sodium amytal, she appeared to be untreatable, in fact worse than prior to diagnosis of her DID, and in need of permanent institutionalization. Sodium amytal should be considered when other techniques have failed or when temporary access to an unavailable alter is required. Anyone using the medication should be aware that artifactual dissociated states can be created that do not exist outside the narcosis. Any apparent alter contacted under sodium amytal should then be called out and worked with in the usual way in subsequent sessions.

Another caution must be repeated. Sodium amytal is not truth serum. Patients can lie, confabulate, get lost in fantasy, and distort their memories under sodium amytal, just as under verbal hypnosis. Sodium amytal interviews are useful therapeutically only if they yield information that can be followed up on in later sessions. The overall guiding principle for the use of medication in DID is *first do no harm*. The most harm is probably done through prescriptions for antidepressants, neuroleptics, and benzodiazepines for undiagnosed patients thought to have schizoaffective disorder, atypical bipolar mood disorder, borderline personality with brief psychotic episodes, and similar diagnoses. In diagnosed DID patients, the cost-benefit calculations for medication can be complicated, and can vary from time to time within one patient, and between patients. Medications are always adjunctive for patients receiving specific intensive psychotherapy.

If medication is to be prescribed, it should be given in an adequate dosage for an adequate duration, with adequate definition and tracking of target symptoms, as for any patient. There is no scientific justification for wildly idiosyncratic regimes in the treatment of DID, but there is room for a well-planned empirical trial of any medication, if there is a reasonable rationale for its use for a particular problem. No more rigorous guidelines are possible because no real research on the use of medications in DID has been done. The use of medication in DID has been reviewed by Barkin, Braun, and Kluft (1986).

PHYSICAL RESTRAINTS

The use of formal physical restraints in DID has been discussed in detail by Walter Young (1986). I used them sparingly in Canada and have abandoned them in the 1990s. If physical restraint is required regularly, or considerable physical effort is required, an inpatient admission is probably necessary. Except in the rare emergency, the only form of physical restraint the practitioner should use on an outpatient basis is light holding that requires little effort.

There is a spectrum of physical restraint from lightly restraining an alter's arm from scratching, to straitjacketing and sheeting in a seclusion room. It is easy to hold a child's arm gently but firmly, while repeating that self-abuse is not acceptable, and that the office will be kept safe for everyone. Scratching, light head-banging, hitting oneself with a closed fist, and similar behavior can be analyzed for its motivation and meaning with minimal physical energy expenditure by the therapist. Such behavior may have components of abreaction, Schneiderian passivity experience, or testing the therapist.

The next level of self-abusive behavior may require more vigorous holding by the therapist. The patient may flail aimlessly in a way that is easy to contain. Sometimes one has to work a bit hard in outpatient sessions to restrain a head-banging alter, and a therapist's hand may get bumped between head and wall. Once the behavior escalates above this level, though, there should be at least two therapists in every session, and an admission is imminent. A prolonged requirement for mild outpatient restraint is an indicator of something wrong in the therapy.

On the inpatient unit, acting out should be anticipated and planned for. We try to discourage it by setting firm limits and clear consequences, including possible discharge. I am prepared to charge patients with assault or support nurses in making such charges if I feel it is warranted. DID patients do not have a right to assault staff, and they do not *have* to assault staff. DID is neither a necessary nor a sufficient cause of assault, in hospital or out. Many complex DID patients with severe abuse histories pose no behavioral problems at all.

The best kind of physical restraint is preventive. When prevention fails, planning is the next best strategy. In an inpatient setting, the most common form of physical restraint involves staff members carrying an acting-out patient to the seclusion room, where she receives an IM injection. Unpleasant as this is, and as much as it recreates the abuse scenario, without such physical restraint some patients cannot be treated. We have restrained DID patients in this way who have gone on to stable integration.

Physical restraints are a humane and effective treatment modality without which some people would not have the possibility of curative treatment. As much as one tries to present restraint in this manner as a technique for safety, patients are angry and frightened by it. Feelings about the restraint often must be talked about at length in calmer periods, including after discharge.

CONCLUSION

These are the principal techniques of the middle and late phases of the treatment of DID. The assignment of techniques to different phases is somewhat arbitrary and could have been done differently from the presentation in this book. The main point to remember is that all the interventions described here must be embedded in a sound treatment based primarily on general principles of psychotherapy. In this chapter, I have described some techniques that I no longer use in order to explain my rationale for deemphasizing them, and because other therapists might want to use them more often than I do.

CHAPTER SIXTEEN

Other Therapeutic Considerations

This final chapter includes a number of techniques that are not related closely to specific phases of therapy or that are miscellaneous in nature. This does not imply that they are unimportant, but they do not form the core of treatment. In addition, there is a discussion of integration and postintegration work.

Integration rituals are unique to the psychotherapy of dissociative identity disorder (DID). They can be done using whatever imagery is suitable for both patient and therapist. I have provided a detailed description of the kind of integration ritual I usually do, because many therapists do not know how to do this part of the work. Then the chapter concludes with some final remarks about the treatment and the patients.

HOSPITALIZATION

In our series of 236 cases of DID, 74.6% had received inpatient psychiatric treatment. We did not ask specifically, but most of these admissions were probably prior to diagnosis. Once the diagnosis is made, inpatient admissions can be either elective or emergency, but elective admissions have virtually disappeared in the 1990s due to insurance pressures. The two types of hospitalization can involve quite different purposes, goals, and treatment modalities. Like any effective medical intervention, hospitalization of the DID patient can be beneficial or toxic. Some patients should be kept out of hospital as much as possible, even in the face of severe suicidal ideation, because they regress quickly and extremely on the ward.

Many colleagues are envious of our setup, which involves dedicated separate inpatient and day hospital programs. If we admit our patients, one of four subspecialty doctors is their admitting psychiatrist, and they see their outpatient therapists throughout if they are from the local area. We are available as ongoing postdischarge consultants for patients of other professionals. However having hospital beds can be a mixed blessing. Some patients jockey to get into hospital, and this can become a tiresome power struggle that diverts attention from the therapeutic focus. The jockeying can lead to serious acting out. A nonmedical therapist with no available hospital that the patient can perceive as a safe haven simply sidesteps all of this.

Working on a dedicated inpatient unit or day hospital requires an extensive educational and process-oriented effort. Many hours have to be spent with nursing staff, administration, students, residents, therapists, social workers, chaplains, family members and friends, agency workers, medical consultants, and other professionals. Much of this is nonbillable time for the private practitioner. For me, it is time away from writing and research.

Anyone getting ready to begin intensive inpatient therapy of DID should plan very carefully. Administration must support the project. The patients will place a major strain on the emotional resources of nursing staff and the therapists. This is especially true if the unit is a general adult psychiatric ward without much psychotherapy expertise. Few psychiatric nurses have hired on with a job expectation of working with DID patients. Nurses could earn the same pay with far less emotional expenditure than occurs listening to abuse stories and restraining alters. In addition, they are at risk for compensation injuries. These are real and legitimate concerns.

A further complication occurs when unit staff have unresolved abuse histories of their own, which is common. Cycles of overinvolvement, rejection, staff acting out, disbelieving the diagnosis, and burnout may ensue. Nurses are most at risk for such reactions, not because they are more unstable than other staff, but because they have the most intensive and prolonged exposure to the patients. Nurses cannot retire to the quiet of their private offices after a session. Some nurses, after much trial by fire, function at a high level as DID specialists, and are expert at switching alters, supportive care, limit setting, and reading the dynamics of a situation.

Splitting is a major issue, as Braun (1986a) has pointed out. Splitting occurs within the patient, between patient and staff, staff and staff, other patients and other staff, in fact in all imaginable combinations and permutations. Without processing by staff, chaos will occur. Patients will attempt to recreate the abusive environment of childhood, just as they do in their personal relations outside the hospital. I can't emphasize enough the need to meet and talk, meet and talk, meet and talk. The DID psychiatrist can expect to be the repository of large amounts of negative displaced affect. All of this can stimulate serious reconsideration of career planning.

A small team can handle only a small number of DID inpatients at a time. In Canada, with trained nurses, myself, a half-time resident, a full-time nurse, and a social worker, we could handle two DID cases at a time with reasonable comfort, given our research, other commitments, and less expert skills. Three stretched us. At four, some of us would start burning out within a few months, depending on who was doing the most work, and all would be emotionally blunted and detached from work within six months. To handle more patients, more full-time staff and more specialist nurses would have been required. By comparison, we have had up to 30 inpatients at a time in our program in Texas with less stress than I experienced treating 4 in Canada.

Some DID patients who are higher-functioning can bring up the general tone of the other patients, whereas ones who are particularly prone to splitting, manipulation, and acting out can bring the tone down. Some DID patients spend a lot of time with DID copatients, some stick to themselves. When two or three acting-out patients are on the unit at the same time, a behavioral contest for therapist and nursing attention can begin. Some of this is based on legitimate need in the middle of difficult psychotherapeutic work, but much is not. There is no general rule of thumb about how DID patients are going to affect each other on an inpatient unit.

We expect our patients to follow regular unit guidelines and procedures. They do not have special rooms, they eat with the other patients, and the consequences for unacceptable conduct are generally the same as for other patients. Switching is allowed out on the unit, and child alters are allowed to be in executive control outside sessions. If spontaneous switching occurs, it is not a problem in and of itself. Problems are caused by observable behavior, irrespective of who is in executive control. In one instance, a behavioral problem might be solved by having the host come back, in another by having the host take a break inside.

We specify the amount of individual psychotherapy as much as possible, which is not less than three hours per week. Nursing staff are available for supportive and general nursing care, but not individual psychotherapy. This arrangement limits unrealistic demands for nursing time, reduces switching, and results in a better-organized milieu. The greater the need for behavioral control, the tighter are these rules. Admissions are usually for suicidal ideation, suicide attempts, or internal chaos and anxiety, so out-of-control behavior is always a possibility.

Kluft (1984a, 1991b, 1995) and Ross (1996a) have provided guidelines for inpatient management of DID. Especially on the ward, DID patients must be managed as well as treated. I disagree with Kluft on the advisability of a private room because I think it increases the specialness of the patient, encourages autism, reduces grounding in the present and, in any case,

A variant of group therapy is the inner group therapy described by David Caul (1984). This involves getting the alters to hold conferences and talk with each other, with the therapist acting as a facilitator. Inner group therapy is a cultivated and refined variant of a technique that is used to some extent by all therapists. The concepts and strategies of non-DID group therapy can be brought to bear on the internal group in such work.

The same holds true for family therapy of the adult DID patient (Millette, 1988; Sachs, Frischolz, & Wood, 1988; Schwartz, 1987). The structure, dynamics, and roles of the external family may be recreated in the internal world of the DID family member, and the interactions between external family members observed in family therapy may provide hints about the organization of the DID personality system. The denial and scapegoating of any abuse family are present in the DID case, with the added complication of amnesia in other family members, including at times the perpetrator. I have very little direct experience with formal family therapy of DID and refer the reader to papers by Lynn and Robert Benjamin (1992, 1994a, 1994b, 1994c, 1994d).

Another type of group is the DID support group. In such groups, which have a professional facilitator, patients do not talk about their "stuff," and they limit the conversation to review of daily difficulties, straightforward suggestions, and mutual support. This more informal group can be healthy and helpful, and is suitable for day hospital, intensive outpatient, and regular outpatient phases of therapy. Its benefits have more than made up for any minor complications it may have caused in our hands in Texas.

Group therapy is very useful in the hospital-based treatment of DID, and can also be used at community agencies and in private practice. I have no experience with closed outpatient groups in which the same group members meet for prolonged periods, but I assume that this structure tilts the group toward analysis of group process and away from the rotating individual therapy mode. With selected, more stable, higher functioning outpatients this might work—with our inpatients, who are 50% Medicare and who have a median length of stay of 13 days, much more structure is required. Overall, it is much better to err on the side of too much structure and control in trying to set up and run DID groups, than to foster chaos and regression.

INVOLVING OTHER SUPPORT AGENCIES

The only publication that deals specifically with other agencies is by Roberta Sachs (1986). Besides individual, marital, and family therapists, Sachs lists parenting programs, parents anonymous, incest groups, assertiveness training groups, the clergy, peer networks, alcohol and substance abuse groups, leisure activity or special talent groups, vocational counselors, tutorial groups, and 24-hour hotlines. Except for parents anonymous, we have used all of these modalities and agencies. It is impossible to work with complex multiples and not become involved in interaction with such agencies. Many patients, especially those on disability, depend heavily on them.

To the list, I could add police, lawyers, child-care agencies, universities and colleges, welfare agencies, insurance companies, other hospitals, foster parents, employers, and nonacademic training programs. The list is testimony to the complex, flexible, technically eclectic approach that is required in the treatment of DID. Sometimes the interactions can become extremely complicated because the patient has created an outside system as dissociated and conflicted as her internal world.

A great deal of educational effort is required when the agency or outside person knows the diagnosis, and strategic obfuscation when it is a secret. Some agencies can't handle the diagnosis and cause unnecessary problems for the patient when it is divulged. Other agencies can't accommodate the diagnosis within their bureaucracy, so an alternate diagnosis is required. This requires creative form-filling without outright lying.

I assessed a 15-year-old girl who feels "little" when she is with her 17-year-old boyfriend. By "little" she meant feeling warm, loved, protected, and special. She had no sense of actually being little or younger at such times, and has no dissociative disorder. She felt "little" when with her boyfriend, who beat her when he was drunk.

This girl's mother left when she was three. After that, she slept with her father, was with him all the time, and had a pathologically intimate relationship with him. There was no memory of incest, and no clear evidence of a dissociative barrier in place when I assessed her. At age 7, she was replaced by a pregnant 17-year-old stepmother. By age 14, she was out of the house and into a foster home. The last time she was beaten up by her boyfriend, a month prior to my assessment, she was placed in protective custody in a locked institution, where she remained. She would not press charges against the boyfriend, who had experienced no consequences for his abusive behavior, and who grew up in a home in which his alcoholic father beat his mother. The child-care agency made no gross errors in this case, the girl has been acting out intensively, and no single person was at fault, but the outcome to that date was that the victim was in custody.

When DID patients have to navigate their way through social institutions, they can encounter a great deal of pathological acting out. They may stimulate acting out by social systems that are primed to be abusive. Most of the time, social agencies provide invaluable support—but not always. The therapist may find himself responding to a parallel process in which the agency has the same transference toward him as the patient does. Sometimes the DID patient will have an unrealistic expectation of the therapist's power to influence external systems, and will attribute lack of change to lack of will on the therapist's part. The external interactions may mirror the patient's internal world and conflicts. Most interactions with other agencies are straightforward and can be handled as for any patient. The complications require street smarts and the therapist's understanding of systems. Encounters with pathological social systems can be part of the patient's schooling in how to survive in the modern world and can provide an opportunity to practice nondissociative coping strategies.

INVOLVING SPOUSES, FRIENDS, AND FAMILY

Working with spouses and friends is usually more rewarding than working with agencies because it is more like therapy. Spouses may participate intensively in therapy, or may take an informed and supportive but less involved stance. Either can be satisfactory. The spouses need to know the diagnosis and be educated as to etiology, treatment, and prognosis. In a nonmedical community-based agency that does not work diagnostically, the same thing can be achieved without using the terms DID or personality.

Formal marital therapy can be conducted using the principles that the therapist would use with a nondissociative couple. These must be supplemented with the techniques described in previous chapters if alters are to be worked with directly during the marital sessions. One approach is to wait until the patient is further along in individual therapy, and can work coconsciously in marital therapy without overt switching. I have worked with couples in which the nondissociative spouse, always the man, has been at ease with switches in session and at home. Often the switching has been going on at home for a long time.

Complex transactional sequences can occur. For example, a hypersexual alter can come out and engage in highly provocative and pleasurable foreplay. Suddenly there is a switch to a crying child. The erotically aroused husband begins to comfort the child, hoping for a quick switch back to the sexual state, when suddenly a hostile verbally abusive alter takes executive control and tears a strip off him. Then the host returns, amnesic for the entire sequence, and wonders out loud what is wrong with the husband.

In some couples, there can be both subtle and overt reinforcement of the dissociation by the husband. This can result in an ongoing incestuous relationship between child alters, who perceive the husband as a paternal protector, and the husband, even if the couple has intercourse only when the wife's adult alters are in control. Complex recreations of the original incestuous family can occur. These are compounded if the husband also has DID. In such a couple, both spouses would require individual therapy, and couple therapy would also be necessary. Communication and coordination between the therapists would take a lot of time and processing in such a case.

Another scenario is the couple in which the wife has DID and the husband appears to be understanding and supportive. Sometimes the husband is secretly reinforcing the dissociation by having unhealthy sex with a sadomasochistic alter for whom the host is amnesic: The husband in such couples may deliberately manipulate the system and insert amnesia instructions. Other husbands reinforce the sick role and lack of treatment progress in a more subtle and unwitting fashion because they fear loss of the sexually active alters. Others like playing with the children and give the system the message that the children should never be integrated, and others simply don't want their wives to become independent.

Most of the time, the approach involves educational and supportive work with the husband and intensive individual therapy with the wife. Supportive husbands can also act as effective cotherapists but this may blur their role as husbands, so must be managed carefully. Another marital relationship is one in which overt physical, sexual, and emotional abuse is occurring: this must be dealt with at a practical level as in any nondissociative abusive marriage. One has to track the patient's cognitions and abuse dynamics across the personality system.

Working with couples includes working with homosexual marriages. These are neither inherently wonderful nor inherently unhealthy. Lesbian lovers can be controlling, infantalizing, or abusive. They can also be tender, understanding, and truly intimate. There are extrinsic problems in the homosexual marriage because of society's response to such relationships, but the same basic relationship issues seem to occur as in the heterosexual relationship. The DID member of the couple has trouble with touch, trust, intimacy, orgasm, limits, dependency, and other issues, whether the other member is male or female. I have seen healthy, adult, intimate relationships in lesbian couples with one DID member, and also in which both members have DID.

In one case I treated in Canada, I had a specific problem that was preventing me from discharging the patient. The patient spontaneously awoke every morning with a psychotic alter in executive control. With a little difficulty, the host could be called out by the nursing staff, and the patient could go to work on a day pass. I had to teach her roommate, with whom she had a platonic relationship, to call out the host, and this had to be practiced on overnight passes before discharge was possible. Spouses, friends, and relatives can be taught specific skills like this depending on what problems must be solved.

Friends can act as part-time nursing staff both inside and outside the hospital on an informal basis. Their main function is to be there and to be themselves. I tell friends and relatives this, and emphasize that their role is not to be the primary therapist. Church groups and other support groups may help avoid admissions by caring for the patient during a rough period. These support people sometimes need a little help adjusting their degree of involvement, and in striking a balance between supporting and smothering. Patients need to stand on their own as much as possible.

Some friends provide useful observations and hypotheses about what is going on at different stages of therapy. I treat the friends as intelligent observers who are with the patient far more than I am, and who have made extensive in vivo observations. The DID therapist is usually delighted to get such help, on the grounds that $N + 1$ heads are better than N heads. Consistent with the spirit of the rest of the therapy, spouses, relatives, and friends are involved in the therapy in a flexible, pragmatic fashion. Most of the time I don't feel any need to attempt extremely fancy systemic interpretations of what is going on.

In some cases, relatives can be involved briefly to give the therapist a firsthand feel for the family system. The main work of therapy can then be to help the patient extricate herself from an untreatable, abusive extended family. In some cases, working with the relatives might involve assisting the police in their arrest. There is no standard stance or goal that is taken with every case. I am sketching this aspect of the therapy in brief because it is based primarily on common sense and general principles of therapy. Some cases require only individual sessions with the patient and no direct contact with anyone else.

The only way of working with relatives and friends I won't agree to is the situation in which the wife doesn't want her husband to know she is in therapy. I would not contract for such a therapy except in unusual circumstances, if ever, and I never have. The therapy contract would create a pathological secret, for one thing, and it would make it impossible to deal effectively with crises. If the patient ever had to be admitted, how would that be done? The secret would be very unfair for the husband. Particularly for a male therapist seeing a female patient, such secrecy would give "seeing" the wrong meaning.

The more community supports and informed loved ones can be involved in the patient's life, the better for the patient, therapist, and therapy. As in other disorders, prognosis seems to improve the better the support system.

INTEGRATION AND POSTINTEGRATON WORK

I am discussing developing new behaviors and coping skills, integration, and postintegration work in a single section because they are inextricably intertwined with each other. Integration has several meanings. In one sense, integration is a slow process that occurs throughout therapy and for years afterward. In another sense, no one is ever integrated, because we all experience some degree of dissociation and have all been highly dissociated at some time in our lives. For example, every woman who has given birth has been in an extreme dissociative state.

Integration can also be used as a synonym for fusion. I don't use the term fusion, purely out of personal preference. Integration in the sense of fusion is a discrete event that occurs at a specific moment in time. It is the joining together of two or more alter personalities to become a single entity. Integrations can occur spontaneously, they can be done deliberately by the patient by herself, or they can be assisted by the therapist using a verbal integration ritual. Usually, I integrate only two personalities at a time, and usually, one of the alters is integrated into the host. However, any possible integration pattern may be suitable in any given case.

In polyfragmented cases, large numbers of fragments can be integrated together at one time to form a more substantial unit. These integration products can in turn be integrated together. This process produces increasingly large fusion products that are eventually combined to form a single self. One can imagine a flowchart with a number of levels: there are several hundred entities at the top, increasingly fewer at each level down, and one person at the bottom.

Integrations are intrinsically meaningful psychic events. I remember in medical school having the opportunity to be first assist on a number of intracranial procedures, and second assist on several. During one procedure, the neurosurgeon commented that the moment of peak intensity for him was always the moment of penetration of the dura. I had observed this in the previous operations. The operating theater is usually a sociable place, with technical conversation, as well as bantering and tension-relieving interchanges. The atmosphere is casual, informal, and secular.

In the moments surrounding the opening of the dura, which is a tough membrane surrounding the brain and separating it from the skull, there is a change. Everyone becomes quiet, serious, and still. Then the living brain is revealed, and the operation proceeds. People are moving around and talking again. The penetration of the dura is the only moment of this nature I have experienced in medicine, except for DID integration rituals.

The actual integration ritual is a landmark for a long process that has finally come to fruition. Before two alters can integrate, they must do a large amount of work. They have shared memories, feelings, hopes, and fears, and learned to work together for the benefit of the whole organism. The actual integration is a ceremony like a wedding, which formalizes everything that has gone before, through the courtship, engagement, practical planning, and all the subtle adjustments and negotiations required to get from the couple's first meeting to the wedding day.

Like a wedding, the integration is the end of one phase and the beginning of another. It is not the end of the therapy. I do integration rituals as follows, having spoken with both alters and confirmed that they are ready:

> You're sitting there now as comfortable and relaxed as possible, with your eyes closed, and I want you to listen to the sound of my voice. Just concentrate on the sound of my voice, and that will help you to relax and prepare for the joining together of Susan and Mary. Even now as I speak that process of joining together has begun, Mary opening herself to Susan, and Susan opening herself to Mary, so that the two can be blended and joined together to become one.
>
> Nothing will be lost and nothing will be left behind. Everything that was separate before as a separate Mary and a separate Susan will be blended and joined together to become the one Susan, stronger, more whole, and better able to deal with life. Nothing is lost and nothing is left behind. All the thoughts, and memories,

and feelings, all the skills, and attitudes that were separate before are blending and joining together to become one Susan.

Nothing is lost and nothing is left behind. Susan opening herself to Mary and Mary opening herself to Susan, blending and joining together to become one, a complete and final blending and joining together of everything that was separate before. We are thankful that there was a separate Mary and a separate Susan, because we know that helped Susan survive. All the others that are listening and watching give thanks now, thanks that Mary was there to help, and thanks that she is now blending together with Susan to make a stronger, more complete personality.

That blending and joining together is becoming complete now. A complete and final blending and joining together of everything that was separate before, complete and final and permanent. Nothing left behind and nothing lost. And for this we give thanks. In a few moments now when you open your eyes it will be Susan who is there, and there will never again be a separate Susan and a separate Mary like there was before. There will be the one Susan, stronger, more whole, more complete, and ready for the work that is to come, ready for the future integrations. And this is good.

In just a moment now, you will open your eyes and the integration of Mary and Susan will be complete. As soon as you're ready, you can open your eyes.

The patient then lifts up her head, opens her eyes, and I ask her how it went. If she says that it went well, I congratulate her and ask her what she would like to do now. Some patients like to be alone for a while, some want a hug or a handshake, others may just get on with business. The integration ritual usually is a little bit longer than the text I have just given because of more repetition. So far no patients have complained that they dislike this style of integration ritual.

Not every integration is successful. This is almost always because the integration was premature and not enough preparatory work had been done. A number of different technical difficulties can occur. Sometimes the integration only goes halfway, and the alter gets stuck. In this situation, the host can't take full executive control and neither can the alter. This has happened a couple of times for over 1,000 alters integrated, and I have dealt with it by repeating the ritual, or by reversing it, finding out what the problem was, solving it, and redoing the integration later.

Sometimes alters will leave a few traumatic memories behind. I've never been able to figure out where these are housed. They seem to be held in a general, nonpersonified unconscious and eventually leak back at some point. Various forms of interference can occur, consisting of noise, depersonalization, fear, or other phenomena that break the alters' concentration and discourage them from proceeding. This is usually due to an alter in the background who hasn't been worked with. Sometimes an alter can get cold feet at the last minute, so the integration has to be postponed.

Some therapists make use of trial integrations to desensitize the alters to the process. I don't do this much, but I don't see anything wrong with it. I prefer to do all the necessary work and shoot for permanent fusion the first time, but some patients may not accept this approach. Trial integrations can be set up on a try-it-and-see basis for minutes, hours, or days. The patient can be instructed to deintegrate whenever she feels the need to. This procedure involves some tricky trance logic, because an alter may make an independent decision to deintegrate, which shouldn't be possible if she is integrated. When you ask the deintegrated alter how this happened, she may explain "I just decided" and not be bothered by the logical difficulties. The same applies to the spontaneous breakdown of what were intended to be permanent fusions.

Kluft (1988e) wrote the most comprehensive literature on integration in the 1980s, and this work has not been significantly extended by anyone in the field. Kluft's paper is mandatory reading for everyone treating DID. It builds on his earlier writings on the topic (Kluft, 1982, 1984a, 1985e, 1985g, 1986b). I have reviewed his criteria for integration in Chapter Nine. He has written more extensively than anyone else on the reasons for relapse following complete integration (Kluft, 1986b).

Patients can relapse for a number of reasons. The most common causes are:

1. Discovery of a new layer of alters (not a true relapse).
2. Reemergence of previously fused alters.
3. Creation of new personality states.
4. Feigned integration (also not a true relapse).
5. Recurrence of dissociative symptoms short of emergence of a full alter personality.

One reason for relapse is further trauma. If the trauma is severe enough, the drive to reactivate an old personality or create a new one will be strong. In fact, it may be unethical to remove all the dissociative defenses in the face of known ongoing trauma, because dissociation is such an effective and protective strategy. Any form of trauma can be involved including death, illness, assault, natural disaster, accident, or war.

Patients may feign integration to please the therapist or as a flight into health. The reasons for this have to be discussed and resolved. Sometimes dissociation can be resorted to transiently out of habit, when the patient could have coped nondissociatively with a little more effort. Some patients may not be prepared to face life as single people, and will deliberately relapse with no intention of doing further work. In practice, this could be the best possible outcome for some people. I would personally count such an adaptation as a partial treatment success. Probably the most common cause of relapse is that not enough work has been done in therapy. This need not be anyone's fault, or a sign of procedural error by the therapist.

When new alters are discovered, this can be discouraging; and when there are many layers, it can seem like an infinite regression. The therapist starts wondering if he is being conned, and whether the new layer really has been there since childhood. One patient was like this, and just wasn't getting better the way she should. The reasons for the layers, and the failure to recover, became clear when ongoing sexual abuse was finally disclosed. One should suspect ongoing trauma in a patient who isn't getting better at the expected pace. Extreme layering and an infinite series of alters should raise the question of whether the patient has a large factitious pathway component.

I am not going to write in detail about postintegration therapy because it is the therapy of an individual person. The techniques and principles are no longer dissociative or subspecialist in nature. Much of the work is educational and supportive, with a lot of strategizing and problem solving. Sometimes the integrated patient will have a personality disorder, and sometimes not. If the patient still has posttraumatic stress disorder following an apparent complete integration, this may be a clue to the existence of another layer of alters, and further trauma.

The first year following integration is tough. The patients say that in many ways it is tougher than having DID, and it is certainly very different. When things get difficult, you can't check out and let somebody else handle it. The issues of therapy tend to be broad and general, including sexuality, coping with stress, religion, work, relationships, and common human problems. Upgrading, retraining, and further education may be embarked on. Some relationships will have to end, some will be strengthened, and new ones will form. Some of the abuse-derived cognitive errors will need further work.

As far as termination is concerned, I don't have any fixed time frame, and I don't think there can be one. I personally wouldn't see someone for five years postintegration, because I think others could do that work as effectively, freeing me for dissociative work with someone else. I wouldn't have any problem with a year. Between those two markers, I would go on a case-by-case basis. This is distinct from follow-up, which goes on forever. I am referring to active supportive therapy, which can be hard work. The intensity is not the same as that of the active phase though. The best arrangement is if the patient terminates with the therapist through a gradual reduction in frequency of sessions.

Some patients may have ongoing concurrent psychiatric disorders after the remission of their dissociative disorder. This could include anxiety, mood, or other problems, which then might require treatment in their own right. Again, no special skills in dissociative work will be required. Watching a formerly severely impaired person functioning effectively, and deriving personal fulfillment from her life, is a wonderful reward for the therapist. The recovered DID patient sounds a hopeful note in a disturbed civilization. For example, I have never seen or heard about an integrated DID patient who had an active ongoing substance abuse problem.

CONCLUSION

There are many little tricks and techniques, derived from a welter of schools of psychotherapy, that can be used in the treatment of DID. Every therapist will have his own favorite interventions. The only one I want to comment on in conclusion is chatting. I was struck at a workshop by comments on chatting made by a fellow Canadian, Marlene Hunter. I was also struck by how appreciative the audience was of her remarks. Chatting is an excellent therapeutic intervention. I regularly make small talk with my patients, at various points throughout the sessions. I also tell jokes.

Therapy needs to be a natural conversation between two people. It shouldn't be fettered with unnecessary and rigid rules and rituals. Chatting is good not just for a minute or two at the beginning of a session, but as a normal experience for the patient. It creates comfort and trust, and gives the patient the experience of being regarded as a normal human being. When I reflect on which of my endowments I think is most valuable for my patients, I usually conclude that it is my seeing them as normal people. The best thing a therapist can do for a patient is spontaneously and naturally perceive her as a normal human being. This is how I see DID patients. For me, switching is a natural, normal, human thing to be doing, if you have been severely traumatized as a child.

The phenomenology of DID is not weird or bizarre, if you know how to see it. The patients are intensely human, and their symptoms are rooted in thousands of years of history. This perception is best communicated in idle, everyday conversation, which is therefore not idle. The most important technique in the treatment of DID is not to be caught up in techniques. Although it is necessary to talk about the person with DID as a patient or client, the important thing is that she is neither. The DID patient is a suffering human being who can get better given the correct form of psychoanalysis.

Dissociative Identity Disorder in the Twenty-First Century

The decade beginning in 1980 saw an exponential increase in the diagnosis of dissociative identity disorder in North America. In the 1990s, the same thing began to occur in Europe, Turkey, Japan, Puerto Rico, Australia, and New Zealand. This growth was accompanied by a similar increase in the volume of professional literature, and the number of conferences, workshops, meetings, journals, newsletters, specialized treatment programs, self-help groups, and professional organizations. Yet mainstream academic psychiatry continued to remain relatively untouched by the resurgence of interest in dissociation. What lies ahead in the twenty-first century? Will dissociation fall into obscurity again, as it did early in the twentieth century? Or will it become an established part of mainstream psychiatry, psychology, and social work, on an equal footing with anxiety and depression?

I predict with more confidence than I did in 1989 that the latter outcome will occur. It appears that undiagnosed DID affects about 5% of inpatients on general adult psychiatry units: This means that there is a large reservoir of undiagnosed cases currently in the mental health system. These patients are probably high utilizers of mental health care services without consistent benefit from conventional treatment. I predict that the positive cost-benefit of the diagnosis and treatment of DID will be appreciated by managed care companies before it is finally conceded by academia. The definitive research supporting this conclusion will be generated in the private sector through joint ventures between clinicians, hospital chains, and insurers.

Over the next 10 years, the already substantial body of clinical research on dissociation will be much expanded, and the trauma theme will become more predominant throughout the mental health field. If DID and trauma do enter the mainstream in this way, there will be a number of effects on general psychiatry. One is that the funding for psychotherapy outcome research will increase. DID will provide a much-needed counter to the excessive enthusiasm for biomedical reductionist psychiatry that has dominated the 1980s and 1990s. From a public health, societal point of view, bioreductionist psychiatry has been overfunded in the past two decades. DID will stimulate new thinking in biological psychiatry, and will steer research toward the psychobiology of trauma, and away from the endogenous biology of separate psychiatric diseases.

The study of dissociation could result in revised exclusion criteria for clinical drug trials, studies of biological markers, family studies, and a wide range of research in mental health. It is not good science to fail to mention severe, chronic childhood trauma as either an inclusion or exclusion criterion for a drug study. I suspect that much of the research data gathered by psychiatry over the past 20 years is contaminated by the inclusion of unrecognized trauma-dissociation patients. Exclusion of these people from heterogeneous groups of subjects would result in cleaner data.

DID will help bring the focus in psychiatry back onto real childhood events that would be disturbing and traumatic for anyone who experienced them. The field has expended too much energy on endogenous biological and psychological models. A willingness to diagnose and treat DID on the part of academic psychiatry might also help bridge the chasm between university-based physicians and community-based nonmedical mental health professionals. DID is a severe mental illness with a psychosocial etiology, and therefore it straddles both domains.

Specialists in dissociative disorders should look outside psychiatry to establish collaborations with anthropologists and other researchers who have studied phenomena related to North American clinical DID. For example, ideas of Luria (1968/1987, 1972/1987) and Jaynes (1976) could stimulate interesting approaches to clinical dissociation, especially disorders of memory and auditory hallucinations.

If dissociation falls back into obscurity and the preceding predictions turn out to have been wishful thinking, that will be unfortunate because DID patients reveal what is happening in our society at large. We should not forget the fragmentation that so many men and women with DID have healed in therapy, because our culture as a whole suffers from DID, and is in need of treatment. The DID patient can teach us about fragmentation in our history, our worldview, and ourselves.

The Dissociative Disorders Interview Schedule— DSM-IV Version

The Dissociative Disorders Interview Schedule (DDIS) is a highly structured interview that makes *DSM-IV* diagnoses of somatization disorder, borderline personality disorder, and major depressive disorder, as well as all the dissociative disorders. It inquires about positive symptoms of schizophrenia, secondary features of DID, extrasensory experiences, substance abuse, and other items relevant to the dissociative disorders.

The DDIS can usually be administered in 30 to 45 minutes.

CONSENT FORM FOR THE DISSOCIATIVE DISORDERS INTERVIEW SCHEDULE

I agree to be interviewed as part of a research project on dissociative disorders. Dissociative disorders involve problems with memory.

I understand that the interview contains some personal questions about my sexual and psychological history; however, all information that I give will be kept confidential. My name will not appear on the research questionnaire.

I understand that my answers will have no direct effect on how I am treated in the future.

I understand that the overall results of this research will be published and these results will be available to authorities or therapists involved with me.

I understand that the interviewer and other researchers cannot offer me treatment.

I understand that the purpose of this interview is for research and that I cannot expect any direct benefit to myself other than knowing that I have helped the researchers understand dissociative disorders better.

I agree to answer the interviewer's questions as well as I can but I know that I am free not to answer any particular questions I do not want to answer.

Although I have signed my name to this form, I know that it will be kept separate from my answers and that my answers cannot be connected to my name, except by the interviewer and his/her research colleagues.

I also understand that I may be asked to participate in further dissociative disorders interviews in the future, but that I will be free to say no. If I do say no, this will have no consequences for me and any authorities or therapists involved with me will not be told of my decision not to be interviewed again.

Signed: _____   Witness: _____

Date: _____

DEMOGRAPHIC DATA FOR DISSOCIATIVE DISORDERS INTERVIEW SCHEDULE

Age: [   ]

Sex: Male = 1   Female = 2   [   ]

Marital   Single = 1   Married (including common-law) = 2

Status: Separated/Divorced = 3   Widowed = 4   [   ]

Number of Children: (If no children, score 0)   [   ]

Occupational Status: Employed = 1   Unemployed = 2   [   ]

Have you been in jail in the past?

Yes = 1   No = 2   Unsure = 3   [   ]

Physical diagnoses currently active: [   ]

                                                              [   ]

                                                              [   ]

Current and past diagnoses must consist of written diagnoses provided by the referring physician or available in the patient's chart (give *DSM-IV* codes if possible, if not write *DSM-IV* diagnoses to the right of the brackets).

Psychiatric diagnoses currently active: [   ]

                                                              [   ]

                                                              [   ]

Psychiatric diagnoses currently in remission: [   ]

                                                        [   ]

DISSOCIATIVE DISORDERS INTERVIEW SCHEDULE
DSM-IV VERSION

Questions in the Dissociative Disorders Interview Schedule must be asked in the order they occur in the Schedule. All the items in the Schedule, including all the items in the *DSM-IV* diagnostic criteria for dissociative disorders, somatization disorder, and borderline personality disorder must be inquired about. The wording of the questions should be exactly as written in order to standardize the information gathered by different interviewers. The interviewer should not read the section headings aloud. The interviewer should open the interview by thanking the subject for his/her participation and then should say:

"Most of the questions I will ask can be answered Yes, No, or Unsure. A few of the questions have different answers and I will explain those as we go along."

I. *Somatic Complaints*

1. Do you suffer from headaches?
Yes = 1 No = 2 Unsure = 3   [ ]

If subject answered No to question 1, go to question 3:

2. Have you been told by a doctor that you have migraine headaches?
Yes = 1 No = 2 Unsure = 3   [ ]

Interviewer should read the following to the subject:

"I am going to ask you about a series of physical symptoms now. To count a symptom as present and to answer yes to these questions, the following must be met:

a) No physical disorder or medical condition has been found to account for the symptom.
b) If there is a related general medical condition, the problems the symptom causes in terms of occupational or social impairment are more than would be expected.
c) The symptom is not caused by a street drug or medication."

Interviewer should now ask the subject, "Have you ever had the following physical symptoms for which doctors could find no physical explanation?"

The interviewer should review criteria a–c for the subject immediately following the first positive response to ensure that the subject has understood.

3. Abdominal pain (other than when menstruating)
Yes = 1 No = 2 Unsure = 3   [ ]
4. Nausea (other than motion sickness)
Yes = 1 No = 2 Unsure = 3   [ ]
5. Vomiting (other than motion sickness)
Yes = 1 No = 2 Unsure = 3   [ ]
6. Bloating (gassy)
Yes = 1 No = 2 Unsure = 3   [ ]
7. Diarrhea
Yes = 1 No = 2 Unsure = 3   [ ]
8. Intolerance of (gets sick on) several different foods
Yes = 1 No = 2 Unsure = 3   [ ]
9. Back pain
Yes = 1 No = 2 Unsure = 3   [ ]
10. Joint pain
Yes = 1 No = 2 Unsure = 3   [ ]
11. Pain in extremities (the hands and feet)
Yes = 1 No = 2 Unsure = 3   [ ]
12. Pain in genitals other than during intercourse
Yes = 1 No = 2 Unsure = 3   [ ]
13. Pain during urination
Yes = 1 No = 2 Unsure = 3   [ ]
14. Other pain (other than headaches)
Yes = 1 No = 2 Unsure = 3   [ ]
15. Shortness of breath when not exerting oneself
Yes = 1 No = 2 Unsure = 3   [ ]
16. Palpitations (a feeling that your heart is
beating very strongly)
Yes = 1 No = 2 Unsure = 3   [ ]
17. Chest pain
Yes = 1 No = 2 Unsure = 3   [ ]
18. Dizziness
Yes = 1 No = 2 Unsure = 3   [ ]
19. Difficulty swallowing
Yes = 1 No = 2 Unsure = 3   [ ]
20. Loss of voice
Yes = 1 No = 2 Unsure = 3   [ ]
21. Deafness
Yes = 1 No = 2 Unsure = 3   [ ]
22. Double vision
Yes = 1 No = 2 Unsure = 3   [ ]
23. Blurred vision
Yes = 1 No = 2 Unsure = 3   [ ]
24. Blindness
Yes = 1 No = 2 Unsure = 3   [ ]
25. Fainting or loss of consciousness
Yes = 1 No = 2 Unsure = 3   [ ]
26. Amnesia
Yes = 1 No = 2 Unsure = 3   [ ]

27. Seizure or convulsion
Yes = 1 No = 2 Unsure = 3   [ ]
28. Trouble walking
Yes = 1 No = 2 Unsure = 3   [ ]
29. Paralysis or muscle weakness
Yes = 1 No = 2 Unsure = 3   [ ]
30. Urinary retention or difficulty urinating
Yes = 1 No = 2 Unsure = 3   [ ]
31. Long periods with no sexual desire
Yes = 1 No = 2 Unsure = 3   [ ]
32. Pain during intercourse
Yes = 1 No = 2 Unsure = 3   [ ]

**Note: If subject is male ask question 33 and
then go to question 38. If female, go to question 34.**

33. Impotence
Yes = 1 No = 2 Unsure = 3   [ ]
34. Irregular menstrual periods
Yes = 1 No = 2 Unsure = 3   [ ]
35. Painful menstruation
Yes = 1 No = 2 Unsure = 3   [ ]
36. Excessive menstrual bleeding
Yes = 1 No = 2 Unsure = 3   [ ]
37. Vomiting throughout pregnancy
Yes = 1 No = 2 Unsure = 3   [ ]
38. Have you had many physical symptoms over a
period of several years beginning before the age
of 30 that resulted in your seeking treatment or which
caused occupational or social impairment?
Yes = 1 No = 2 Unsure = 3   [ ]
39. Were the physical symptoms you described
deliberately produced by you?
Yes = 1 No = 2 Unsure = 3   [ ]

II. *Substance Abuse*
40. Have you ever had a drinking problem?
Yes = 1 No = 2 Unsure = 3   [ ]
41. Have you ever used street drugs extensively?
Yes = 1 No = 2 Unsure = 3   [ ]
42. Have you ever injected drugs intravenously?
Yes = 1 No = 2 Unsure = 3   [ ]
43. Have you ever had treatment for a drug or
alcohol problem?
Yes = 1 No = 2 Unsure = 3   [ ]

III. *Psychiatric History*
44. Have you ever had treatment for an emotional problem
or mental disorder?
Yes = 1 No = 2 Unsure = 3   [ ]

45. Do you know what psychiatric diagnoses, if any, you have been given in the past?
Yes = 1 No = 2 Unsure = 3   [   ]

46. Have you ever been diagnosed as having:
  a) depression   [   ]
  b) mania   [   ]
  c) schizophrenia   [   ]
  d) anxiety disorder   [   ]
  e) other psychiatric disorder (specify) _____   [   ]
     Yes = 1 No = 2 Unsure = 3

If subject did not volunteer a diagnosis for 46(e) go to question 48.

47. If the subject volunteered diagnoses for (e), did the subject volunteer any of the following:
  a) dissociative amnesia   [   ]
  b) dissociative fugue   [   ]
  c) dissociative identity disorder (multiple personality disorder)   [   ]
  d) depersonalization disorder   [   ]
  e) dissociative disorder not otherwise specified   [   ]
     Yes = 1 No = 2 Unsure = 3

48. Have you ever been prescribed psychiatric medication?
Yes = 1 No = 2 Unsure = 3   [   ]

49. Have you ever been prescribed one of the following medications?
  a) antipsychotic   [   ]
  b) antidepressant   [   ]
  c) lithium   [   ]
  d) antianxiety or sleeping medication   [   ]
  e) other (specify) _____   [   ]
     Yes = 1 No = 2 Unsure = 3

50. Have you ever received ECT, also know as electroshock treatment?
Yes = 1 No = 2 Unsure = 3   [   ]

51. Have you ever had therapy for emotional, family, or psychological problems, for more than 5 sessions in one course of treatment?
Yes = 1 No = 2 Unsure = 3   [   ]

52. How many therapists, if any, have you seen for emotional problems or mental illness in your life?
Unsure = 89   [   ]

If subject answered No to both questions 51 and 52, go to question 54.

53. Have you ever had a treatment for an emotional problem or mental illness which was ineffective?
Yes = 1 No = 2 Unsure = 3   [   ]

IV. *Major Depressive Episode*

The purpose of this section is to determine whether the subject has ever had or currently has a major depressive episode.

54. Have you ever had a period of depressed mood lasting at least two weeks in which you felt depressed, blue, hopeless, low, or down in the dumps?
Yes = 1 No = 2 Unsure = 3   [ ]

If subject answered No to question 54, go to question 62.

If subject answered Yes or Unsure, interviewer should ask, "During this period did you experience the following symptoms nearly every day for at least two weeks?"

55. Poor appetite or significant weight loss (when not dieting) or increased appetite or significant weight gain.
Yes = 1 No = 2 Unsure = 3   [ ]
56. Sleeping too little or too much.
Yes = 1 No = 2 Unsure = 3   [ ]
57. Being physically and mentally slowed down, or agitated to the point where it was noticeable to other people.
Yes = 1 No = 2 Unsure = 3   [ ]
58. Loss of interest or pleasure in usual activities, or decrease in sexual drive.
Yes = 1 No = 2 Unsure = 3   [ ]
59. Loss of energy or fatigue nearly every day.
Yes = 1 No = 2 Unsure = 3   [ ]
60. Feelings of worthlessness, self-reproach, or excessive or inappropriate guilt nearly every day.
Yes = 1 No = 2 Unsure = 3   [ ]
61. Difficulty concentrating or difficulty making decisions.
Yes = 1 No = 2 Unsure = 3   [ ]
62. Recurrent thoughts of death, suicidal thoughts, wishes to be dead, or attempted suicide.
Yes = 1 No = 2 Unsure = 3   [ ]
If you have made a suicide attempt, did you:
a) take an overdose   [ ]
b) slash your wrists or other body areas   [ ]
c) inflict cigarette burns or other self injuries   [ ]
d) use a gun, knife, or other weapons   [ ]
e) attempt hanging   [ ]
f) use another method   [ ]
      Yes = 1   No = 2   Unsure = 3

63. If you have had an episode of depression as
described above, is it: [   ]
currently active, first occurrence = 1
currently in remission   = 2
currently active, recurrence   = 3
uncertain   = 4
due to a specific organic cause   = 5

V. *Positive Symptoms of Schizophrenia (Schneiderian First-Rank
Symptoms)*

64. Have you ever experienced the following
Yes = 1 No = 2 Unsure = 3
a) voices arguing in your head   [   ]
b) voices commenting on your actions   [   ]
c) having your feelings made or controlled by
someone or something outside you   [   ]
d) having your thoughts made or controlled by
someone or something outside you   [   ]
e) having your actions made or controlled by
someone or something outside you   [   ]
f) influences from outside you playing on or
affecting your body such as some external
force or power   [   ]
g) having thoughts taken out of your mind   [   ]
h) thinking thoughts which seemed to be someone
else's   [   ]
i) hearing your thoughts out loud   [   ]
j) other people being able to hear your thoughts as
if they're out loud   [   ]
k) thoughts of a delusional nature that were very
out of touch with reality   [   ]

**If subject answered No to all schizophrenia
symptoms, go to question 67, otherwise,
interviewer should ask:**

"If you have experienced any of the above symptoms
are they clearly limited to one of the following:"

65. Occurred only under the influence of drugs, or
alcohol.
Yes = 1 No = 2 Unsure = 3   [   ]
66. Occurred only during a major depressive episode.
Yes = 1 No = 2 Unsure = 3   [   ]

VI. *Trances, Sleepwalking, Childhood Companions*
67. Have you ever walked in your sleep?
Yes = 1 No = 2 Unsure = 3   [   ]

**If subject answered No to question 67, go to
question 69.**

68. If you have walked in your sleep, how many
times roughly?
1–10 = 1 11–50 = 2 > 50 = 3 Unsure = 4   [ ]

69. Have you ever had a trancelike episode where
you stare off into space, lose awareness of what
is going on around you and lose track of time?
Yes = 1 No = 2 Unsure = 3   [ ]

**If subject answered No to question 69, go to
question 71.**

70. If you have had this experience, how many times,
roughly?
1–10 = 1   11–50 = 2   >50 = 3   Unsure = 4   [ ]

71. Did you have imaginary playmates as a child?
Yes = 1 No = 2 Unsure = 3   [ ]

**If subject answered No to question 71, go to
question 73.**

72. If you had imaginary playmates, how old were you
when they stopped?
Unsure = 0   [ ]

**If subject still has imaginary companions,
score subject's current age.**

VII. *Childhood Abuse*
73. Were you physically abused as a child or adolescent?
Yes = 1 No = 2 Unsure = 3   [ ]

**If subject answered No to question 73, go to
question 78.**

74. Was the physical abuse independent of episodes
of sexual abuse?
Yes = 1 No = 2 Unsure = 3   [ ]

75. If you were physically abused, was it by:
a) father   [ ]
b) mother   [ ]
c) stepfather   [ ]
d) stepmother   [ ]
e) brother   [ ]
f) sister   [ ]
g) male relative   [ ]
h) female relative   [ ]
i) other male   [ ]
j) other female   [ ]
Yes = 1 No = 2 Unsure = 3

76. If you were physically abused, how old were you
when it started?
Unsure = 89. **If less than 1 year, score 0.**   [ ]

77. If you were physically abused how old were you
when it stopped?
Unsure = 89 **If less than 1 year, score 0. If
ongoing, score subject's current age.**   [   ]
78. Were you sexually abused as a child or adolescent?
Sexual abuse includes rape, or any type of unwanted
sexual touching or fondling that you may have
experienced.
Yes = 1 No = 2 Unsure = 3   [   ]

**If the subject answered No to question 78, go
to question 85. If the subject answered Yes or
Unsure to question 78, the interviewer should
state the following before asking further
questions on sexual abuse:**

"The following questions concern detailed examples
of the types of sexual abuse you may or may not have
experienced. Because of the explicit nature of these
questions, you have the option not to answer any or all
of them. The reason I am asking these questions is to
try to determine the severity of the abuse that you
experienced. You may answer Yes, No, Unsure or not
give an answer to each question."

79. If you were sexually abused was it by:
  a) father   [   ]
  b) mother   [   ]
  c) stepfather   [   ]
  d) stepmother   [   ]
  e) brother   [   ]
  f) sister   [   ]
  g) male relative   [   ]
  h) female relative   [   ]
  i) other male   [   ]
  j) other female   [   ]
  Yes = 1 No = 2 Unsure = 3 No Answer = 4

**If subject is female, skip question 80. If male, skip
question 81.**

80. If you are male and were sexually abused, did the abuse
involve:
  a) hand to genital touching   [   ]
  b) other types of fondling   [   ]
  c) intercourse with a female   [   ]
  d) anal intercourse with a male—you active   [   ]
  e) you performing oral sex on a male   [   ]
  f) you performing oral sex on a female   [   ]
  g) oral sex done to you by a male   [   ]

    h) oral sex done to you by a female [ ]
    i) anal intercourse—you passive [ ]
    j) enforced sex with animals [ ]
    k) pornographic photography [ ]
    l) other (specify) _____ [ ]
    Yes = 1 No = 2 Unsure = 3 No Answer = 4

81. If you are female and were sexually abused, did the abuse involve:
    a) hand to genital touching [ ]
    b) other types of fondling [ ]
    c) intercourse with a male [ ]
    d) simulated intercourse with a female [ ]
    e) you performing oral sex on a male [ ]
    f) you performing oral sex on a female [ ]
    g) oral sex done to you by a male [ ]
    h) oral sex done to you by a female [ ]
    i) anal intercourse with a male [ ]
    j) enforced sex with animals [ ]
    k) pornographic photography [ ]
    l) other (specify) _____ [ ]
    Yes = 1 No = 2 Unsure = 3 No Answer = 4

82. If you were sexually abused, how old were you when it started?
    Unsure = 89. **If less than 1 year, score 0.** [ ]

83. If you were sexually abused, how old were you when it stopped?
    Unsure = 89 **If less than 1 year, score 0. If ongoing, score subject's current age.** [ ]

84. How many separate incidents of sexual abuse were you subjected to up until the age of 18?
    1–5 = 1 6–10 = 2 11–50 = 3 > 50 = 4
    Unsure = 5 [ ]

85. How many separate incidents of sexual abuse were you subjected to after the age of 18?
    0 = 1 1–5 = 2 6–10 = 3 11–50 = 4 > 50 = 5
    Unsure = 6 [ ]

VIII. *Features Associated with Dissociative Identity Disorder*

For questions 86–95, if subject answers Yes, ask subject to specify whether it is occasionally, fairly often, or frequently, excluding question 93.

86. Have you ever noticed that things are missing from your personal possessions or where you live?
    Never = 1 Occasionally = 2 Fairly Often = 3
    Frequently = 4 Unsure = 5 [ ]

87. Have you ever noticed that there are things present where you live, and you don't know where they came

from or how they got there (e.g., clothes jewelry, books, furniture)?
Never = 1 Occasionally = 2 Fairly Often = 3
Frequently = 4 Unsure = 5   [ ]

88. Have you ever noticed that your handwriting changes drastically or that there are things around in handwriting you don't recognize?
Never = 1 Occasionally = 2 Fairly Often = 3
Frequently = 4 Unsure = 5   [ ]

89. Do people ever come up and talk to you as if they know you but you don't know them, or only know them faintly?
Never = 1 Occasionally = 2 Fairly Often = 3
Frequently = 4 Unsure = 5   [ ]

90. Do people ever tell you about things you've done or said, that you can't remember, not counting times you have been using drugs or alcohol?
Never = 1 Occasionally = 2 Fairly Often = 3
Frequently = 4 Unsure = 5   [ ]

91. Do you ever have blank spells or periods of missing time that you can't remember, not counting times you have been using drugs or alcohol?
Never = 1 Occasionally = 2 Fairly Often = 3
Frequently = 4 Unsure = 5   [ ]

92. Do you ever find yourself coming to in an unfamiliar place, wide awake, not sure how you got there, and not sure what has been happening for the past while, not counting times when you have been using drugs or alcohol?
Never = 1 Occasionally = 2 Fairly Often = 3
Frequently = 4 Unsure = 5   [ ]

93. Are there large parts of your childhood after age 5 which you can't remember?
Yes = 1 No = 2 Unsure = 3   [ ]

94. Do you ever have memories come back to you all of a sudden, in a flood or like flashbacks?
Never = 1 Occasionally = 2 Fairly Often = 3
Frequently = 4 Unsure = 5   [ ]

95. Do you ever have long periods when you feel unreal, as if in a dream, or as if you're not really there, not counting when you are using drugs or alcohol?
Never = 1 Occasionally = 2 Fairly Often = 3
Frequently = 4 Unsure = 5   [ ]

96. Do you hear voices talking to you sometimes or talking inside your head?
Yes = 1 No = 2 Unsure = 3   [ ]

If subject answered No to question 96, go to question 98.

97. If you hear voices, do they seem to come from inside you?
Yes = 1 No = 2 Unsure = 3   [ ]
98. Do you ever speak about yourself as "we" or "us"?
Yes = 1 No = 2 Unsure = 3   [ ]
99. Do you ever feel that there is another person or persons inside you?
Yes = 1 No = 2 Unsure = 3   [ ]

If subject answered No to question 99, go to question 102.

100. Is there another person or persons inside you that has a name?
Yes = 1 No = 2 Unsure = 3   [ ]
101. If there is another person inside you, does he or she ever come out and take control of your body?
Yes = 1 No = 2 Unsure = 3   [ ]

IX. *Supernatural/Possession/ESP Experiences/Cults*
102. Have you ever had any kind of supernatural experience?
Yes = 1 No = 2 Unsure = 3   [ ]
103. Have you ever had any extrasensory perception experiences such as:
a) mental telepathy   [ ]
b) seeing the future while awake   [ ]
c) moving objects with your mind   [ ]
d) seeing the future in dreams   [ ]
e) déjà vu (the feeling that what is happening to you has happened before)   [ ]
f) other (specify) _____   [ ]
Yes = 1 No = 2 Unsure = 3
104. Have you ever felt you were possessed by a:
a) demon   [ ]
b) dead person   [ ]
c) living person   [ ]
d) some other power or force   [ ]
Yes = 1 No = 2 Unsure = 3
105. Have you ever had any contact with:
a) ghosts   [ ]
b) poltergeists (cause noises or objects to move around)   [ ]
c) spirits of any kind   [ ]
Yes = 1 No = 2 Unsure = 3
106. Have you ever felt you know something about past lives or incarnations of yours?
Yes = 1 No = 2 Unsure = 3   [ ]
107. Have you ever been involved in cult activities?
Yes = 1 No = 2 Unsure = 3   [ ]

X. *Borderline Personality Disorder*

> **Interviewer should state,** "For the following nine questions, please answer Yes only if you have been this way much of the time for much of your life. Have you experienced":

108. Impulsive or unpredictable behavior in at least two areas that are potentially self-damaging, e.g., spending, sex, substance use, reckless driving, binge eating?
Yes = 1 No = 2 Unsure = 3   [ ]

109. A pattern of intense, unstable personal relationships characterized by your alternating between extremes of positive and negative feelings?
Yes = 1 No = 2 Unsure = 3   [ ]

110. Intense anger or lack of control of anger, e.g., frequent displays of temper, constant anger, recurrent physical fights?
Yes = 1 No = 2 Unsure = 3   [ ]

111. Unstable identity, self-image, or sense of self.
Yes = 1 No = 2 Unsure = 3   [ ]

112. Frequent mood swings: noticeable shifts from normal mood to depression, irritability or anxiety, usually lasting only a few hours and rarely more than a few days?
Yes = 1 No = 2 Unsure = 3   [ ]

113. Frantic efforts to avoid real or imagined abandonment?
Yes = 1 No = 2 Unsure = 3   [ ]

114. Recurrent suicidal behavior, e.g., suicidal attempts, self-mutilation, or threats of suicide?
Yes = 1 No = 2 Unsure = 3   [ ]

115. Chronic feelings of emptiness?
Yes = 1 No = 2 Unsure = 3   [ ]

116. Transient, stress-related paranoia or severe dissociative symptoms?
Yes = 1 No = 2 Unsure = 3   [ ]

XI. *Dissociative Amnesia*

117. Have you ever experienced inability to recall important personal information, particularly of a traumatic or stressful nature, that is too extensive to be explained by ordinary forgetfulness?
Yes = 1 No = 2 Unsure = 3   [ ]

If subject answered No or Unsure to question 117, go to 120.

118. If you answered Yes to the previous question was the disturbance due to known physical disorder (e.g.,

blackouts during alcohol intoxication, or stroke),
substance abuse, or another psychiatric disorder?
Yes = 1 No = 2   Unsure = 3   [ ]
119. Did the symptoms cause you significant distress
or impairment in social or occupational function?
Yes = 1 No = 2 Unsure = 3   [ ]

XII. *Dissociative Fugue*
120. Have you ever experienced sudden unexpected
travel away from your home or customary place of
work, with inability to recall your past?
Yes = 1 No = 2 Unsure = 3   [ ]
121. During this period, did you experience confusion
about your identity or assume a partial or complete
new identity?
Yes = 1 No = 2 Unsure = 3   [ ]

**If subject answered No to one or both of
questions 120 and 121, go to 124.**

122. If you answered Yes to both the previous two
questions was the disturbance due to a known
physical disorder (e.g., blackouts during alcohol
intoxication or stroke)?
Yes = 1 No = 2 Unsure = 3   [ ]
123. Did the symptoms cause you significant distress
or impairment in occupational or social function?
Yes = 1 No = 2 Unsure = 3   [ ]

XIII. *Depersonalization Disorder*
124. **Interviewer should say,** "I am now going to ask you a
series of questions about depersonalization.
Depersonalization means feeling unreal, feeling as
if you're in a dream, seeing yourself from outside
your body or similar experiences."
a) Have you had one or more episodes of
depersonalization sufficient to cause
problems in your work or social life?
Yes = 1 No = 2 Unsure = 3   [ ]
b) Have you ever had the feeling that your feet
and hands or other parts of your body have
changed in size?
Yes = 1 No = 2 Unsure = 3   [ ]
c) Have you ever experienced seeing yourself
from outside your body?
Yes = 1 No = 2 Unsure = 3   [ ]
d) Have you ever had a strong feeling of
unreality that lasted for a period of time, not
counting when you are using drugs or alcohol?
Yes = 1 No = 2 Unsure = 3   [ ]

**If subject did not answer Yes to any of
124 (a)–(d), go to question 127.**

125. If you answered Yes to any of the previous
     questions about depersonalization was the
     disturbance due to another disorder, such as
     Schizophrenia, Anxiety Disorder, or epilepsy,
     substance abuse, or a general medical condition?
     Yes = 1 No = 2 Unsure = 3   [ ]
126. During the periods of depersonalization, did
     you stay in touch with reality and maintain
     your ability to think rationally?
     Yes = 1 No = 2 Unsure = 3   [ ]

XIV. *Dissociative Identity Disorder*
127. Have you ever felt like there are two or more distinct
     identities or personalities within yourself, each of which
     has its own pattern of perceiving, thinking, and relating
     to self and others?
     Yes = 1 No = 2 Unsure = 3   [ ]

**If subject answered No to question 127, go to
question 131.**

128. Do at least two of the identities or personalities
     recurrently take control of your behavior?
     Yes = 1 No = 2 Unsure = 3   [ ]

**Interviewer should score question 129 based
on the subject's response to Question 117,
and should not read question 129 aloud.**

129. Have you experienced inability to recall important
     personal information that is too extensive to be
     explained by ordinary forgetfulness?
     Yes = 1 No = 2 Unsure = 3   [ ]
130. Is the problem with different identities or
     personalities due to substance abuse (e.g.,
     alcohol blackouts) or a general medical condition?
     Yes = 1 No = 2 Unsure = 3   [ ]

XV. *Dissociative Disorder Not Otherwise Specified*
131. Subject appears to have a dissociative disorder
     but does not satisfy the criteria for a specific
     dissociative disorder. Examples include trancelike
     states, derealization unaccompanied by
     depersonalization, and those more prolonged
     dissociated states that may occur in persons who
     have been subjected to periods of prolonged and intense
     coercive persuasion (brainwashing, thought reform, and
     indoctrination while captive).
     Yes = 1 No = 2 Unsure = 3   [ ]

XVI. *Concluding Item*
    132. During the interview, did the subject display unusual,
        illogical, or idiosyncratic thought processes?
        Yes = 1 No = 2 Unsure = 3   [   ]

        **Interviewer should make a brief concluding
        statement telling subject that there are no more
        questions and thanking the subject for his/her
        participation.**

SCORING THE DISSOCIATIVE DISORDERS INTERVIEW SCHEDULE

The Dissociative Disorders Interview Schedule (DDIS), is divided into 16 sections. Each section is scored independently. All *DSM-IV* diagnoses are made according to the rules in *DSM-IV.*

There is no total score for the entire interview. However, average scores for 166 dissociative identity disorder (DID) subjects on selected subsections are given below (Ross, Anderson, et al., 1992).

Following presentation of scoring rules for each section, you will find a description of a typical profile for a DID patient. The DDIS has been administered to over 500 subjects with a confirmed false positive diagnosis of DID in 1% of cases. The sensitivity of the DDIS for the diagnosis of DID in 196 clinically diagnosed cases was 95.4%.

I. *Somatic Complaints*

This is scored according to *DSM-IV* rules. To receive a diagnosis of somatization disorder by *DSM-IV* rules, one must be positive for at least four pain symptoms, two gastrointestinal symptoms, one sexual symptom, and one pseudoneurological symptom:

1. Pain—questions 9–14, 17, 32, 35
2. Gastrointestinal—questions 3–8
3. Sexual—questions 31, 33–37
4. Pseudoneurological—questions 19–30

One must also answer "yes" to question 38 and "no" to question 39.

A history of somatization disorder distinguishes DID from schizophrenia, eating disorders, and controls, but not from panic disorder. The average number of symptoms positive from questions 3–37 for DID was 14.1. Out of 166 subjects, 39.8% met *DSM-III-R* criteria for somatization disorder: these data have not been reanalyzed by *DSM-IV* criteria.

II.   Substance Abuse

We score the subject as positive for substance abuse if he or she answers "yes" to any question in this section. A history of substance abuse differentiates DID from schizophrenia, eating disorders, panic disorder, and controls: 51.2% of 166 DID subjects were positive.

III.   Psychiatric History

This is a descriptive section that does not yield a score as such. In a questionnaire study (Ross, Norton, & Wozney, 1989) we found that in 236 cases of DID, the average patient had received 2.74 other psychiatric diagnoses besides DID.

IV.   Major Depressive Episode

This is scored according to *DSM-IV* rules, which underwent only minor changes in wording from *DSM-III-R*. To be positive, the subject must answer "yes" to question 54. He or she must answer "yes" to 4 questions from 55 through 62.

A history of depression does not discriminate DID from other diagnostic groups: Out of 166 subjects, 89.8% had been clinically depressed at some time.

V.   Positive Symptoms of Schizophrenia (Schneiderian First-Rank Symptoms)

In this section, we score the total number of "yes" responses. The total number of positive Schneiderian symptoms discriminates DID from all groups tested including schizophrenia. The average number of positive symptoms in 166 subjects was 6.5.

VI.   Trances, Sleepwalking, Childhood Companions

Each of these items is scored independently. The subject is positive for sleepwalking if he or she answers "yes" to question 67, positive for trances if "yes" to 69, positive for imaginary playmates if "yes" to 71. Each of these items discriminates DID from schizophrenia, eating disorder, panic disorder, and controls.

VII.   Childhood Abuse

The subject is scored positive for physical abuse if he or she answers "yes" to question 73. Other data are descriptive. A history of physical abuse discriminates DID from schizophrenia, eating disorders, and panic disorder.

The subject is positive for sexual abuse if he or she answers "yes" to question 78. Sexual abuse also discriminates DID from the other three groups. Out of 166 subjects, 84.3% reported sexual abuse, 78.3% physical abuse, and 91.0% physical and/or sexual abuse.

VIII.   Features Associated with Dissociative Identity Disorder

The responses in this section are added up to give a total score. A positive response in this section is either "yes" or else "fairly often" or "frequently," depending on the structure of the question. "Never" and "occasionally" are scored as negative.

Secondary features discriminate DID from panic disorder, eating disorders, and schizophrenia. The average number of features positive in 166 subjects with DID was 10.2.

IX.   Supernatural/Possession/ESP Experiences/Cults

In this section, the positive answers are added up to give a total score. These experiences discriminate DID from the other groups. The average number of positive responses for 166 subjects was 5.3.

X.   Borderline Personality Disorder

This is scored by *DSM-IV* rules. The subject must be positive for 5 items to meet the criteria for borderline personality. Borderline personality does not discriminate DID from other groups tested to date, except for panic disorder and controls. However, the average number of borderline criteria positive does discriminate DID from schizophrenia, eating disorders, and panic disorder. The average for 166 DID subjects was 5.1.

XI.   Dissociative Amnesia

This is scored by *DSM-IV* rules. The subject must be positive for question 117, negative for question 118, and positive for question 119.

XII. Dissociative Fugue

This is scored by *DSM-IV* rules. The subject must be positive for questions 120 and 121, negative for 122, and positive for 123.

XIII. Depersonalization Disorder

This is scored by *DSM-IV* rules. The subject must be positive for question 124(a), negative for 125, and positive for 126. Questions 124(b)–(d) are examples of depersonalization that are not required for the *DSM-IV* diagnosis. This diagnosis discriminates DID from other groups very poorly.

XIV. Dissociative Identity Disorder

This is scored by *DSM-IV* rules. The subject must be positive for questions 127–130 to receive a diagnosis of DID.

XV. Dissociative Disorder Not Otherwise Specified

This is scored positive based on the interviewer's judgment. A patient can be positive for dissociative disorder not otherwise specified only if he or she does not have any other dissociative disorder.

XVI. Concluding Item

This is a descriptive question and is not scored.

Most DID patients will exhibit the DDIS profile but some will score lower than usual in some or all sections.

Individuals with dissociative disorder not otherwise specified have the same profile, but to a lesser degree than those with full DID. It is not unusual for subjects to meet criteria for both dissociative amnesia and depersonalization disorder and to have elevated symptom profiles in the rest of the DDIS: These people usually have a chronic, complex dissociative disorder that is not well classified by the *DSM-IV* system. One might diagnose them as having a partial form of DID and classify them as dissociative disorder not otherwise specified, but this is not allowed by *DSM-IV* rules. One should bear in mind that subjects who are positive for dissociative amnesia and depersonalization disorder but negative for DID on the DDIS might actually have DID, in which case they have received a false negative diagnosis of DID from the DDIS.

Therapist Dissociative Checklist

Client's Initials _____   Age _____

Client Number _____   Sex   M   or   F
                                            (please circle)

1. Time period for which you are rating the checklist:

From (date) _____ To (date) _____

2. Please indicate which phase (s) of therapy you have been working in during this time period (see guidelines for the therapist).

   a. Preintegration:

   Initial _____   Middle _____   Late _____

   b. Postintegration _____

3. How long have you been seeing the client in therapy?

_____ months or weeks (please circle)

4. How often have you been seeing the client since you last filled out this form or since you started working with the client?

_____ average number of hours/week

_____ average number of sessions/week

5. Has the Dissociative Disorders Interview Schedule (DDIS) been administered?

yes or no (please circle)

6. Has the Dissociative Experience Scale (DES) been administered?

yes or no (please circle)

Therapist Dissociative Checklist

Please indicate with a checkmark (√) how often the following techniques have been used or addressed during the given time period (see guidelines for the therapist).

	Never	Occasion-ally	Fairly Often	Frequently
	0	1	2	3
1. Establish Trust				
2. Establishing Safety				
3. Developing a Treatment Alliance				
4. Discussing Diagnosis				
5. Education and Information Processing				
6. Stated Goal of Integration				
7. Contacting Alter Personalities				
8. Gathering a History of the Personality System				
9. Mapping the Personality System				

	Never	Occasion-ally	Fairly Often	Frequently
	0	1	2	3
10. Treatment Contracting or Renegotiating				
11. Establishing Interpersonality Communication				
12. Establishing Coconsciousness				
13. Disclosing Abuse and Traumatic Memories				
14. Abreacting Abuse Memories				
15. Debriefing of Memories and Feelings				
16. Age-Appropriate Activities with Child Alters				
17. Working with Aggressive/ Persecutory Alters				
18. Cognitive Restructuring Techniques				
19. Negotiation				
20. Using Metaphors, Rituals, Imagery, or Dreams				
21. Hypnosis				
22. Relaxation Techniques				
23. Age Progression				
24. Age Regression				
25. Writing Exercises				

	Never	Occasion-ally	Fairly Often	Frequently
	0	1	2	3
26. Audiovisual				
27. Using Expressive Arts				
28. Medications				
29. Physical Restraints				
30. Hospitalization				
31. Group Therapy				
32. Involving Other Support Agencies				
33. Involving Spouses, Friends, or Relatives				
34. Limit-setting				
35. Developing New Behaviors and Coping Skills				
36. Integration				
37. Postintegration Work				
38. Other (please list)				
_____				
_____				
_____				

GUIDELINES FOR THE THERAPIST DISSOCIATIVE CHECKLIST

Phases of Therapy

Initial   The assessment and planning phase of therapy. In the treatment of DID, it involves contacting alters, mapping the system, developing a treatment alliance.

Middle	The working phase of therapy. In the treatment of DID, it involves establishing interpersonality communication, breaking down amnesic barriers, disclosing memories.
Late	The evaluation and consolidation of gains made in the middle phase of therapy and further reworking of conflicts. In treatment of DID, it involves preparation for and carrying out of the integration of alters.
Postintegration	The work following the resolution of the major abuse issues and memories, such as developing and applying new coping skills, adjusting to new feelings and memories. In treatment of DID, it involves grieving the loss of alters.

Treatment Techniques

For further discussion of some of these techniques, see Ross and Gahan's (1988b) "Techniques in the Treatment of Multiple Personality Disorder."

1. *Establishing Trust.* Addressing the issue of trust directly or applying specific interventions in developing trust.
2. *Establishing Safety.* Directly addressing the issue of safety or applying specific interventions in developing safety.
3. *Developing a Treatment Alliance.* Beginning to establish a working relationship with the client and defining mutually agreed upon goals; the client making a commitment to treatment.
4. *Discussing Diagnosis.* Presenting the client with a diagnosis and explanation of his/her dissociative process.
5. *Education and Information Processing.* Educating clients about dissociative disorders, offering clients reading materials or additional resources.
6. *Stated Goal of Integration.* Explicitly stating to the client that a goal of treatment is integration.
7. *Contacting Alter Personalities.* Making direct contact with alter personalities.
8. *Gathering History.* Learning the history of each alter, for example, who they are, when they came about, why they appeared, where they fit in the personality system, what function they serve.
9. *Mapping the Personality System.* Representing in a drawing or chart how the client perceives his/her personality system or internal world.
10. *Treatment Contracting or Renegotiating.* Formulating a written or verbal treatment agreement between the therapist and the client to determine duration of treatment, identify consequences for

self-destructive or violent behavior, and identify other types of treatment expectations.

11. *Establishing Interpersonality Communication.* Establishing internal communication between the personality states; sharing information and knowledge among the personalities, including indirect work with alter personalities.

12. *Establishing Coconsciousness.* Using techniques designed to allow the host personality to remember when the other alters are "out" and to remove amnesic barriers.

13. *Disclosing Abuse and Traumatic Memories.* Revealing sexual, physical, and emotional abuse or other traumatic memories that have been dissociated; usually occurred in childhood or adolescence and were not previously known to the host personality or to the presenting part of the client.

14. *Abreacting Abuse Memories.* Reexperiencing abusive events both physically and emotionally as if they are happening in the present.

15. *Debriefing of Memories and Feelings.* Exploring and processing thoughts, memories, and feelings surrounding the abuse.

16. *Age-Appropriate Activities with Child Alters.* Adjusting treatment approaches or interventions to correspond with the developmental stage of a younger personality.

17. *Working with Aggressive or Persecutory Alters.* Adjusting treatment approaches or adopting specific interventions when directly talking to or working with aggressive or persecutory personalities.

18. *Cognitive Restructuring Techniques.* Using cognitive therapy strategies to challenge the alter personalities' distorted beliefs and perceptions, especially of being separate selves, including cognitive dissonance (see Ross & Gahan, 1988a).

19. *Negotiations.* Encouraging decision making and discussions among the alters about positions in the system, conflicts, or decisions of daily living, for example, taking a vote among the alters.

20. *Using Metaphors, Rituals, Imagery, or Dreams.* Using creative elements such as metaphors, rituals, imagery or dreams in the therapy process to recover memories, ensure safety, or process information.

21. *Hypnosis.* Using formal induction of hypnosis to contact alter personalities, integrate personalities, reduce symptoms, or accomplish other purposes.

22. *Relaxation Techniques.* Applying specific relaxation techniques or exercises to help the client relax.

23. *Age Progression.* Using hypnotic suggestions to age progress an alter to an older age.

24. *Age Regression.* Using hypnotic suggestions to age regress an alter to a younger age.

25. *Writing Exercises.* Using diaries or journals to assist in the recovery of memories or to assist in processing memories, thoughts, and feelings; or using writing as a way to communicate with alter personalities who may be reluctant to come out.

26. *Audiovisual.* Using audio or videotaping to assist in convincing the client of the diagnosis, to help reduce the client's fears of the other parts, or to assist the client to get to know the other parts across amnesic barriers.

27. *Using Expressive Arts.* Using music, drawing, or movement as an alternative to verbalizing feelings and expressing self.

28. *Medications.* Using medications as an adjunct to therapy to relieve symptoms of depression or anxiety.

29. *Physical Restraints.* Physically restraining the client to avoid injury to self and others.

30. *Hospitalization.* Requiring inpatient treatment to protect the client's safety or to work through a crisis in therapy.

31. *Group Therapy.* Using group therapy as an adjunct to individual therapy, for example, an incest group.

32. *Involving Other Support Agencies.* Involving outside agencies such as social services, AA groups, assertiveness training, vocational counselors, or social support groups as a part of the therapy process to help the client meet various needs.

33. *Involving Spouses, Friends, or Relatives.* Educating friends and relatives and involving them as support persons when a client is in the therapy process.

34. *Limit Setting.* Setting limits around the pacing of therapy, behavior, personal boundaries for the client and therapist, or the uncovering of painful material.

35. *Developing New Behaviors and Coping Skills.* Learning and practicing new responses, changing old coping patterns, and developing new ways of dealing with conflict without dissociating.

36. *Integration.* Joining together the various personalities into a single self; different personalities will be ready to join at different times throughout therapy.

37. *Postintegration Work.* May include grieving the loss of the alters, adjusting to new feelings, accepting new memories, increasing self-confidence and self-esteem, and exploring future plans.

38. *Other Techniques.* List any other treatment techniques or approaches used in working with the client who experiences any form of dissociative disorder including DID.

Dissociative Disorders Unit Master Treatment Plan

I. Diagnosis

    1. Dissociative Amnesia   _____
    2. Dissociative Fugue   _____
    3. Depersonalization Disorder   _____
    4. Dissociative Identity Disorder   _____
    5. Dissociative Disorder Not Otherwise Specified   _____
    6. Major Depressive Disorder   _____
    7. Borderline Personality Disorder   _____
    8. Substance Abuse   _____
    9. Somatization Disorder   _____

II. Problems

    1. Suicidal Ideation or Attempt   _____
    2. Homicidal Ideation or Attempt   _____
    3. Severe Anxiety   _____
    4. Severe Depression   _____
    5. Severe Posttraumatic Symptoms   _____
    6. Nonsuicidal Self-Harm   _____
    7. Chaotic, Disorganized, or Regressed Behavior   _____
    8. Inability to Function at Work or Home   _____
    9. Dangerous Behavior, Victim of Ongoing Abuse   _____

10. Abusive Behavior Toward Others _____
11. Other Specific Problems _____

III. Interventions

  1. Suicidal Ideation
    i. Ensure safety.
    ii. Map personality system. _____
    iii. Identify involved persecutor personality
      and its motivation. _____
    iv. Reframe persecutor's behavior in system
      as positive. _____
    v. Contract with persecutor for no self-harm
      for a specified period of time. _____
    vi. Devise alternative behaviors to meet the
      persecutor's objectives. _____
    vii. Determine whether persecutor is carrying
      out behavior by itself or controlled or motivated
      by another personality. _____
    viii. Contract with persecutor to be called out in
      future sessions. _____
    ix. Reframe persecutor alter(s) as positive for
      rightened child alters and host. _____
    x. Empathize with persecutor's own pain, fear,
      and dysphoria. _____
    xi. Encourage dialogue between persecutor
      and host. _____

  2. Homicidal Ideation
    i. Ensure safety. _____
    ii. Map personality system. _____
    iii. Identify homicidal personality and its motivation. _____
    iv. Reframe alters' behavior as positive in intention
      (e.g., to protect other alters and the body) if
      possible. _____
    v. Contract with homicidal personality for no
      violence for a specified period of time. _____
    vi. Devise alternative behaviors to meet the
      homicidal personality's objectives. _____
    vii. Determine whether homicidal personality is
      carrying out behavior by itself or is motivated
      or controlled by another personality. _____
    viii. Contract with homicidal personality to be called
      out in future sessions. _____
    ix. Reframe homicidal alter's behavior as positive
      for other relevant alters and host. _____
    x. Empathize with the homicidal alter's own pain,
      fear, and dysphoria. _____
    xi. Encourage dialogue between homicidal
      alter and host. _____

3. Severe Anxiety
    (Strategies may apply to both generalized anxiety
    and panic attacks)
    i. Anxiolytic medication. _____
    ii. Relaxation audiotape. _____
    iii. Relaxation/meditation/grounding techniques. _____
    iv. Modify caffeine intake and other physiological
        contributors. _____
    v. Modify identifiable environmental stressors on
       unit contributing to anxiety or work on
       desensitizing patient to them. _____
    vi. Map personality system. _____
    vii. Identify alter(s) in system who are most
         anxious and from whom the anxiety is originating. _____
    viii. Identify specific memories/fears/personality
          system conflicts contributing to anxiety. _____
    ix. Identify protector/soothing alters who can
        reduce anxiety from inside and contract with
        them taking vii and viii into account. _____
    x. Put extremely anxious alters to sleep
       inside temporarily. _____
    xi. If anxiety is due to potentially violent
        alters threatening to come out, review
        strategies for suicidal and homicidal ideation. _____
    xii. If anxiety is due to an emerging memory,
         refer to strategies for posttraumatic symptoms. _____

4. Severe Depression
    i. Review and /or readminister Beck
       Depression Inventory. _____
    ii. Assess suicidal ideation and ensure safety. _____
    iii. Map personality system. _____
    iv. Identify whether depression is affecting
        most of the personality system or only a
        few alters. _____
    v. Antidepressant medication. _____
    vi. Modify environmental stressors contributing
        to depression. _____
    vii. Set limits on lethargic, withdrawn behavior;
         reinforce nondepressed behavior. _____

    If Only the Host Personality Is Depressed

    viii. Establish communication, coconsciousness
          between host and nondepressed alters. _____
    ix. Help nondepressed alters and host to share
        executive control in a way that improves
        overall function. _____
    x. Determine whether any alters are deliberately
       making the host depressed—if so, refer to
       strategies for suicidal ideation. _____

    xi. Modify cognitive errors contributing to
depression. Always remember that wherever
you find depression, anger is not far away.   _____

5. Severe Posttraumatic Symptoms
    i. Ensure safety during any abreactions.   _____
    ii. Map personality system.   _____
    iii. Medication.   _____
    iv. Relaxation audiotape.   _____
    v. Relaxation/meditation/grounding techniques.   _____
    vi. Modify identifiable environmental triggers on
unit contributing to PTSD symptoms if feasible.   _____
    vii. Identify specific alters from whom memories
are emerging.   _____
    viii. Determine the general nature of the memories
involved in the current symptom.   _____
    ix. Identify protector/soothing alters inside who
can reduce the flashbacks, rate of memory
recovery, and level of arousal from the inside.   _____
    x. Stage recovery of memories through dreams,
journals, art therapy, internal visualization
without full abreaction.   _____
    xi. Contract with any persecutors amplifying the
PTSD symptoms to reduce the rate of flashbacks.   _____

These interventions are focused on the
hyperarousal component of PTSD; the psychic
numbing component is much less likely to be a
focus of inpatient treatment.

6. Nonsuicidal Self-Harm
The difference between suicide attempts and deliberate self-
harm is often unclear and both can occur together in the same
behavior. Deliberate self-harm involves burning, scratching,
head-banging, picking, minor cutting, and other behaviors
clearly not intended to cause death. The persecutor's motivation is usually to punish the host, let out the bad feelings,
relieve tension or depersonalization, appease angry alters temporarily, experience a euphonic rush, show outside people that
the pain is real, or simply to see blood. The interventions are
the same as for suicidal ideation in principle but the content is
not focused on a desire to die.
    i. Ensure safety.   _____
    ii. Map personality system.   _____
    iii. Identify involved persecutor personality and its
motivation.   _____
    iv. Reframe persecutor's behavior in system as
positive.   _____
    v. Contract with persecutor for no self-harm for
a specified period of time.   _____

      vi. Devise alternative behaviors to meet the
persecutor's objectives. _____
     vii. Determine whether persecutor is carrying out
behavior by itself or is motivated or controlled
by another personality. _____
    viii. Contract with persecutor to be called out in
future sessions. _____
     ix. Reframe persecutor alter(s) as positive for
frightened child alters and host. _____
      x. Empathize with persecutor's own pain, fear,
and dysphoria. _____
     xi. Encourage dialogue between persecutor
and host. _____

7. Chaotic, Disorganized, or Regressed Behavior
      i. Ensure safety. _____
     ii. Map system. _____
    iii. Identify involved personality and the reason for
its behavior (fear, abreaction, infantile alter,
hallucinating alter). _____
    iv. Call out a behaviorally controlled alter. _____
     v. Talk through to other alters—ask for a switch
or soothing from inside. _____
    vi. If iii–v are unsuccessful after a few minutes,
escort to patient's room or quiet room. _____
    vii. Do not allow patient out of room until
behavior is controlled; iii–v may be repeated in
patient's room or quiet room. _____
   viii. Medication. _____

          If Behavior is Due to Uncontrolled Rapid
Switching

     ix. Medication. _____
      x. Talk to system as a whole and explain the
need for reduced switching. _____
     xi. If ix–x ineffective, escort to patient's room or
quiet room. _____
    xii. Do not allow patient out of room until behavior
is controlled. _____

8. Inability to Function at Work or Home
      i. Map system. _____
     ii. Identify alters who have carried out these
functions in the past or could perform them
in the future. _____
    iii. Contract with these alters to work toward
being in control at necessary times. _____
    iv. Identify other problems from problem list that
are contributing to this problem and choose
relevant interventions. _____

9. Dangerous Behavior, Victim of Ongoing Abuse
   i. Map system. _____
   ii. Identify alters involved in behavior and their
       motivation. _____
   iii. Reframe alter's behavior in system as positive. _____
   iv. Identify how behavior is a reenactment of
       childhood trauma. _____
   v. Devise alternative behaviors to meet the
      alter personality's objectives. _____
   vi. Modify social factors contributing to entrapment
       in abuse or make appropriate referrals. _____
   vii. Interview others involved in abusive behavior
        if feasible. _____

10. Abusive Behavior Toward Others
    i. Ensure safety. _____
    ii. Inform child protection, police, or other
        agencies as required. _____
    iii. Medication. _____
    iv. Map system. _____
    v. Identify alters involved in behavior and
       their motivation. _____
    vi. Reframe abusive alters' behavior as a
        reenactment of childhood traumas if feasible. _____
    vii. Reframe abusive alters' behavior as positive
         in intention if feasible (e.g., protecting child alters). _____
    viii. Contract for no assaultive behavior. _____
    ix. Devise alternative strategies to meet alters'
        objectives. _____
    x. Set behavioral limits and consequences. _____
    xi. Encourage dialogue between assaultive
        alters and host. _____
    xii. Instruct all alters that responsibility and
         consequences for behavior belong to the
         person as a whole. _____

11. Other Specific Problems
    i. Identify problem. _____
    ii. Map system. _____
    iii. Specify necessary interventions. _____

References

Aldridge-Morris, R. (1989). *Multiple personality. An exercise in deception.* London: Erlbaum.

Alexander, V. K. (1956). A case study of a multiple personality. *Journal of Abnormal and Social Psychology, 52,* 272–276.

Allen, J. G., & Smith, W. H. (1995). *Diagnosis and treatment of dissociative disorders.* Northvale, NJ: Jason Aronson.

Allison, R. B. (1974). A new treatment approach for multiple personalities. *American Journal of Clinical Hypnosis, 17,* 15–32.

Allison, R. B. (1984). Difficulties diagnosing the multiple personality syndrome in a death penalty case. *International Journal of Clinical and Experimental Hypnosis, 32,* 102–117.

Allison, R. B. (1985). The possession syndrome on trial. *American Journal of Forensic Psychiatry, 6,* 46–56.

Altrocchi, J. (1991). "We don't have that problem here": MPD in New Zealand. *Dissociation, 5,* 104–108.

American Medical Association Council on Scientific Affairs. (1995). Report on memories of childhood abuse. *International Journal of Clinical and Experimental Hypnosis, 43,* 114–117.

American Psychiatric Association. (1980). *Diagnostic and statistical manual of mental disorders* (3rd ed.). Washington, DC: Author.

American Psychiatric Association. (1987). *Diagnostic and statistical manual of mental disorders* (3rd ed., rev.). Washington, DC: Author.

American Psychiatric Association. (1994a). *Diagnostic and statistical manual of mental disorders* (4th ed.). Washington, DC: Author.

American Psychiatric Association. (1994b). Statement on memories of sexual abuse. *International Journal of Clinical and Experimental Hypnosis, 42,* 261–264.

Anderson, G. (1988). Understanding multiple personality disorder. *Journal of Psychosocial Nursing, 26,* 26–30.

Anderson G., & Ross, C. A. (1988a). A model for psychiatric nurses in working with patients who have multiple personality disorder. *Canadian Journal of Psychiatric Nursing, 29,* 13–18.

Anderson, G., & Ross, C. A. (1988b). Strategies for working with a patient who has multiple personality disorder. *Archives of Psychiatric Nursing, 11,* 236–243.

Anderson, G., Yasenik, L., & Ross, C. A. (1993). Dissociative experiences and disorders among women who identify themselves as sexual abuse survivors. *Child Abuse and Neglect, 17,* 677–686.

Andorfer, J. C. (1985). Multiple personality in the human information-processor: A case history and theoretical formulation. *Journal of Clinical Psychology, 41,* 309–324.

Atlas, G. (1988). Multiple personality disorder misdiagnosed as mental retardation. *Dissociation, 1*(1), 77–83.

Atwood, G. E. (1978). The impact of *Sybil* on a patient with multiple personality. *American Journal of Psychoanalysis, 38,* 277–279.

Barach, P. M. M. (1991). Multiple personality disorder as an attachment disorder. *Dissociation, 3,* 117–123.

Barkin, R., Braun, B. G., & Kluft, R. P. (1986). The dilemma of drug therapy for multiple personality disorder. In B. G. Braun (Ed.), *Treatment of multiple personality disorder* (pp. 107–132). Washington, DC: American Psychiatric Press.

Barrett, D. (1994). Dreaming as a normal model for multiple personality disorder. In S. J. Lynn & J. W. Rhue (Eds.), *Dissociation. Clinical and theoretical perspectives* (pp. 123–135). New York: Guilford.

Barrett, D. (1995). The dream character as a prototype for the multiple personality alter. *Dissociation, 8,* 61–68.

Barton, C. (1994a). Backstage in psychiatry: The multiple personality disorder controversy. *Dissociation, 7,* 167–172.

Barton, C. (1994b). More from backstage: A rejoinder to Merskey. *Dissociation, 7,* 176–177.

Beahrs, J. (1982). *Unity and multiplicity.* New York: Brunner/Mazel.

Beck, A. T. (1976). *Cognitive therapy and the emotional disorders.* New York: New American Library.

Beck, A. T., & Emery, G. (1985). *Anxiety disorders and phobias: A cognitive perspective.* New York: Basic Books.

Beck, A. T., Rush, A. J., Shaw, B. F., & Emery, G. (1979). *Cognitive therapy of depression.* New York: Guilford.

Benjamin, L. R., & Benjamin, R. (1992). An overview of family treatment in dissociative disorders. *Dissociation, 5,* 236–241.

Benjamin, L. R., & Benjamin, R. (1993). Interventions with children in dissociative families: A family treatment model. *Dissociation, 6,* 54–65.

Benjamin, L. R., & Benjamin, R. (1994a). A group for partners and parents of MPD clients, Part III: Martial types and dynamics. *Dissociation, 7,* 191–196.

Benjamin, L. R., & Benjamin, R. (1994b). Issues in the treatment of dissociative couples. *Dissociation, 7,* 229–238.

Benjamin, L. R., & Benjamin, R. (1994c). Utilizing parenting as a clinical focus in the treatment of dissociative disorders. *Dissociation, 7,* 239–245.

Benjamin, L. R., & Benjamin, R. (1994d). Various perspectives on parenting and their implications for the treatment of dissociative disorders. *Dissociation, 7,* 246–260.

Benner, D. G., & Evans, C. (1984). Unity and multiplicity in hypnosis, commisurotomy, and multiple personality disorder. *Journal of Mind and Behavior, 5,* 423–432.

Benner, D. G., & Joscelyne, B. (1984). Multiple personality as a borderline disorder. *Journal of Nervous and Mental Disease, 172,* 98–104.

Benson, D. F. (1986). Interictal behavior disorders in epilepsy. *Psychiatric Clinics of North America, 9,* 283–292.

Benson, D. F., Miller, B. L., & Signer, S. F. (1986). Dual personality associated with epilepsy. *Archives of Neurology, 43,* 471–474.

Berg, S., & Melin, E. (1975). Hypnotic susceptibility in old age: Some data from residential homes for old people. *International Journal of Clinical and Experimental Hypnosis, 23,* 184–189.

Berger, D., Sato, S., Ono, Y., Tezuka, I., Shirahase, J., Kuboki, T., & Suematsu, H. (1994). Dissociation and child abuse histories in an eating disorder cohort in Japan. *Acta Psychiatrica Scandinavica, 90,* 274–280.

Bernstein, E. M., & Putnam, F. W. (1986). Development, reliability, and validity of a dissociation scale. *Journal of Nervous and Mental Disease, 174,* 727–735.

Binet, A. (1977a). *Alterations of personality.* Washington, DC: University Publications of America. (Original work published 1896)

Binet, A. (1977b). *On double consciousness.* Washington, DC: University Publications of America. (Original work published 1890)

Blake, W. (1966). *Complete writings.* Oxford, England: Oxford University Press.

Bliss, E. L. (1980). Multiple personalities. A report of 14 cases with implications for schizophrenia. *Archives of General Psychiatry, 37,* 1388–1397.

Bliss, E. L. (1983). Multiple personalities, related disorders and hypnosis. *American Journal of Clinical Hypnosis, 26,* 114–123.

Bliss, E. L. (1984a). A symptom profile of patients with multiple personalities, including MMPI results. *Journal of Nervous and Mental Disease, 172,* 197–202.

Bliss, E. L. (1984b). Hysteria and hypnosis. *Journal of Nervous and Mental Disease, 172,* 203–206.

Bliss, E. L. (1984c). Spontaneous self-hypnosis in multiple personality disorder. *Psychiatric Clinics of North America, 7,* 135–148.

Bliss, E. L. (1985). Sexual criminality and hypnotizability. *Journal of Nervous and Mental Disease, 173,* 522–526.

Bliss, E. L. (1986). *Multiple personality, allied disorders, and hypnosis.* New York: Oxford University Press.

Bliss, E. L. (1988). Professional skepticism about multiple personality. *Journal of Nervous and Mental Disease, 176,* 533–534.

Bliss, E. L., & Jeppsen, A. (1985). Prevalence of multiple personality among inpatients and outpatients. *American Journal of Psychiatry, 142,* 250–251.

Bliss, E. L., & Larson, E. M. (1985). Sexual criminality and hypnotizability. *Journal of Nervous and Mental Disease, 173,* 522–526.

Boon, S., & Draijer, N. (1993). *Multiple personality disorder in the Netherlands.* Amsterdam: Swets & Zeitlinger.

Boor, M. (1982). The multiple personality epidemic: Additional cases and inferences regarding diagnosis, etiology, dynamics and treatment. *Journal of Nervous and Mental Disease, 170,* 302–304.

Boor, M., & Coons, P. M. (1983). A comprehensive bibliography of literature pertaining to multiple personality. *Psychological Reports, 53,* 295–310.

Borges, E. M. (1995). A social critique of biological psychiatry. In C. A. Ross & A. Pam (Eds.), *Pseudoscience in biological psychiatry. Blaming the body* (pp. 211–240). New York: Wiley.

Bornn, E. M. (1988, October). Multiple personality disorder. *Canadian Nurse,* 16–19.

Bowers, M. K., Brecher-Marer, S., Newton, B. W., Piotrowski, Z., Spyer, T. C., Taylor, W. S., & Watkins, J. G. (1971). Therapy of multiple personality. *International Journal of Clinical and Experimental Hypnosis, 19,* 57–65.

Bowman, E. S., Blix, S., & Coons, P. M. (1985). Multiple personality in adolescence: Relationship to incestual experiences. *Journal of the American Academy of Child Psychiatry, 24,* 109–114.

Bowman, E. S., Coons, P. M., Jones, R. S., & Oldstrom, M. (1987). Religious psychodynamics' in multiple personalities: Suggestions for treatment. *American Journal of Psychotherapy, 41,* 542–553.

Brandsma, J. M., & Ludwig, A. M. (1974). A case of multiple personality: Diagnosis and therapy. *International Journal of Clinical and Experimental Hypnosis, 22,* 216–233.

Branscomb, L. P., & Fagan, J. (1992). Development and validation of a scale measuring childhood dissociation in adults: The childhood dissociative predictor scale. *Dissociation, 5,* 80–86.

Braude, S. E. (1995). *First person plural. Multiple personality and the philosophy of mind* (Rev. ed.). London: Rowman & Littlefield.

Braun, B. G. (1983a). Neurophysiologic changes due to integration: A preliminary report. *American Journal of Clinical Hypnosis, 26,* 84–92.

Braun, B. G. (1983b). Psychophysiologic phenomena in multiple personality and hypnosis. *American Journal of Clinical Hypnosis, 26,* 124–137.

Braun, B. G. (1984). Hypnosis creates multiple personality: Myth or reality? *International Journal of Clinical and Experimental Hypnosis, 32,* 191–197.

Braun, B. G. (1985). The transgenerational incidence of dissociation and multiple personality disorder: A preliminary report. In R. P. Kluft (Ed.), *Childhood antecedents of multiple personality disorder* (pp. 167–196). Washington, DC: American Psychiatric Press.

Braun, B. G. (1986a). Issues in the psychotherapy of multiple personality disorder. In B. G. Braun (Ed.), *Treatment of multiple personality disorder* (pp. 1–28). Washington, DC: American Psychiatric Press.

Braun, B. G. (1986b). *Treatment of multiple personality disorder.* Washington, DC: American Psychiatric Press.

Braun, B. G. (1988a). The BASK (behavior, affect, sensation, knowledge) model of dissociation. *Dissociation, 1*(1), 4–23.

Braun, B. G. (1988b). The BASK model of dissociation. Clinical applications. *Dissociation, 1*(2), 16–23.

Braun, B. G., & Sachs, R. G. (1985). The development of multiple personality disorder: Predisposing, precipitating, and perpetuating factors. In R. P. Kluft (Ed.), *Childhood antecedents of multiple personality disorder* (pp. 37–64). Washington, DC: American Psychiatric Press.

Brende, J. O., & Benedict, B. D. (1980). The Vietnam combat delayed stress response syndrome: Hypnotherapy of "dissociative symptoms." *American Journal of Clinical Hypnosis, 23,* 34–40.

Breuer, J., & Freud, S. (1986). *Studies on hysteria.* New York: Pelican Books. (Original work published 1895)

Buck, O. D. (1983). Multiple personality as a borderline state. *Journal of Nervous and Mental Disease, 171,* 62–65.

Caddy, G. P. (1985). Cognitive behavior therapy in the treatment of multiple personality. *Behavior Modification, 9,* 267–292.

Cardena, E. (1994). The domain of dissociation. In S. J. Lynn & J. W. Rhue (Eds.), *Dissociation. Clinical and theoretical perspectives* (pp. 15–31). New York: Guilford.

Carlson, E. B. (1989). Integrating research on dissociation and hypnotizability: Are there two pathways to hypnotizability? *Dissociation, 2,* 32–38.

Carlson, E. B. (1994). Studying the interaction between physical and psychological states with the Dissociative Experiences Scale. In D. Spiegel (Ed.), *Dissociation. Culture, mind, and body* (pp. 41–58). Washington, DC: American Psychiatric Press.

Carlson, E. B., & Armstrong, J. (1994). The diagnosis and assessment of dissociative disorders. In S. J. Lynn & J. W. Rhue (Eds.), *Dissociation. Clinical and theoretical perspectives* (pp. 159–174). New York: Guilford.

420   References

Carlson, E. B., & Putnam, F. W. (1989). Integrating research on dissociation and hypnotizability: Are there two pathways to hypnotizability? *Dissociation, 2,* 32–38.

Carlson, E. B., & Putnam, F. W. (1993). An update on the Dissociative Experiences Scale. *Dissociation, 6,* 16–27.

Carlson, E. B., Putnam, F. W., Ross, C. A., Torem, M., Coons, P., Bowman, E. S., Chu, J., Dill, D. L., Loewenstein, R. J., & Braun, B. G. (1993). Predictive validity of the Dissociative Experiences Scale. *American Journal of Psychiatry, 150,* 1030–1036.

Carlson, E. T. (1981). The history of multiple personality in the United States: I. The beginnings. *American Journal of Psychiatry, 138,* 666–668.

Carlson, E. T. (1984). The history of multiple personality in the United States: Mary Reynolds and her subsequent reputation. *Bulletin of the History of Medicine, 58,* 72–82.

Caul, D. (1984). Group and videotape techniques for multiple personality disorder. *Psychiatric Annals, 14,* 46–50.

Caul, D., Sachs, R. G., & Braun, B. G. (1986). Group therapy in treatment of multiple personality disorder. In B. G. Braun (Ed.), *Treatment of multiple personality disorder* (pp. 143–156). Washington, DC: American Psychiatric Press.

Chu, J. A. (1988). Ten traps for therapists in the treatment of trauma survivors. *Dissociation, 1,* 24–32.

Chu, J. A., & Dill, D. L. (1990). Dissociative symptoms in relation to childhood physical and sexual abuse. *American Journal of Psychiatry, 147,* 887–892.

Clark, E. E. (1960). *Indian legends of the Pacific Northwest.* Toronto: McClelland & Stewart.

Clary, W. F., Burstin, K. J., & Carpenter, J. S. (1984). Multiple personality and borderline personality disorder. *Psychiatric Clinics of North America, 7,* 89–99.

Cocores, J. A., Bender, A. L., & McBride, E. (1984). Multiple personality, seizure disorder, and the electroencephalogram. *Journal of Nervous and Mental Disease, 172,* 436–438.

Cohen, B. M., & Cox, C. T. (1995). *Telling without talking. Art as a window into the world of multiple personality.* New York: W. W. Norton.

Cohen, B. M., Giller, E., & Lynn, W. (1991). *Multiple personality disorder from the inside out.* Baltimore: Sidran Press.

Cohen, L., Berzoff, J., & Elin, M. (1995). *Dissociative identity disorder: Theoretical and treatment controversies.* Northvale, NJ: Jason Aronson.

Comstock, C. (1987). Internal self helpers or centers. *Integration, 3*(1), 3–12.

Confer, W. N., & Ables, B. S. (1983). *Multiple personality: Etiology, diagnosis and treatment.* New York: Human Sciences Press.

Congdon, M. H., Hain, J., & Stevenson, I. (1961). A case of multiple personality illustrating the transition from role-playing. *Journal of Nervous and Mental Disease, 132,* 497–504.

Coons, P. M. (1980). Multiple personality: Diagnostic considerations. *Journal of Clinical Psychiatry, 41,* 330–336.

Coons, P. M. (1984). The differential diagnosis of multiple personality. *Psychiatric Clinics of North America, 7,* 51–67.

Coons, P. M. (1985). Children of parents with multiple personality disorder. In R. P. Kluft (Ed.), *Childhood antecedents of multiple personality disorder* (pp. 151–165). Washington, DC: American Psychiatric Press.

Coons, P. M. (1986a). Child abuse and multiple personality disorder: Review of the literature and suggestions for treatment. *Child Abuse and Neglect, 10,* 455–465.

Coons, P. M. (1986b). Dissociative disorders: Diagnosis and treatment. *Indiana Medicine, 79,* 410–415.

Coons, P. M. (1986c). The prevalence of multiple personality disorder. *Newsletter of the International Society for the Study of Multiple Personality and Dissociation, 4*(3), 6–8.

Coons, P. M. (1986d). Treatment progress in 20 patients with multiple personality disorder. *Journal of Nervous and Mental Disease, 174,* 715–721.

Coons, P. M. (1988a). Misuse of forensic hypnosis: A hypnotically elicited false confession with the apparent creation of multiple personality. *International Journal of Clinical and Experimental Hypnosis, 36,* 1–11.

Coons, P. M. (1988b). Psychophysiologic investigation of multiple personality disorder: A review. *Dissociation, 1*(1), 47–53.

Coons, P. M. (1992). Dissociative disorder not otherwise specified: A clinical investigation of 50 cases with suggestions for typology and treatment. *Dissociation, 5,* 187–195.

Coons, P. M. (1994). Confirmation of childhood abuse in child and adolescent cases of multiple personality disorder and dissociative disorder not otherwise specified. *Journal of Nervous and Mental Disease, 182,* 461–464.

Coons, P. M., Bowman, E. S., & Milstein, V. (1988). Multiple personality disorder: A clinical investigation of 50 cases. *Journal of Nervous and Mental Disease, 176,* 519–527.

Coons, P. M., & Bradley, K. (1985). Group psychotherapy with multiple personality patients. *Journal of Nervous and Mental Disease, 173,* 515–521.

Coons, P. M., & Fine, C. (1988). Accuracy of the MMPI in identifying multiple personality disorder. In B. G. Braun (Ed.), *Proceedings of the Fifth International Conference on Multiple Personality/Dissociative States* (p. 102). Chicago: Rush-Presbyterian-St. Luke's Medical Center.

Coons, P. M., & Milstein, V. (1984). Rape and post-traumatic stress in multiple personality. *Psychological Reports, 55,* 839–845.

Coons, P. M., & Milstein, V. (1986). Psychosexual disturbances in multiple personality: Characteristics, etiology, and treatment. *Journal of Clinical Psychiatry, 47,* 106–110.

Coons, P. M., Milstein, V., & Marley, C. (1982). EEG studies of two multiple personalities and a control. *Archives of General Psychiatry, 39,* 823–825.

Coons, P. M., & Sterne, A. L. (1986). Initial and follow-up psychological testing on a group of patients with multiple personality disorder. *Psychological Reports, 58,* 43–49.

Copeland, C. L., & Kitching, E. H. (1937). A case of profound dissociation of the personality. *Journal of Mental Science, 83,* 719–726.

Crabtree, A. (1985). *Multiple man: Explorations in possession and multiple personality.* Toronto: Collins.

Crabtree, A. (1986). Explanations of dissociation in the first half of the twentieth century. In J. M. Quen (Ed.), *Split minds split brains* (pp. 85–107). New York: New York University Press.

Crabtree, A. (1993). *From Mesmer to Freud: Magnetic sleep and the roots of psychological healing.* New Haven, CT: Yale University Press.

Curtis, J. C. (1988, February). Exposing multiple personality disorder. *Diagnosis,* 85–87, 90–95.

Cutler, B., & Reed, J. (1975). Multiple personality: A single case study with a 15-year follow-up. *Psychological Medicine, 5,* 18–26.

Damgaard, J., Van Benschoten, S., & Fagan, J. (1985). An updated bibliography of literature pertaining to multiple personality. *Psychological Reports, 57,* 131–137.

Darves-Bornoz, J., Degovianni, A., & Gaillard, P. (1995). Why is dissociative identity disorder infrequent in France? *American Journal of Psychiatry, 152,* 1530–1531.

Dell, P. F. (1988a). Not reasonable skepticism but extreme skepticism. *Journal of Nervous and Mental Disease, 176,* 537–538.

Dell, P. F. (1988b). Professional skepticism about multiple personality. *Journal of Nervous and Mental Disease, 176,* 528–531.

Dell, P. F., & Eisenhower, J. W. (1990). Adolescent multiple personality disorder. *Journal of the American Academy of Child and Adolescent Psychiatry, 29,* 359–366.

Derogatis, L. R., Lipman, R. S., Rickels, K., Uhenhuth, E. H., & Covi, L. (1973). SCL-90: An outpatient psychiatric rating scale-preliminary report. *Psychopharmacology Bulletin, 9,* 13–28.

Draijer, N., & Boon, S. (1993). The validation of the Dissociative Experiences Scale against the criterion of the SCID-D using receiver operating characteristics (ROC) analysis. *Dissociation, 6,* 28–37.

Drew, B. L. (1988). Multiple personality disorder: An historical perspective. *Archives of Psychiatric Nursing, 2,* 227–230.

Dunn, G. E., Paolo, A. M., & Ryan, J. J. (1993). Dissociative symptoms in a substance abuse population. *American Journal of Psychiatry, 150,* 1043–1047.

Dunn, G. E., Paolo, A. M., Ryan, J. J., & Van Fleet, J. N. (1994). Belief in the existence of multiple personality disorder among psychologists and psychiatrists. *Journal of Clinical Psychology, 50,* 454–457.

Dyck, P. B., & Gillette, G. M. (1987). Development of a dissociative symptom inventory. In B. G. Braun (Ed.), *Proceedings of the Fourth International Conference on Multiple Personality/Dissociative States* (p. 143). Chicago: Rush-Presbyterian-St. Luke's Medical Center.

Dysken, M. W., Chang, S. S., Casper, R. C., & Davis, J. M. (1979). Barbiturate-facilitated interviewing. *Biological Psychiatry, 14,* 421–432.

Dysken, M. W., Kooser, J. A., Haraszti, J. S., & Davis, J. M. (1979). Clinical usefulness of sodium amobarbital interviewing. *Archives of General Psychiatry, 36,* 789–794.

Eliade, M. (1964). *Shamanism.* Princeton, NJ: Princeton University Press.

Ellason, J. W., & Ross, C. A. (1995a). Positive and negative symptoms in dissociative identity disorder and schizophrenia. *Journal of Nervous and Mental Disease, 183,* 236–241.

Ellason, J. W., & Ross, C. A. (1995b). *Two-year followup of inpatients with dissociative identity disorder.* Unpublished manuscript.

Ellason, J. W., & Ross, C. A. (1996). Million Clinical Multiaxial Inventory-II followup of patients with dissociative identity disorder. *Psychological Reports, 78,* 707–716.

Ellason, J. W., Ross, C. A., & Anderson, G. (1996). *Borderline and non-borderline subsets of dissociative identity disorder.* Unpublished manuscript.

Ellason, J. W., Ross, C. A., & Fuchs, D. (1995). Assessment of dissociative identity disorder with the Millon Clinical Multiaxial Inventory-II. *Psychological Reports, 76,* 895–905.

Ellason, J. W., Ross, C. A., Mayran, L. W., & Sainton, K. (1994). Convergent validity of the new form of the Dissociative Experiences Scale. *Dissociation, 7,* 101–103.

Ellason, J. W., Ross, C. A., Sainton, K., & Mayran, L. (1996). Axis I and II comorbidity and childhood trauma history in chemical dependency. *Bulletin of the Menninger Clinic, 60,* 39–51.

Ellenberger, H. (1970). *The discovery of the unconscious.* New York: Basic Books.

Emery, G., Hollon, S. D., & Bedrosian, R. C. (1981). *New directions in cognitive therapy.* New York: Guilford.

Estabrooks, G. H. (1943). *Hypnotism.* New York: E. P. Dutton.

Estabrooks, G. H. (1947). *Spiritism.* New York: E. P. Dutton.

Estabrooks, G. H. (1957). *Hypnotism* (2nd ed.). New York: E. P. Dutton.

Estabrooks, G. H. (1971, April). Hypnosis comes of age. *Science Digest,* 44–50.

Evers-Szostak, M., & Sanders, S. (1992). The Children's Perceptual Alteration Scale (CPAS): A measure of children's dissociation. *Dissociation, 5,* 91–97.

Fagan, J., & McMahon, P. (1984). Incipient multiple personality in children. *Journal of Nervous and Mental Disease, 172,* 26–36.

Fahy, T. A. (1988). The diagnosis of multiple personality disorder: A critical review. *British Journal of Psychiatry, 153,* 597–606.

Fast, I. (1974). Multiple identities in borderline personality organization. *British Journal of Medical Psychology, 47,* 291–300.

Feldman, M. D., & Ford, C. V. (1994). *Patient or pretender: Inside the strange world of factitious disorders.* New York: Wiley.

Fine, C. G. (1988). The work of Antoine Despine: The first scientific report on the diagnosis and treatment of a child with multiple personality disorder. *American Journal of Clinical Hypnosis, 31,* 33–39.

Frances, A., & Spiegel, D. (1987). Chronic pain masks depression, multiple personality disorder. *Hospital and Community Psychiatry, 38,* 933–935.

Franklin, J. (1990). Dreamlike thought and dream mode processes in the formation of personalities in MPD. *Dissociation, 3,* 7–80.

Fraser, G. A. (1991). The dissociative table technique: A strategy for working with ego states in dissociative disorders and ego-state therapy. *Dissociation, 4,* 205–213.

Fraser, G. A., & Lapierre, Y. D. (1986). Lactate-induced panic attacks in dissociative states (multiple personalities). In B. G. Braun (Ed.), *Proceedings of the Third International Conference on Multiple Personality/Dissociative States* (p. 124). Chicago: Rush-Presbyterian-St. Luke's Medical Center.

Freeland, A., Manchanda, R., Chiu, S., Sharma, V., & Merskey, H. (1993). Four cases of supposed multiple personality disorder: Evidence of iatrogenesis. *Canadian Journal of Psychiatry, 38,* 245–247.

Freeman, A. (Ed.). (1983). *Cognitive therapy with couples and groups.* New York: Plenum.

French, O., & Chodoff, P. (1987). More on multiple personality disorder [letter to the editor]. *American Journal of Psychiatry, 144,* 123–125.

Freyd, J. (1993, August 7). *Theoretical and personal perspectives on the delayed memory debate.* Paper presented at Controversies Around Recovered Memories of Incest and Ritualistic Abuse, A Continuing Education Conference for Mental Health Professionals, Ann Arbor, MI.

Frischholz, E. J., Braun, B. G., Sachs, R. G., Hopkins, L., Shaeffer, D. M., Lewis, J., Leavitt, F., Pasquotto, J. N., & Schwartz, D. R. (1990). The Dissociative Experiences Scale: Further replication and validation. *Dissociation, 3,* 151–153.

Frischholz, M. A. (1985). The relationship among dissociation, hypnosis, and child abuse in the development of multiple personality disorder. In R. P. Kluft (Ed.), *Childhood antecedents of multiple personality disorder* (pp. 99–126). Washington, DC: American Psychiatric Press.

Gabel, S. (1990). Dreams and dissociation theory: Speculations on beneficial aspects of their linkage. *Dissociation, 3,* 38–47.

Gainer, K. (1994). Dissociation and schizophrenia: An historical review of conceptual development and relevant treatment approaches. *Dissociation, 7,* 261–271.

Ganaway, G. K. (1995). Hypnosis, childhood trauma, and dissociative identity disorder: Toward an integrative theory. *International Journal of Clinical and Experimental Hypnosis, 38,* 127–144.

Gilbertson, A., Torem, M., Cohen, R., Newman, I., & Radojicic, C. (1992). Susceptibility of common self-report measures of dissociation to malingering. *Dissociation, 5,* 216–220.

Gleaves, D. H., Eberenz, K. P., Warner, M. S., & Fine, G. (1995). Measuring clinical and nonclinical dissociation: A comparison of the Dissociative Experiences Scale (DES) and the Questionnaire of Experiences of Dissociation (QED). *Dissociation, 8,* 24–31.

Goettman, C., Greaves, G. B., & Coons, P. M. (1992). *Multiple personality and dissociation, 1791–1991. A complete bibliography.* Lutherville, MD: Sidran Press.

Golub, D. (1995). Cultural variations in multiple personality disorder. In L. Cohen, J. Berzoff, & M. Elin (Eds.), *Dissociative identity disorder: Theoretical and treatment controversies* (pp. 285–326). Northvale, NJ: Jason Aronson.

Goodwin, D. W., Crane, J. B., & Guze, S. B. (1969). Phenomenological aspects of the alcoholic "blackout." *British Journal of Psychiatry, 115,* 1033–1038.

Goodwin, J. (1985). Credibility problems in multiple personality disorder patients and abused children. In R. P. Kluft (Ed.), *Childhood antecedents of multiple personality disorder* (pp. 1–19). Washington, DC: American Psychiatric Press.

Goodwin, J. (1988). Munchausen's syndrome as a dissociative disorder. *Dissociation, 1*(1), 54–60.

Goodwin, J., & Attias, R. (1988). Eating disorder as a multimodal response to child abuse. In B. G. Braun (Ed.), *Proceedings of the Fifth International Conference on Multiple Personality/Dissociative States* (p. 29). Chicago: Rush-Presbyterian-St. Luke's Medical Center.

Goodwin, J., Cheeves, K., & Connell, V. (1988). Defining a syndrome of severe symptoms in patients with severe incestuous abuse. *Dissociation, 1*(4), 11–16.

Gordon, M. C. (1972). Age and performance differences of male patients on modified Stanford hypnotic susceptibility scales. *International Journal of Clinical and Experimental Hypnosis, 20,* 152–155.

Gray, G. T., & Braun, B. G. (1986). Report on the 1985 questionnaire multiple personality disorder. In B. G. Braun (Ed.), *Proceedings of the Third International Conference on Multiple Personality/Dissociative States* (p. 111). Chicago: Rush-Presbyterian-St. Luke's Medical Center.

Greaves, G. B. (1980). Multiple personality. 165 years after Mary Reynolds. *Journal of Nervous and Mental Disease, 168,* 577–596.

Greaves, G. B. (1988). Common errors in the treatment of multiple personality disorder. *Dissociation, 1,* 61–66.

Gruenewald, D. (1971). Hypnotic techniques without hypnosis in the treatment of dual personality. *Journal of Nervous and Mental Disease, 153,* 41–46.

Gruenewald, D. (1977). Multiple personality and splitting phenomena: A reconceptulization. *Journal of Nervous and Mental Disease, 153,* 41–46.

Gruenewald, D. (1984). On the nature of multiple personality: Comparisons with hypnosis. *International Journal of Clinical and Experimental Hypnosis, 32,* 170–190.

Gruenewald, D. (1988). [Review of the book *Multiple personality, allied disorders, and hypnosis.*] *International Journal of Clinical and Experimental Hypnosis, 36,* 53–56.

Gunderson, J. G., Carpenter, W. T., & Strauss, J. S. (1975). Borderline and schizophrenic patients: A comparative study. *American Journal of Psychiatry, 132,* 1257–1264.

Gunderson, J. G., & Kolb, J. E. (1978). Discriminating features of borderline patients. *American Journal of Psychiatry, 135,* 792–796.

Gunderson, J. G., Kolb, J. E., & Austin, V. (1981). The diagnostic interview for borderlines. *American Journal of Psychiatry, 138,* 896–903.

Gunderson, J. G., & Singer, M. T. (1975). Defining borderline patients: An overview. *American Journal of Psychiatry, 132,* 1–10.

Hacking, I. (1991). Double consciousness in Britain 1815–1875. *Dissociation, 4,* 134–146.

Hacking, I. (1995). *Rewriting the soul. Multiple personality and the sciences of memory.* Princeton, NJ: Princeton University Press.

Hall, R. C. W., LeCann, A. F., & Schoolar, J. C. (1978). Amobarbital treatment of multiple personality. *Journal of Nervous and Mental Disease, 166,* 666–670.

Hammond, D. C., Garver, R. B., Mutter, C. B., Crasilneck, H. B., Frischholz, E., Gravitz, M. A., Hibler, N. S., Olson, J., Scheflin, A., Spiegel, H., & Wester, W. (1994). *Clinical hypnosis and memory: Guidelines for clinicians and for forensic hypnosis.* American Society of Clinical Hypnosis Press.

Harner, M. J. (Ed.). (1973). *Hallucinogens and shamanism.* New York: Oxford University Press.

Harriman, P. L. (1942a). The experimental induction of a multiple personality. *Psychiatry, 5,* 179–186.

Harriman, P. L. (1942b). The experimental production of some phenomena related to multiple personality. *Journal of Abnormal and Social Psychology, 37,* 244–255.

Harriman, P. L. (1943). A new approach to multiple personalities. *American Journal of Orthopsychiatry, 13,* 638–643.

Hassan, S. (1988). *Combatting cult mind control.* Rochester, VT: Park Street Press.

Hattori, Y. (1995). *Multiple personality disorder.* Tokyo: PHP.

Hattori, Y., & Ross, C. A. (1995). *Dissociative experiences among Japanese college students.* Unpublished data.

Haule, J. R. (1986). Pierre Janet and dissociation: The first transference theory and its origins in hypnosis. *American Journal of Clinical Hypnosis, 29,* 86–94.

Hawthorne, J. (1983). *Multiple personality and the disintegration of literary character.* New York: St. Martin's.

Heber, S., Fleisher, W. P., Ross, C. A., & Stanwick, R. (1989). Dissociation in alternative helpers and traditional therapists: A comparative study. *American Journal of Psychotherapy, 43,* 562–574.

Hicks, R. E. (1985). Discussion: A clinician's perspective. In R. P. Kluft (Ed.), *Childhood antecedents of multiple personality disorder* (pp. 239–258). Washington, DC: American Psychiatric Press.

Hilgard, E. R. (1977). *Divided consciousness: Multiple controls in human thought and action.* New York: Wiley.

Hilgard, E. R. (1984). The hidden observer and multiple personality. *International Journal of Clinical and Experimental Hypnosis, 132,* 248–253.

Hilgard, E. R. (1987). Multiple personality and dissociation. In *Psychology in America: A historical survey* (pp. 303–315). San Diego: Harcourt Brace Jovanovich.

Hilgard, E. R. (1988). Professional skepticism about multiple personality. *Journal of Nervous and Mental Disease, 176,* 532.

Hilgard, E. R. (1994). Neodissociation theory. In S. J. Lynn & J. W. Rhue (Eds.), *Dissociation. Clinical and theoretical perspectives* (pp. 32–51). New York: Guilford.

Hoch, P. H., & Polatin, P. (1949). Pseudoneurotic forms of schizophrenia. *Psychiatric Quarterly, 23,* 248–276.

Hocking, S. J. (1992). *Living with your selves.* Rockville, MD: Launch Press.

Horen, S. A., Leichner, P. P., & Lawson, J. S. (1995). Prevalence of dissociative symptoms and disorders in an adult psychiatric inpatient population in Canada. *Canadian Journal of Psychiatry, 40,* 185–191.

Horevitz, R. P., & Braun, B. G. (1984). Are multiple personalities borderline? *Psychiatric Clinics of North America, 7,* 69–87.

Hornstein, N. L. (1993). Recognition and differential diagnosis of dissociative disorders in children and adolescents. *Dissociation, 6,* 136–144.

Hornstein, N. L., & Putnam, F. W. (1992). Clinical phenomenology of child and adolescent dissociative disorders. *Journal of the American Academy of Child and Adolescent Psychiatry, 31,* 1077–1085.

Hornstein, N. L., & Tyson, S. (1991). Inpatient treatment of children with multiple personality/dissociative disorders and their families. *Psychiatric Clinics of North America, 14,* 631–638.

Horton, P., & Miller, D. (1972). The etiology of multiple personality. *Comprehensive Psychiatry, 13,* 151–159.

Howland, J. S. (1975). The use of hypnosis in the treatment of a case of multiple personality. *Journal of Nervous and Mental Disease, 161,* 138–142.

Huber, M. (1995). *Multiple personlichkeiten.* Frankfurt: Fischer Taschenbuch Verlag.

International Society for the Study of Dissociation. (1994). *Guidelines for treating dissociative identity disorder (multiple personality disorder) in adults (1994).* Skokie, IL: Author.

James, W. (1983). *The principles of psychology.* Cambridge, MA: Harvard University Press. (Original work published 1890)

Janet, P. (1965). *The major symptoms of hysteria.* New York: Hafner. (Original work published 1907)

Janet, P. (1977). *The mental state of hystericals.* Washington, DC: University Publications of America. (Original work published 1901)

Jaynes, J. (1976). *The origin of consciousness in the breakdown of the bicameral mind.* Toronto: University of Toronto Press.

Jones, E. (1953). *Sigmund Freud: Life and work* (Vol. 1). London: Hogarth Press.

Jorn, N. (1982). Repression in a case of multiple personality disorder. *Perspectives in Psychiatric Care, 20,* 105–110.

Jung, C. G. (1977). On the psychology and pathology of so-called occult phenomena. In C. G. Jung, *Psychology and the occult* (pp. 6–91). Princeton, NJ: Princeton University Press. (Original work published 1902)

Kales, A., Soldatos, C. R., Caldwell, A. B., Kales, J. D., Humphrey, F. J., Charney, D. S., & Schweitzer, P. K. (1980). Somnambulism: Clinical characteristics and personality patterns. *Archives of General Psychiatry, 37,* 1406–1410.

Kampman, R. (1976). Hypnotically induced multiple personality: An experimental study. *International Journal of Clinical and Experimental Hypnosis, 24,* 215–227.

Kenny, M. G. (1981). Multiple personality and spirit possession. *Psychiatry, 44,* 337–358.

Kenny, M. G. (1986). *The passion of Ansel Bourne: Multiple personality in American culture.* Washington, DC: Smithsonian Institution Press.

Kernberg, O. J. (1975). *Borderline conditions and pathological narcissism.* New York: Jason Aronson.

Keyes, D. (1981). *The minds of Billy Milligan.* New York: Random House.

Kilhstrom, J. F. (1994). One hundred years of hysteria. In S. J. Lynn & J. W. Rhue (Eds.), *Dissociation. Clinical and theoretical perspectives* (pp. 365–394). New York: Guilford.

Kirmayer, L. J. (1994). Pacing the void: Social and cultural dimensions of dissociation. In D. Spiegel (Ed.), *Dissociation. Culture, mind, and body* (pp. 91–122). Washington, DC: American Psychiatric Press.

Klein, M. K., & Doane, B. K. (1994). *Psychological concepts and dissociative disorders.* Hillsdale, NJ: Erlbaum.

Kline, M. V. (1984). Multiple personality: Facts and artifacts in relation to hypnotherapy. *International Journal of Clinical and Experimental Hypnosis, 32,* 198–209.

Kluft, E. S. (1993). *Expressive and functional therapies in the treatment of multiple personality disorder.* Springfield, IL: Charles C. Thomas.

Kluft, R. P. (1982). Varieties of hypnotic interventions in the treatment of multiple personality. *American Journal of Clinical Hypnosis, 24,* 230–240.

Kluft, R. P. (1983). Hypnotherapeutic crisis intervention in multiple personality. *American Journal of Clinical Hypnosis, 26,* 73–83.

Kluft, R. P. (1984a). Aspects of the treatment of multiple personality disorder. *Psychiatric Annals, 14,* 51–55.

Kluft, R. P. (1984b). Multiple personality in childhood. *Psychiatric Clinics of North America, 7,* 121–134.

Kluft, R. P. (1984c). Treatment of multiple personality disorder. *Psychiatric Clinics of North America, 7,* 9–29.

Kluft, R. P. (Ed.). (1985a). *Childhood antecedents of multiple personality disorder.* Washington, DC: American Psychiatric Press.

Kluft, R. P. (1985b). Childhood multiple personality disorder: Predictors, clinical findings, and treatment results. In R. P. Kluft (Ed.), *Childhood antecedents of multiple personality disorder* (pp. 167–196). Washington, DC: American Psychiatric Press.

Kluft, R. P. (1985c). Hypnotherapy of childhood multiple personality disorder. *American Journal of Clinical Hypnosis, 27,* 201–210.

Kluft, R. P. (1985d). Making the diagnosis of multiple personality disorder (MPD). In F. F. Flach (Ed.), *Directions in Psychiatry, 5*(23), 1–10. New York: Hatherleigh.

Kluft, R. P. (1985e). The natural history of multiple personality disorder. In R. P. Kluft (Ed.), *Childhood antecedents of multiple personality disorder* (pp. 197–238). Washington, DC: American Psychiatric Press.

Kluft, R. P. (1985f). The treatment of multiple personality disorder (MPD): Current concepts. In F. F. Flach (Ed.), *Directions in Psychiatry, 5*(24), 1–10. New York: Hatherleigh.

Kluft, R. P. (1985g). Using hypnotic inquiry protocols to monitor treatment progress and stability in multiple personality disorder. *American Journal of Clinical Hypnosis, 28,* 63–75.

Kluft, R. P. (1986a). High-functioning multiple personality patients. *Journal of Nervous and Mental Disease, 174,* 722–726.

Kluft, R. P. (1986b). Personality unification in multiple personality disorder: A follow-up study. In B. G. Braun (Ed.), *Treatment of multiple personality disorder* (pp. 29–60). Washington, DC: American Psychiatric Press.

Kluft, R. P. (1986c). Preliminary observations on age regression in multiple personality disorder patients before and after integration. *American Journal of Clinical Hypnosis, 28,* 147–156.

Kluft, R. P. (1986d). The prevalence of multiple personality [Letter to the editor]. *American Journal of Psychiatry, 143,* 802–803.

Kluft, R. P. (1986e). Treating children who have multiple personality disorder. In B. G. Braun (Ed.), *Treatment of multiple personality disorder* (pp. 79–105). Washington, DC: American Psychiatric Press.

Kluft, R. P. (1987a). An update on multiple personality disorder. *Hospital and Community Psychiatry, 38,* 363–373.

Kluft, R. P. (1987b). First-rank symptoms as a diagnostic clue to multiple personality disorder. *American Journal of Psychiatry, 144,* 293–298.

Kluft, R. P. (1987c). On the use of hypnosis to find lost objects: A case report of a tandem hypnotic technique. *American Journal of Clinical Hypnosis, 29,* 242–248.

Kluft, R. P. (1987d). The simulation and dissimulation of multiple personality disorder. *American Journal of Clinical Hypnosis, 30,* 104–118.

Kluft, R. P. (1987e, October 24). *The process of personality unification in a multiple.* Paper presented at the conference on Multiple Personality in the 1980s, Toronto, Ontario, Canada.

Kluft, R. P. (1988a). Editorial: Ubi sumus? quo vademis? *Dissociation, 1*(3), 1–2.

Kluft, R. P. (1988b). On giving consultations to therapists treating multiple personality disorder: Fifteen years' experience-Part I. *Dissociation, 1*(3), 1–2.

Kluft, R. P. (1988c). On giving consultations to therapists treating multiple personality: Fifteen years' experience-Part II. *Dissociation, 1*(3), 30–35.

Kluft, R. P. (1988d). On treating the older patient with multiple personality disorder: "Race against time" or "make haste slowly?" *American Journal of Clinical Hypnosis, 30,* 257–266.

Kluft, R. P. (1988e). The postunification treatment of multiple personality disorder: First findings. *American Journal of Psychotherapy, 42,* 212–228.

Kluft, R. P. (1991a). Clinical presentations of multiple personality disorder. *Psychiatric Clinics of North America, 14,* 605–630.

Kluft, R. P. (1991b). Hospital treatment of multiple personality disorder. *Psychiatric Clinics of North America, 14,* 695–719.

Kluft, R. P. (1994). Clinical observations on the use of the CSDS Dimensions of Therapeutic Movement Instrument (DTMI). *Dissociation, 7,* 272–283.

Kluft, R. P. (1995). Current controversies surrounding dissociative identity disorder. In L. Cohen, J. Berzoff, & M. Elin (Eds.), *Dissociative identity disorder. Theoretical and treatment controversies* (pp. 347–377). Northvale, NJ: Jason Aronson.

Kluft, R. P., Braun, B. G., & Sachs, R. (1984). Multiple personality, intra-familial abuse and family psychiatry. *International Journal of Family Psychiatry, 5,* 283–301.

Kluft, R. P., & Fine, C. G. (1993). *Clinical perspectives on multiple personality disorder.* Washington, DC: American Psychiatric Press.

Kluft, R. P., Steinberg, M., & Spitzer, R. L. (1988). *DSM-III-R* revisions in the dissociative disorders: An exploration of their derivation and rationale. *Dissociation, 1*(1), 39–46.

Knudsen, H., Draijer, N., Haselrud, J., Boe, T., & Boon, S. (1995). *Dissociative disorders in Norwegian psychiatric inpatients.* Paper presented at the Spring meeting of the International Society for the Study of Dissociation, Amsterdam, The Netherlands.

Krasad, A. (1985). Multiple personality syndrome. *British Journal of Hospital Medicine, 34,* 301–303.

Krippner, S. (1986). Cross-cultural approaches to multiple personality disorder: Therapeutic practices in Brazilian spiritism. *The Humanistic Psychologist, 14,* 176–193.

Krippner, S. (1994). Cross-cultural perspectives on dissociative disorders. In S. J. Lynn & J. W. Rhue (Eds.), *Dissociation. Clinical and theoretical perspectives* (pp. 338–361). New York: Guilford.

Kuhn, T. (1962). *The structure of scientific revolutions.* Chicago: University of Chicago Press.

Larmore, K., Ludwig, A. M., & Cain, R. L. (1977). Multiple personality-An objective case study. *British Journal of Psychiatry, 131,* 35–40.

Lasky, R. (1978). The psychoanalytic treatment of a case of multiple personality. *Psychoanalytic Review, 65,* 355–380.

Latz, T. T., Kramer, S. I., & Hughes, D. L. (1995). Multiple personality disorder among female inpatients in a state hospital. *American Journal of Psychiatry, 152,* 1343–1348.

Laurence, J. R., Nadon, R., Nogrady, H., Perry, C. (1986). Duality, dissociation, and memory creation in highly hypnotizable subjects. *International Journal of Clinical and Experimental Hypnosis, 34,* 295–310.

Leavis, Q. D. (1968). Henry Sidgwick's Cambridge. In F. R. Leavis (Ed.), *A Selection from Scrutiny* (Vol. 1, pp. 31–41). Cambridge, England: Cambridge University Press.

Leavitt, H. C. (1947). A case of hypnotically produced secondary and tertiary personalities. *Psychoanalytic Review, 34,* 274–295.

Leeper, D. H., Page, B., & Hendricks, D. E. (1992). *The prevalence of dissociative disorders in a drug and alcohol abusing population of a residential treatment facility in a military medical center.* Unpublished manuscript.

Lego, S. (1988). Multiple personality disorder: An interpersonal approach to etiology, treatment, and nursing care. *Archives of Psychiatric Nursing, 2,* 231–235.

Lewis, I. M. (1971). *Ecstatic religion: An anthropological study of spirit possession and shamanism.* Baltimore: Penguin Books.

Lewis, G. R. (1976). Criteria for the discerning of spirits. In J. W. Mongomery (Ed.), *Demon possession* (pp. 346–363). Minneapolis: Bethany House.

Lewis-Fernandez, R. (1994). Culture and dissociation: A comparison of *ataque de nervios* among Puerto Ricans and possession syndrome in India. In D. Spiegel (Ed.), *Dissociation. Culture, mind, and body* (pp. 123–167). Washington, DC: American Psychiatric Press.

Lifton, R. J. (1961). *Thought reform and the psychology of totalism.* New York: W. W. Norton.

Links, P. S. (1988). Symposium: Borderline personality disorder. *Canadian Journal of Psychiatry, 33*(5), 335–374.

Liotti, G. (1992). Disorganized/disoriented attachment in the etiology of the dissociative disorders. *Dissociation, 5,* 196–204.

Lipton, S. D., & Kezur, E. (1948). Dissociated personality: Status of a case after five years. *Psychiatric Quarterly, 22,* 252–256.

Loewenstein, R. J. (1993a). Anna O: Reformulation as a case of multiple personality disorder. In J. M. Goodwin (Ed.), *Rediscovering childhood trauma. Historical casebook and clinical applications* (pp. 139–167). Washington, DC: American Psychiatric Press.

Loewenstein, R. J. (1993b). Psychogenic amnesia and psychogenic figure: A comprehensive review. In D. Spiegel (Ed.), *Dissociative disorders. A clinical review* (pp. 45–77). Lutherville, MD: Sidran Press.

Loewenstein, R. J., Hamilton, J., Alagna, S., Reid, N., & de Vries, M. (1987). Experiential sampling in the study of multiple personality disorder. *American Journal of Psychiatry, 144,* 19–24.

Loewenstein, R. J., Hornstein, N., & Farber, D. (1988). Open trial of clonazepam in the treatment of posttraumatic stress symptoms in multiple personality disorder. *Dissociation 1*(3), 3–12.

Loewenstein, R. J., & Putnam, F. W. (1988). A comparison study of dissociative symptoms in patients with complex partial seizures, multiple personality disorder, and posttraumatic stress disorder. *Dissociation, 1*(4), 17–23.

Loewenstein, R. J., & Putnam, F. W. (1990). The clinical phenomenology of males with multiple personality disorder: A report of 21 cases. *Dissociation, 3,* 135–143.

Lotterman, A. C. (1985). Prolonged psychotic states in borderline personality disorder. *Psychiatric Quarterly, 57,* 33–46.

Lovitt, R., & Lefkof, G. (1985). Understanding multiple personality with the comprehensive Rorschach system. *Journal of Personality Assessment, 49,* 289–294.

Ludolph, P. S. (1985). How prevalent is multiple personality? and Reply of E. L. Bliss [Letters to the editor]. *American Journal of Psychiatry, 142,* 1526–1527.

Ludwig, A. M., Brandsma, J. M., Wilbur, C. B., Benfeldt, F., & Jameson, D. H. (1972). The objective study of a case of multiple personality, or, are four heads better than one? *Archives of General Psychiatry, 26,* 298–310.

Luria, A. R. (1987). *The mind of a mnemonist.* Cambridge, MA: Harvard University Press. (Original work published 1968)

Luria, A. R. (1987). *The man with a shattered world.* Cambridge, MA: Harvard University Press. (Original work published 1972)

Lynn, S. J., & Rhue, J. W. (1988). Fantasy proneness: Hypnosis, developmental antecedents, and psychopathology. *American Psychologist, 43,* 35–44.

Lynn, S. J., & Rhue, J. W. (1994). *Dissociation. Clinical and theoretical perspectives.* New York: Guilford.

Mai, F. (1995). Psychiatrists' attitudes to multiple personality disorder: A questionnaire study. *Canadian Journal of Psychiatry, 40,* 154–157.

Mai, F. M., & Merskey, H. (1980). Briquet's treatise on hysteria. *Archives of General Psychiatry, 37,* 1401–1405.

Malenbaum, R., & Russell, A. T. (1987). Case report: Multiple personality disorder in an 11 year old boy and his mother. *Journal of the American Academy of Child and Adolescent Psychiatry, 26,* 436–439.

Marcol, L. R., & Trujillo, M. (1978). The sodium amytal interview as a therapeutic modality. *Current Psychiatric Therapies, 18,* 129–136.

Marcum, J. M., Wright, K., & Bissell, W. G. (1986). Chance discovery of multiple personality disorder in a depressed patient by amobarbital interview. *Journal of Nervous and Mental Disease, 174,* 489–792.

Margolis, C. G. (1988). [Review of the book *Psychiatric clinics of North America: Vol. 7. Symposium on Multiple Personality.*] *International Journal of Clinical and Experimental Hypnosis, 36,* 56–60.

Markowitz, J., & Viederman, M. (1986). A case report of dissociative pseudodementia. *General Hospital Psychiatry, 8,* 87–90.

Marks, J. (1979). *The search for the Manchurian candidate.* New York: W. W. Norton.

Marmer, S. S. (1980). Psychoanalysis of multiple personality. *International Journal of Psychoanalysis, 61,* 439–459.

Martinez-Taboas, A. (1989). Preliminary observations on multiple personality disorder in Puerto Rico. *Dissociation, 2*, 128–131.

Martinez-Taboas, A. (1991). Multiple personality disorder in Puerto Rico: Analysis of fifteen cases. *Dissociation, 4*, 189–192.

Martinez-Taboas, A. (1995). A sociocultural analysis of Merskey's approach. In L. Cohen, J. Berzoff, & M. Elin (Eds.), *Dissociative identity disorder. Theoretical and treatment controversies* (pp. 57–63). Northvale, NJ: Jason Aronson.

Masterson, J. F. (1976). *Psychotherapy of the borderline adult.* New York: Brunner/Mazel.

Mathew, R. J., Jack, R. A., & West, W. S. (1985). Regional cerebral blood flow in a patient with multiple personality. *American Journal of Psychiatry, 142*, 504–505.

Mayer, R. (1988). *Through divided minds.* New York: Doubleday.

McHugh, P. R. (1994, December 10). *The do's and dont's for the clinician managing memories of abuse.* Paper presented at the Memory and Reality: Reconciliation. Scientific, Clinical and Legal Issues of False Memory Syndrome Conference, Baltimore, MD.

McHugh, P. R. (1995). Resolved: Multiple personality disorder is an individually and socially created artifact. Affirmative. *Journal of the American Academy of Child and Adolescent Psychiatry, 34*, 957–959. Rebuttal, 962–963.

McKee, J. B., & Wittkower, E. D. (1962). A case of double personality with death of the imaginary partner. *Canadian Psychiatric Association Journal, 7*, 134–139.

McMahon, P. P., & Fagan, J. (1993). Play therapy with children with multiple personality disorder. In R. P. Kluft & C. G. Fine (Eds.), *Clinical perspectives on multiple personality disorder* (pp. 253–276). Washington, DC: American Psychiatric Press.

Meichenbaum, D. (1977). *Cognitive-behavior modification.* New York: Plenum.

Merskey, H. (1994). The artifactual nature of multiple personality disorder. Comments on Charles Barton's "Backstage in psychiatry: The multiple personality disorder controversy." *Dissociation, 7*, 173–175.

Merskey, H. (1995). The manufacture of personalities: The production of multiple personality disorder. In L. Cohen, J. Berzoff, & M. Elin (Eds.), *Dissociative identity disorder: Theoretical and treatment controversies* (pp. 3–32). Northvale, NJ: Jason Aronson.

Mesulam, M.-M. (1981). Dissociative states with abnormal temporal lobe EEG: Multiple personality and the illusion of possession. *Archives of Neurology, 38*, 176–181.

Michelson, L. K., & Ray, W. J. (1996). *Handbook of dissociation.* New York: Plenum.

Miller, A. (1984). Hypnotherapy in a case of dissociated incest. *International Journal of Clinical and Experimental Hypnosis, 34*, 13–28.

Millette, C. (1988). Using subparts in a case of multiple personality. In S. R. Lankton & J. K. Zeig (Eds.), *Treatment of special populations with Ericksonian approaches* (pp. 104–119). New York: Brunner/Mazel.

Millon, T. (1977). *Millon clinical multiaxial inventory manual.* Minneapolis, MN: National Computer Systems.

Montgomery, J. W. (Ed.). (1976). *Demon possession.* Minneapolis, MN: Bethany House.

Morgan, A. H., & Hilgard, E. R. (1973). Age differences in susceptibility to hypnosis. *International Journal of clinical and Experimental Hypnosis, 21*, 78–85.

Morrison, J. (1989). Childhood sexual histories of women with somatization disorder. *American Journal of Psychiatry, 146*, 239–241.

Murphy, P. E. (1994). Dissociative experiences and dissociative disorders in a non-clinical university group. *Dissociation, 7*, 28–34.

Myers, F. W. H. (1920). *Human personality and its survival of bodily death.* London: Longmans, Green. (Original work published 1903)

Naples, M., & Hackett, T. P. (1978). The amytal interview: History and current uses. *Psychosomatics, 19*, 98–105.

Nemiah, J. C. (1980). Obsessive-compulsive disorder. In H. I. Kaplan, A. M. Freedman, & B. J. Sadock (Eds.), *Comprehensive textbook of psychiatry* (3rd ed., Vol. 2, pp. 1504–1516). Baltimore: Williams & Wilkins.

Nietzsche, F. (1956). *The birth of tragedy and the genealogy of morals*. New York: Doubleday. (Original work published 1872)

North, C. S., Ryall, J., Ricci, D. A., & Wetzel, R. D. (1993). *Multiple personalities, multiple disorders. Psychiatric classification and media influence*. New York: Oxford University Press.

Norton, G. R., Ross, C. A., & Novotny, M. (1990). Factors that predict scores on the Dissociative Experiences Scale. *Journal of Clinical Psychology, 46*, 273–277.

O'Brien, P. (1985). The diagnosis of multiple personality syndromes: Overt, covert, and latent. *Comprehensive Therapy, 11*, 59–66.

O'Connor, J. (1988, September 2). Therapists should consider novel approaches in child abuse treatment cases. *Psychiatric News, 23*(17), 20, 27.

Oesterreich, T. K. (1974). *Possession demoniacal and other*. Secaucus, NJ: Citadel Press. (Original work published 1921)

Ofshe, R., & Watters, E. (1994). *Making monsters. False memories, psychotherapy, and sexual hysteria*. New York: Charles Scribner's.

Orne, M. T., Dinges, D. F., & Orne, E. C. (1984). On the differential diagnosis of multiple personality in the forensic context. *International Journal of Clinical and Experimental Hypnosis, 32*, 118–169.

Packard, R. C., & Brown, F. (1986). Multiple headaches in a case of multiple personality disorder. *Headaches, 26*, 99–102.

Paley, A. -M. N. (1988). Growing up in chaos: The dissociative response. *American Journal of Psychoanalysis, 48*, 72–83.

Paley, K. S. (1992). Dream wars: A case study of a woman with multiple personality disorder. *Dissociation, 5*, 111–116.

Pellegrini, A. J., & Putnam, P. (1984). The amytal interview in the diagnosis of late onset psychosis with cultural features presenting as catatonic stupor. *Journal of Nervous and Mental Disease, 172*, 502–504.

Perry, J. C., & Jacobs, D. (1982). Overview: Clinical applications of the amytal interview in psychiatric emergency settings. *American Journal of Psychiatry, 139*, 552–559.

Peterson, G. (1990). Diagnosis of childhood multiple personality disorder. *Dissociation, 3*, 3–9.

Peterson, G. (1991). Children coping with trauma: Diagnosis of "dissociation identity disorder." *Dissociation, 4*, 152–164.

Peterson, G., & Putnam, F. W. (1994). Preliminary results of the field trial of proposed criteria for dissociative disorder of childhood. *Dissociation, 7*, 212–220.

Phillips, D. W. (1994). Initial development and validation of the Phillips Dissociation Scale (PDS) of the MMPI. *Dissociation, 7*, 92–100.

Piper, A. (1990). Multiple personality disorder [letter to the editor]. *Canadian Journal of Psychiatry, 35*, 195–196.

Piper, A. (1994a). Treatment of multiple personality disorder. At what cost? *American Journal of Psychotherapy, 48*, 392–400.

Piper, A. (1994b). Multiple personality disorder. *British Journal of Psychiatry, 164*, 600–612.

Piper, A. (1995a). A skeptical look at multiple personality disorder. In L. Cohen, J. Berzoff, & M. Elin (Eds.), *Dissociative identity disorder: Theoretical and treatment controversies* (pp. 135–173). Northvale, NJ: Jason Aronson.

Piper, A. (1995b). Reply to Ross. *American Journal of Psychotherapy, 49*, 315–316.

Pollock, G. H. (1984). Anna O: Insight, hindsight, and foresight. In M. Rosenbaum & M. Muroff (Eds.), *Anna O. Fourteen contemporary reinterpretations* (pp. 26–33). New York: Free Press.

Pope, H. G., & Hudson, J. I. (1992). Is childhood sexual abuse a risk factor for bulimia nervosa? *American Journal of Psychiatry, 149*, 241–248.

Prince, M. (1978). *The dissociation of a personality*. New York: Oxford University Press. (Original work published 1905)

Putnam, F. W. (1984a). The psychophysiologic investigation of multiple personality disorder. *Psychiatric Clinics of North America, 7,* 31–39.

Putnam, F. W. (1984b). The study of multiple personality disorder: General strategies and practical considerations. *Psychiatric Annals, 14,* 58–61.

Putnam, F. W. (1985). Dissociation as a response to extreme trauma. In R. P. Kluft (Ed.), *Childhood antecedents of multiple personality disorder* (pp. 65–97). Washington, DC: American Psychiatric Press.

Putnam, F. W. (1986a). The scientific study of multiple personality disorder. In J. M. Quen (Ed.), *Split minds split brains* (pp. 109–125). New York: New York University Press.

Putnam, F. W. (1986b). The treatment of multiple personality: State of the art. In B. G. Braun (Ed.), *Treatment of multiple personality disorder* (pp. 178–198). Washington, DC: American Psychiatric Press.

Putnam, F. W. (1988). The switch process in multiple personality disorder. *Dissociation 1*(1), 24–32.

Putnam, F. W. (1989). *Diagnosis and treatment of multiple personality disorder.* New York: Guilford.

Putnam, F. W. (1995). Resolved: Multiple personality disorder is an individually and socially created artifact. Negative. *Journal of the American Academy of Child and Adolescent Psychiatry, 34,* 960–962. Rebuttal, 963.

Putnam, F. W., Guroff, J. J., Silberman, E. K., Barban, L., & Post, R. M. (1986). The clinical phenomenology of multiple personality disorder: Review of 100 recent cases. *Journal of Clinical Psychiatry, 47,* 285–293.

Putnam, F. W., Loewenstein, R. J., Silberman, E. K., & Post, R. M. (1984). Multiple personality in a hospital setting. *Journal of Clinical Psychiatry, 45,* 172–175.

Putnam, F. W., & Peterson, G. (1994). Further validation of the child dissociative checklist. *Dissociation, 7,* 204–211.

Quen, J. M. (Ed.). (1986). *Split minds split brains.* New York: New York University Press.

Ray, W. J. (1996). Dissociation in normal populations. In L. K. Michelson & W. J. Ray (Eds.), *Handbook of dissociation* (pp. 51–68). New York: Plenum.

Ray, W. J., & Faith, M. (1995). Dissociative experiences in a college age population: Follow-up with 1190 subjects. *Personal and Individual Differences, 18,* 223–230.

Reagor, P. A., Kasten, J., & Morelli, N. (1992). A checklist for screening dissociative disorders in children and adolescents. *Dissociation, 5,* 4–19.

Richards, D. G. (1991). A study of the correlations between subjective psychic experiences and dissociative experiences. *Dissociation, 4,* 83–91.

Riley, K. (1988). Measures of dissociation. *Journal of Nervous and Mental Disease, 176,* 449–450.

Riley, R. L., & Mead, J. (1988). The development of symptoms of multiple personality disorder in a child of three. *Dissociation, 1*(3), 43–46.

Rivera, M. (1987). Multiple personality: An outcome of child abuse. *Canadian Woman Studies, 8,* 18–23.

Rivera, M. (1988). *All of them to speak: Feminism, poststructuralism, and multiple personality.* Unpublished doctoral dissertation, University of Toronto, Toronto, Ontario, Canada.

Rivera, M. (1989). Linking the psychological and the social: Feminism, poststructuralism and multiple personality. *Dissociation, 2,* 24–31.

Rivera, M. (1991). Multiple personality and the social systems: 185 cases. *Dissociation, 4,* 79–82.

Robins, L. N., Helzer, J. E., Croughan, J., & Ratcliff, K. S. (1981). National Institute of Mental Health diagnostic interview schedule. *Archives of General Psychiatry, 38,* 381–389.

Robins, L. N., Helzer, J. E., Weissman, M. M., Orvaschel, H., Gruenberg, E., Burke, J. D., & Reiger, D. A. (1984). Lifetime prevalence of psychiatric disorders in three communities. *Archives of General Psychiatry, 41,* 949–958.

Rogo, D. S. (1986a). *Mind over matter: The case for psychokinesis.* Wellingborough, Northamptonshire, England: Aquarian Press.

Rogo, D. S. (1986b). *On the track of the poltergeist.* Englewood Cliffs, NJ: Prentice-Hall.

Rosenbaum, M. (1980). The role of the term schizophrenia in the decline of diagnoses of multiple personality. *Archives of General Psychiatry, 37,* 1383–1385.

Rosenbaum, M., & Weaver, G. M. (1980). Dissociated state: Status of a case after 38 years. *Journal of Nervous and Mental Disease, 168,* 597–603.

Rosenzweig, S. (1988). The identity and idiodynamics of the multiple personality "Sally Beauchamp": A confirmatory supplement. *American Psychologist, 43,* 45–48.

Ross, C. A. (1981). Basic research by medical students. *Journal of the Royal Society of Medicine, 74,* 7–10.

Ross, C. A. (1984). Diagnosis of multiple personality during hypnosis: A case report. *International Journal of Clinical and Experimental Hypnosis, 32,* 222–235.

Ross, C. A. (1985). *DSM-III:* Problems in diagnosing partial forms of multiple personality disorder. *Journal of the Royal Society of Medicine, 75,* 933–936.

Ross, C. A. (1986a). Biological tests for mental illness: Their use and misuse. *Biological Psychiatry, 21,* 431–435.

Ross, C. A. (1986b, July 8). The insanity of the insanity defense. *The Medical Post,* p. 10.

Ross, C. A. (1987). Inpatient treatment of multiple personality disorder. *Canadian Journal of Psychiatry, 32,* 779–781.

Ross, C. A. (1988, January). Multiple personality disorder in Canada. *Psychiatry in Canada,* 11–13.

Ross, C. A. (1989). *Multiple personality disorder: Diagnosis, clinical features, and treatment.* New York: Wiley.

Ross, C. A. (1990a). Twelve cognitive errors about multiple personality disorder. *American Journal of Psychotherapy, 44,* 348–356.

Ross, C. A. (1990b). Comment on Takahashi's: "Is MPD really rare in Japan?" *Dissociation, 3,* 64–65.

Ross, C. A. (1990c). Comment on Garcia's "The concept of dissociation and conversion in the new ICD-10." *Dissociation, 3,* 211–213.

Ross, C. A. (1990d). Multiple personality disorders, reply to Piper [letter to the editor]. *Canadian Journal of Psychiatry, 35,* 449–450.

Ross, C. A. (1991a). Epidemiology of multiple personality disorder and dissociation. *Psychiatric Clinics of North America, 14,* 503–517.

Ross, C. A. (1991b). The dissociated executive self and the cultural dissociation barrier. *Dissociation, 5,* 55–61.

Ross, C. A. (1992). Childhood sexual abuse and psychobiology. *Journal of Child Sexual Abuse, 1,* 95–101.

Ross, C. A. (1994a). Dissociation and physical illness. In D. Spiegel (Ed.), *Dissociation. Culture, mind, and body* (pp. 171–184). Washington, DC: American Psychiatric Press.

Ross, C. A. (1994b). *The Osiris Complex: Case studies in multiple personality disorder.* Toronto: University of Toronto Press.

Ross, C. A. (1994c). Comment on positive associations between dichotic listening errors, complex partial epileptic-like signs, and paranormal beliefs. *Journal of Nervous and Mental Disease, 182,* 56–58.

Ross, C. A. (1995a). *Satanic ritual abuse: Principles of treatment.* Toronto: University of Toronto Press.

Ross, C. A. (1995b). The validity and reliability of dissociative identity disorder. In L. Cohen, J. Berzoff, & M. Elin (Eds.), *Dissociative identity disorder: Theoretical and treatment controversies* (pp. 65–84). Northvale, NJ: Jason Aronson.

Ross, C. A. (1995c). Diagnosis of dissociative identity disorder. In L. Cohen, J. Berzoff, & M. Elin (Eds.), *Dissociative identity disorder: Theoretical and treatment controversies* (pp. 261–284). Northvale, NJ: Jason Aronson.

Ross, C. A. (1995d). Current treatment of dissociative identity disorder. In L. Cohen, J. Berzoff, & M. Elin (Eds.), *Dissociative identity disorder: Theoretical and treatment controversies* (pp. 413–434). Northvale, NJ: Jason Aronson.

Ross, C. A. (1995e). Comment on Piper. *American Journal of Psychotherapy, 49,* 314–315.

Ross, C. A. (1995f). Re: Multiple personality [letter to the editor]. *Canadian Journal of Psychiatry, 40,* 47–48.

Ross, C. A. (1996a). Short-term, problem-oriented inpatient treatment. In J. L. Spira (Ed.), *Treating dissociative identity disorder* (pp. 337–365). San Francisco: Jossey-Bass.

Ross, C. A. (1996b). History, phenomenology, and epidemiology of dissociation. In L. K. Michelson & W. J. Ray (Eds.), *Handbook of dissociation* (pp. 3–24). New York: Plenum.

Ross, C. A. (1996c). Epidemiology of dissociation in children and adolescents. *Child and Adolescent Psychiatric Clinics of North America, 5,* 273–284.

Ross, C. A. (in press-a). Cognitive therapy of dissociative identity disorder. In M. R. Elin, P. Appelbaum, & L. Uyehara (Eds.), *Trauma and memory: Clinical and legal controversies.* Oxford, England: Oxford University Press.

Ross, C. A. (in press-b). Structured interviews. In J. A. Turkus & B. M. Cohen (Eds.), *Multiple personality disorder: Continuum of care.* New York: Jason Aronson.

Ross, C. A., & Anderson, G. (1988). Phenomenological overlap of multiple personality disorder and obsessive compulsive disorder. *Journal of Nervous and Mental Disease, 176,* 295–299.

Ross, C. A., Anderson, G., & Clark, P. (1994). Childhood abuse and the positive symptoms of schizophrenia. *Hospital and Community Psychiatry, 45,* 489–491.

Ross, C. A., Anderson, G., Fleisher, W. P., & Norton, G. R. (1992). Dissociative experiences among psychiatric inpatients. *General Hospital Psychiatry, 14,* 350–354.

Ross, C. A., Anderson, G., Fraser, G. A., Reagor, P., Bjornson, L., & Miller, S. D. (1992). Differentiating multiple personality disorder and dissociative disorder not otherwise specified. *Dissociation, 5,* 88–91.

Ross, C. A., Anderson, G., Heber, S., & Norton, G. R. (1990). Dissociation and abuse in multiple personality patients, prostitutes, and exotic dancers. *Hospital and Community Psychiatry, 41,* 328–330.

Ross, C. A., & Clark, P. (1992). Assessment of childhood trauma and dissociation in an emergency department. *Dissociation, 5,* 163–165.

Ross, C. A., & Dua, V. (1993). Psychiatric health care costs of multiple personality disorder. *American Journal of Psychotherapy, 47,* 103–112.

Ross, C. A., Fast, E., Anderson, G., Auty, A., & Todd, J. (1990). Somatic symptoms in multiple sclerosis and MPD. *Dissociation, 3,* 102–106.

Ross, C. A., & Fraser, G. A. (1987). Recognizing multiple personality disorder. *Annals of the Royal College of Physicians and Surgeons of Canada, 20,* 357–360.

Ross, C. A., & Gahan, P. (1988a). Cognitive analysis of multiple personality disorder. *American Journal of Psychotherapy, 42,* 229–239.

Ross, C. A., & Gahan, P. (1988b). Techniques in the treatment of multiple personality disorder. *American Journal of Psychotherapy, 42,* 40–52.

Ross, C. A., Heber, S., Anderson, G., Norton, G. R., Anderson, B., del Campo, M., & Pillay, N. (1989). Differentiating multiple personality disorder and complex partial seizures. *General Hospital Psychiatry, 11*, 54–58.

Ross, C. A., Heber, S., Norton, G. R., Anderson, D., Anderson, G., & Barchet, P. (1989). The Dissociative Disorders Interview Schedule: A structured interview. *Dissociation, 2*, 169–189.

Ross, C. A., Heber, S., Norton, G. R., & Anderson, G. (1989a). Differences between multiple personality disorder and other diagnostic groups on structured interview. *Journal of Nervous and Mental Disease, 179*(8), 487–491.

Ross, C. A., Heber, S., Norton, G. R., & Anderson, G. (1989b). Somatic symptoms in multiple personality disorder. *Psychosomatics, 30*(2), 154–160.

Ross, C. A., & Joshi, S. (1992a). Paranormal experiences in the general population. *Journal of Nervous and Mental Disease, 180*, 357–361.

Ross, C. A., & Joshi, S. (1992b). Schneiderian symptoms and childhood trauma in the general population. *Comprehensive Psychiatry, 33*, 269–273.

Ross, C. A., Joshi, S., & Currie, R. P. (1990). Dissociative experiences in the general population. *American Journal of Psychiatry, 147*, 1547–1552.

Ross, C. A., Joshi, S., & Currie, R. P. (1991). Dissociative experiences in the general population: A factor analysis. *Hospital and Community Psychiatry, 42*, 297–301.

Ross, C. A., Kronson, J., Koensgen, S., Barkman, K., Clark, P., & Rockman, G. (1992). Dissociative comorbidity in 100 chemically dependent patients. *Hospital and Community Psychiatry, 43*, 840–842.

Ross, C. A., & Matas, M. (1987). A clinical trial of buspirone and diazepam in treatment of generalized anxiety disorder. *Canadian Journal of Psychiatry, 32*, 351–355.

Ross, C. A., Miller, S. D., Bjornson, L., Reagor, P., Fraser, G. A., & Anderson, G. (1990). Schneiderian symptoms in multiple personality disorder and schizophrenia. *Comprehensive Psychiatry, 31*, 111–118.

Ross, C. A., Miller, S. D., Bjornson, L., Reagor, P., Fraser, G. A., & Anderson, G. (1991). Abuse histories in 102 cases of multiple personality disorder. *Canadian Journal of Psychiatry, 36*, 97–101.

Ross, C. A., Miller, S. D., Reagor, P., Bjornson, L., Fraser, G. A., & Anderson, G. (1990). Structured interview data on 102 cases of multiple personality disorder from four centers. *American Journal of Psychiatry, 147*, 596–601.

Ross, C. A., & Norton, G. R. (1987). Signs and symptoms of multiple personality disorder. *Modern Medicine of Canada, 42*, 392–396.

Ross, C. A., & Norton, G. R. (1988). Multiple personality patients with a past diagnosis of schizophrenia. *Dissociation, 1*(2), 39–42.

Ross, C. A., & Norton, G. R. (1989a). Differences between men and women with multiple personality disorder. *Hospital and Community Psychiatry, 40*(2), 186–188.

Ross, C. A., & Norton, G. R. (1989b). Suicide and parasuicide in multiple personality disorder. *Psychiatry, 52*, 365–371.

Ross, C. A., & Norton, G. R. (1989c). Effects of hypnosis on the features of multiple personality disorder. *American Journal of Clinical Hypnosis, 32*, 99–106.

Ross, C. A., Norton, G. R., & Anderson, G. (1988). The dissociative experiences scale: A replication study. *Dissociation, 1*(3), 21–22.

Ross, C. A., Norton, G. R., & Fraser, G. A. (1989). Evidence against the iatrogenesis of multiple personality disorder. *Dissociation, 2*, 61–65.

Ross, C. A., Norton, G. R., & Wozney, K. (1989). Multiple personality disorder: An analysis of 236 cases. *Canadian Journal of Psychiatry, 34*(5), 413–418.

Ross, C. A., & Pam, A. (1995). *Pseudoscience in biological psychiatry. Blaming the body.* New York: Wiley.

Ross, C. A., Ryan, L., Ross, D., & Hardy, L. (1989). Dissociative experiences in adolescents and college students. *Dissociation, 2*, 239–242.

Ross, C. A., Ryan, L., Voigt, H., & Edie, L. (1991). High and low dissociators in a college student population. *Dissociation, 4,* 147–151.

Ross, C. A., Siddiqui, A. R., & Matas, M. (1987). *DSM-III:* Problems in diagnosis of paranoia and obsessive-compulsive disorder. *Canadian Journal of Psychiatry, 32,* 351–355.

Ruedrich, S. L., Chu, C. -C., & Wadle, D. V. (1985). The amytal interview in the treatment of psychogenic amnesia. *Hospital and Community Psychiatry, 36,* 1045–1046.

Rush, F. (1980). *The best kept secret: Sexual abuse of children.* New York: McGraw-Hill.

Russell, B. (1945). *A history of Western philosophy.* New York: Simon & Schuster.

Ryan, L. (1988). *Prevalence of dissociative disorders and symptoms in a university population.* Unpublished doctoral dissertation, California Institute of Integral Studies, San Francisco.

Ryan, L., & Ross, C. A. (1988). Dissociation in adolescents and college students. In B. G. Braun (Ed.), *Proceedings of the Fifth International Conference on Multiple Personality/Dissociative States* (p. 19). Chicago: Rush-Presbyterian-St. Luke's Medical Center.

Sachs, R. G. (1986). The adjunctive role of social support systems in the treatment of multiple personality disorder. In B. G. Braun (Ed.), *Treatment of multiple personality disorder* (pp. 157–174). Washington, DC: American Psychiatric Press.

Sachs, R. G., Frischholtz, E. J., & Wood, J. I. (1988). Marital and family therapy in the treatment of multiple personality disorder. *Journal of Marital and Family Therapy, 14,* 249–259.

Sackheim, D. K., & Devine, S. (1995). Trauma-related syndromes. In C. A. Ross & A. Pam (Eds.), *Pseudoscience in biological psychiatry. Blaming the body* (pp. 255–272). New York: Wiley.

Sanders, S. (1986). The perceptual alteration scale: A scale measuring dissociation. *American Journal of Clinical Hypnosis, 29,* 95–102.

Sarbin, T. R. (1995). On the belief that one body may be host to two or more personalities. *International Journal of Clinical and Experimental Hypnosis, 43,* 163–183.

Saxe, G. N., van der Kolk, B. A., Berkowitz, R., Chinman, G., Hall, K., Lieberg, G., & Schwartz, J. (1993). Dissociative disorders in psychiatric inpatients. *American Journal of Psychiatry, 150,* 1037–1042.

Schafer, D. W. (1981). The recognition and hypnotherapy of patients with unrecognized altered states. *American Journal of Clinical Hypnosis, 23,* 176–183.

Schafer, D. W. (1986). Recognizing multiple personality patients. *American Journal of Psychotherapy, 40,* 500–510.

Schenk, L., & Bear, D. (1981). Multiple personality and related dissociative phenomena in patients with temporal lobe epilepsy. *American Journal of Psychiatry, 138,* 1311–1316.

Schreiber, F. R. (1973). *Sybil.* Chicago: Henry Regnery.

Schultz, R. K., Braun, B. G., & Kluft, R. P. (1985). Creativity and the imaginary companion phenomenon: Prevalence and phenomenology. In *Proceedings of the Second International Conference on Multiple Personality/Dissociative States* (p. 103). Chicago: Rush-Presbyterian-St. Luke's Medical Center.

Schultz, R. K., Braun, B. G., & Kluft, R. P. (1989). Multiple personality disorder: Phenomenology of selected variables in comparison to major depression. *Dissociation, 2,* 45–51.

Schwartz, R. (1987, March–April). Our multiple selves. *Networker,* 25–31, 80–83.

Seltzer, A. (1994). Multiple personality: A psychiatric mis-adventure. *Canadian Journal of Psychiatry, 39,* 442–445.

Seltzer, A. (1995). Re: Multiple personality. The author replies [letter to the editor]. *Canadian Journal of Psychiatry, 40,* 49–50.

Sheehy, M., Goldsmith, L., & Charles, M. A. (1980). A comparative study of borderline patients in a psychiatric outpatient clinic. *American Journal of Psychiatry, 137,* 1374–1379.

Sidis, B., & Goodhart, S. P. (1905). *Multiple personality.* New York: Appleton-Century-Crofts.

Sidtis, J. J. (1986). Can neurological disconnection account for psychiatric dissociation? In J. M. Quen (Ed.), *Split minds split brains* (pp. 127–147). New York: New York University Press.

Siegel, A. E. (1995). Consequences of arriving at the diagnosis of multiple personality disorder. In L. Cohen, J. Berzoff, & M. Elin (Eds.), *Dissociative identity disorder. Theoretical and treatment controversies* (pp. 435–445). Northvale, NJ: Jason Aronson.

Siemens, J. G., & Ross, C. A. (1991). Dissociation and childhood trauma in gastroenterological patients. In B. G. Braun (Ed.), *Dissociative disorders: 1991. Proceedings of the Eighth International Conference on Multiple Personality/Dissociative States* (p. 75). Chicago: Rush-Presbyterian-St. Luke's Medical Center.

Silberman, E. K., Putnam, F. W., Weingartner, H., Braun, B. G., & Post, R. M. (1985). Dissociative states in multiple personality disorder: A quantitative study. *Psychiatry Research, 15,* 253–260.

Silbert, M. H., & Pines, A. M. (1981). Sexual child abuse as an antecedent to prostitution. *Child Abuse and Neglect, 5,* 407–411.

Silbert, M. H., & Pines, A. M. (1982). Entrance into prostitution. *Youth and Society, 13,* 471–500.

Silbert, M. H., & Pines, A. M. (1983). Early sexual exploitation as an influence in prostitution. *Social Work, 28,* 285–290.

Silbert, M. H., & Pines, A. M. (1984). Pornography and sexual abuse of women. *Sex Roles, 10,* 857–868.

Simpson, M. (1995). Gullible's travels, or the importance of being multiple. In L. Cohen, J. Berzoff, & M. Elin (Eds.), *Dissociative identity disorder: Theoretical and treatment controversies* (pp. 87–134). Northvale, NJ: Jason Aronson.

Singer, M. (1995). *Cults in our midst. The hidden menace in our everyday lives.* San Francisco: Jossey-Bass.

Sizemore, C., & Pittillo, E. (1977). *I'm Eve.* New York: Doubleday.

Sneiderman, B. (1988, June 20). Sleepwalk defense has precedent. *Winnipeg Free Press,* p. 7.

Spanos, N. P., Burgess, C. A., & Burgess, M. F. (1995). Past-life identities, UFO abductions, and satanic ritual abuse: The social construction of memories. *International Journal of Clinical and Experimental Hypnosis, 43,* 433–446.

Spanos, N. P., Weekes, J. R., & Bertrand, L. D. (1985). Multiple personality: A social psychological perspective. *Journal of Abnormal Psychology, 94,* 362–376.

Spanos, N. P., Weekes, J. R., Menary, E., & Bertrand, L. D. (1986). Hypnotic interview and age regression procedures in elicitation of multiple personality symptoms: A simulation study. *Psychiatry, 49,* 298–311.

Spiegel, D. (1984). Multiple personality as a post-traumatic stress disorder. *Psychiatric Clinics of North America, 7,* 101–110.

Spiegel, D. (1986a). Dissociating damage. *American Journal of Clinical Hypnosis, 29,* 123–131.

Spiegel, D. (1986b). Dissociation, double binds, and posttraumatic stress in multiple personality disorder. In B. G. Braun (Ed.), *Treatment of multiple personality disorder* (pp. 61–77). Washington, DC: American Psychiatric Press.

Spiegel, D. (1988). The treatment accorded those who treat patients with multiple personality disorder. *Journal of Nervous and Mental Disease, 176,* 535–536.

Spiegel, D. (1993). *Dissociative disorders: A clinical review.* Lutherville, MD: Sidran Press.

Spiegel, D. (1994). *Dissociation. Culture, mind, and body.* Washington, DC: American Psychiatric Press.

Spiegel, D., Hunt, T., & Dondershine, H. E. (1988). Dissociation and hypnotizability in posttraumatic stress disorder. *American Journal of Psychiatry, 145,* 301–305.

Spiegel, D., & Rosenfeld, A. (1984). Spontaneous hypnotic age regression: Case report. *Journal of Clinical Psychiatry, 45,* 522–524.

Spiegel, H., & Spiegel, D. (1978). *Trance and treatment.* New York: Basic Books.

Spira, J. L. (1996). *Treating dissociative identity disorder.* San Francisco: Jossey-Bass.

Spitzer, R. L., Williams, J. B. W., Gibbon, M., & First, M. B. (1990). *Users guide for the structured clinical interview for DSM-III-R.* Washington, DC: American Psychiatric Press.

Steinberg, M. (1987). Diagnostically discriminating questions on the structured clinical interview for *DSM-III-R* dissociative disorder. In B. G. Braun (Ed.), *Proceedings of the Fourth International Conference on Multiple Personality/Dissociative States* (p. 130). Chicago: Rush-Presbyterian-St. Luke's Medical Center.

Steinberg, M. (1993). The spectrum of depersonalization: Assessment and treatment. In D. Spiegel (Ed.), *Dissociative disorders. A clinical review* (pp. 79–103). Lutherville, MD: Sidran Press.

Steinberg, M. (1994). Systematizing dissociation: Symptomatology and diagnostic assessment. In D. Spiegel (Ed.), *Dissociation. Culture, mind, and body* (pp. 59–88). Washington, DC: American Psychiatric Press.

Steinberg, M. (1995). *Handbook for the assessment of dissociation. A clinical guide.* Washington, DC: American Psychiatric Press.

Steinberg, M., Howland, F., & Cicchetti, D. (1986). The structured clinical interview for *DSM-III-R* dissociative disorder: A preliminary report. In B. G. Braun (Ed.), *Proceedings of the Third International Conference on Multiple Personality/Dissociative States* (p. 125). Chicago: Rush-Presbyterian-St. Luke's Medical Center.

Stern, C. R. (1984). The etiology of multiple personalities. *Psychiatric Clinics of North America, 7,* 149–159.

Stevenson, I., & Pasricha, S. (1979). A case of secondary personality with xenoglossy. *American Journal of Psychiatry, 136,* 1591–1592.

Stewart, W. A. (1984). Analytic biography of Ann O. In M. Rosenbaum & M. Muroff (Eds.), *Anna O: Fourteen contemporary reinterpretations* (pp. 50–68). New York: Free Press.

Stoller, R. J. (1973). *Splitting: A case of female masculinity.* New York: Dell.

Suryani, L. K., & Jensen, G. D. (1993). *Trance and possession in Bali. A window on western multiple personality, possession disorder, and suicide.* Oxford, England: Oxford University Press.

Sutcliffe, J. P., & Jones, J. (1962). Personal identity, multiple personality, and hypnosis. *International Journal of Clinical and Experimental Hypnosis, 10,* 231–269.

Taylor, W. S., & Martin, M. F. (1944). Multiple personality. *Journal of Abnormal and Social Psychology, 39,* 281–300.

Thigpen, C. H., & Cleckley, H. M. (1957). *The three faces of Eve.* New York: McGraw-Hill.

Thigpen, C. H., & Cleckley, H. M. (1984). On the incidence of multiple personality disorder. *International Journal of Clinical and Experimental Hypnosis, 32,* 63–66.

Torem, M. S. (1986). Dissociative states presenting as an eating disorder. *American Journal of Clinical Hypnosis, 29,* 137–142.

Torem, M. S. (1987). Ego-state therapy for eating disorders. *American Journal of Clinical Hypnosis, 30,* 94–103.

Torem, M. S. (1988). PTSD presenting as an eating disorder. *Stress Medicine, 4,* 139–142.

Tutkun, H., Yargic, I., & Sar, V. (1995). Dissociative identity disorder: A clinical investigation of 20 cases in Turkey. *Dissociation, 8,* 3–9.

Tyson, G. M. (1992). Childhood MPD/dissociative identity disorder: Applying and extending current diagnostic checklists. *Dissociation, 5,* 20–27.

van der Hart, O., & van der Velden, K. (1987). The hypnotherapy of Dr. Andries Hoek: Uncovering hypnotherapy before Janet, Breuer, and Freud. *American Journal of Clinical Hypnosis, 29,* 264–271.

van der Kolk, B. A. (1987). *Psychological trauma.* Washington, DC: American Psychiatric Press.

Vanderlinden, J. (1993). *Dissociative experiences, trauma and hypnosis. Research findings & clinical applications in eating disorders.* Delft, The Netherlands: Uitgeverij Eburon.

Vanderlinden, J., Van Dyck, R., Vandereycken, W., & Vertommen, H. (1991). Dissociative experiences in the general population in the Netherlands and Belgium: A study with the Dissociation Questionnaire (DIS-Q). *Dissociation, 4,* 180–184.

Vanderlinden, J., Varga, K., Peuskens, J., & Pieters, G. (1995, May). *Dissociative symptoms in a population sample of Hungary.* Paper presented at the Spring Conference of the International Society for the Study of Dissociation, Amsterdam, The Netherlands.

van Ijzendoorn, M. H., & Schuengel, C. (in press). The measurement of dissociation in normal and clinical populations: Meta-analytic validation of the Dissociative Experiences Scale. *Clinical Psychology Review.*

Varma, V. K., Bouri, M., & Wig, N. N. (1981). Multiple personality in India: Comparison with hysterical possession state. *American Journal of Psychotherapy, 35,* 113–120.

Veith, I. (1965). *Hysteria: The history of a disease.* Chicago: University of Chicago Press.

Villoldo, A., & Krippner, S. (1986). *Healing states: A journey into the world of spiritual healing and shamanism.* New York: Simon & Schuster.

Vincent, M., & Pickering, M. R. (1988). Multiple personality disorder in childhood. *Canadian Journal of Psychiatry, 33,* 524–529.

Walker, J., Norton, G. R., & Ross, C. A. (1991). *Panic disorder and agoraphobia: A guide for the practitioner.* Pacific Grove, CA: Brooks/Cole.

Waller, N. G., Putnam, F. W., & Carlson, E. B. (1995). *Types of dissociation and dissociative types: A taxometric analysis of dissociative experiences.* Unpublished manuscript.

Waller, N. G., & Ross, C. A. (1995). *The prevalence of pathological dissociation in the general population.* Unpublished manuscript.

Wasson, R. G. (1973). *Soma: Divine mushroom of immortality.* San Diego: Harcourt Brace Jovanovich.

Waterbury, M. (1991). Abuse histories and prior diagnoses in 123 inner city children with dissociative disorders. In B. G. Braun (Ed.), *Proceedings of the Eighth International Conference on Multiple Personality/Dissociative States* (p. 111). Chicago: Rush-Presbyterian-St. Luke's Medical Center.

Watkins, J. G. (1984). The Bianchi (L. A. Hillside Strangler) case: Sociopath or multiple personality? *International Journal of Clinical and Experimental Hypnosis, 32,* 67–101.

Weinberg, S. K. (1955). *Incest behavior.* New York: Citadel Press.

Weiss, M., Sutton, P. J., & Utecht, A. J. (1985). Multiple personality in a 10 year old girl. *Journal of the American Academy of Child Psychiatry, 24,* 495–501.

Weissberg, M. (1992). *The first sin of Ross Michael Carlson.* New York: Delacorte Press.

West, L. J., & Martin, P. (1994). Pseudo-identity and the treatment of personality change in victims of captivity and cults. In S. J. Lynn & J. W. Rhue (Eds.), *Dissociation. Clinical and theoretical perspectives* (pp. 268–288). New York: Guilford.

Wilbur, C. G. (1984). Multiple personality and child abuse. *Psychiatric Clinics of North America, 7,* 3–7.

Wilbur, C. G. (1985). The effect of child abuse on the psyche. In R. P. Kluft (Ed.), *Childhood antecedents of multiple personality disorder* (pp. 21–35). Washington, DC: American Psychiatric Press.

Wilbur, C. G. (1986). Psychoanalysis and multiple personality disorder. In B. G. Braun (Ed.), *Treatment of multiple personality disorder* (pp. 133–142). Washington, DC: American Psychiatric Press.

Wilson, W. P. (1976). Hysteria and demons, depression and oppression, good and evil. In J. W. Montgomery (Ed.), *Demon possession* (pp. 223–231). Minneapolis, MN: Bethany House.

Winer, D. (1978). Anger and dissociation: A case study of multiple personality. *Journal of Abnormal Psychology, 87,* 368–372.

World Health Organization. (1992). *ICD-10. The ICD-10 classification of mental and behavioral disorders. Clinical descriptions and diagnostic guidelines.* Geneva: Author.

Yank, J. R. (1991). Handwriting variations in individuals with multiple personality disorder. *Dissociation, 4,* 2–12.

Yargic, L. I., Tutkun, H., & Sar, V. (1995). Reliability and validity of the Turkish version of the Dissociative Experiences Scale. *Dissociation, 8,* 10–13.

Young, W. C. (1986). Restraints in the treatment of a patient with multiple personality. *American Journal of Psychotherapy, 40,* 601–606.

Young, W. C. (1987). Emergence of a multiple personality in a posttraumatic stress disorder of adulthood. *American Journal of Clinical Hypnosis, 29,* 249–254.

Young, W. C. (1988). Psychodynamics and dissociation: All that switches is not split. *Dissociation, 1*(1), 33–38.

Author Index

Subject Index